Odyssey of the Voice

Odyssey of the Voice

Jean Abitbol, M.D.

Translated by Patricia Crossley

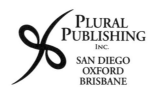

PLURAL
PUBLISHING
INC.
SAN DIEGO
OXFORD
BRISBANE

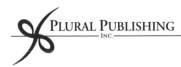

PLURAL PUBLISHING
INC.

5521 Ruffin Road
San Diego, CA 92123

e-mail: info@pluralpublishing.com
Web site: http://www.pluralpublishing.com

49 Bath Street
Abingdon, Oxfordshire OX14 1EA
United Kingdom

"Ouvrage publié avec le concours du Ministère Français chargé de la Culture - Centre National du Livre"

Typeset in 11/13 Garamond by Flanagan's Publishing Services, Inc. Printed in the United States of America by McNaughton and Gunn

For permission to use material from this text, contact us by
Telephone: (866) 758-7251
Fax: (888) 758-7255
e-mail: permissions@pluralpublishing.com

ISBN-13: 978-1-59756-029-0
ISBN-10: 1-59756-029-4
Library of Congress Control Number: 2005909340

Contents

Foreword

Jean Abitbol's unique, new book is an extraordinary synthesis of history, science, and philosophy. Rather than being a medical text, it truly presents an "Odyssey" through historical landmarks in time and their relationships to human communication. It is replete with the latest medical and scientific information about the human voice. However, the literary fabric into which this information is woven includes a synthesis of cultural and vocal history throughout the ages, the evolution of communication as a keystone of human society, and a panoramic vision of the intertwining of voice and intellectual development.

Into this unprecedented exposition, Abitbol has incorporated subtle education about the latest concepts and vocal function and care. He has included not only traditional science and medicine, but also information about alternative medicine as it relates to vocal health. His discussions of special topics are extraordinary, including the chapters on castrati, impersonators, ventriloquists, parrots, and mythology.

This book represents a major contribution not merely to vocal literature, but moreover to literature in general. Abitbol's wisdom, insights, subtlety, and humor have resulted in a truly remarkable work.

Robert T. Sataloff, M.D., D.M.A.
Chairman, The Voice Foundation
Philadelphia, Pennsylvania

Preface: Homo Vocalis

The quest for the human voice, its origins, its story, its challenges and limitations, its emotional impact and conjurations—such is the voyage of discovery I propose to take you on.

A voyage that is not without pitfalls. It will challenge us to understand how life can leave its scars on our voice, to apprehend the passage of time and its impact, to protect this alchemy between mind and body that is the voice.

The outcome of an evolution that has lasted over 4.5 billion years, the physical body of *Homo vocalis* seems perfectly conceived. But if breathing and walking are instinctive to us, the voice is mastered only after years of apprenticeship. It is the end result of an integration and growth process that starts at birth and persists into adulthood.

The newborn, still immature, has first to create his own cerebral circuits before he can speak or sing. He listens! He learns! He expresses himself and thus enters into the world of thoughts. Where does the arrow of time that guides him come from? Where does his voice come from, a voice that today can be reduced to a genetic code? What energy provides it with life? What energy does the voice empower? The voice has no past and no future; it exists only in the present moment. In the chaotic logic of space and time, this precious gift that is the voice is an emotional amplifier.

Where the fingerprint points to a man's guilt, the vocal print evokes his personality and reveals his artistry. It is a reflection of his Self and of his private world of fancy. Much like an explorer or an archeologist, let's set off in search of the origins of the human voice.

During my career as doctor and surgeon, I came across numerous vocal pathologies, some of which were an enigma to me. In order to heal these injured voices, I had to understand them! What makes a voice hoarse? Why does a woman's voice change during her menstrual cycle? How can the normal breaking of the voice at puberty go wrong? How does a polyp appear on a vocal cord?

So many questions, so many clues. If we are to solve this enquiry, we shall inevitably have to understand the tool that enables us to communicate. Understanding the alchemy between man's genetic code and the intangible voice will take us to the frontier between art and science. Man's evolution is the common thread that will help us solve the mystery of the human voice. Between the cell and the larynx, the brain and language, hearing and giving voice, the vocal landscape of *Homo vocalis* takes shape. The first section of this book addresses this very question: *What do we know about the voice?*

The second part focuses on revealing the magic of the voice, *what we do with it* and *how we use it*. Its beauty, its weaknesses, its diversity, its charisma, its psychological impact are a reflection of the scars we carry. The sacred voice, deviant forms of voice—from eunuchs to ventriloquists, the voices of professionals—be they singers, comedians, lawyers, politicians or teachers, voice in its day-to-day usages—in all its forms, the voice is always a reflection of our personality.

But is there such a thing as a normal voice? Should a nodule on the vocal cords automatically be operated on, when it imparts such sensuous charm to a voice? For here we have an imperfection giving rise to vocal seduction.

Does the individuality of one's voice make one its accomplice? Are we the instigators of its problems? Does our voice not reflect our present state? And when all is said and done, is the vocal print not simply the imprint left by the breath of life?

Acknowledgments

$\mathscr{T}$his voyage was first conceived at the start of this millennium. My encounters with others, the emotional charge of the voice, the latest scientific discoveries relating to Man's vibratory mechanism, enabled the writing of this book. The alchemy between my family circle, my friends, patients, artists, musicians and science was its creative source.

I should like to thank those who witnessed the early stirrings and the development of my passion:

My wife, Beatrice, who lovingly, hour by hour, shared my passion.

My son, Patrick, who was able to give me filial and professional advice with pertinence and affection; his wife Elsa, whose comments were always justified and sincere, and my grandson, Sacha, whose first words enriched my inspiration.

My daughter, Delphine, whose tender love, patience, understanding and attentive listening have been a precious help to me.

My parents, Charles and Lise.

My grandmother, mamie Hélène.

My sister Betty and her children, Thierry and Candice, and her companion David.

My sister Caroline, artistic photographer, who observes the present.

For nearly two years, the storyline of this book monopolized me, practically kidnapped me from the family unit. Yet my family was always present for me with objective, valid, and helpful criticism when I struggled with writing difficulties.

Yves Gauguet, my friend on this long voyage, philosopher of the affect, helped me understand the frontiers between art and science, helped me perceive and integrate these few words of Albert Einstein: "Science is nothing without imagination."

Knowledge sources, scientific sources and artists were indispensable to me in my quest to penetrate the intangibility of the voice, its origins, its personality. Special thanks to my scientific friends and colleagues. Dr. Charly Presgurvic, a country doctor I replaced at the start of my career, who enabled me to understand Man beyond his illness, was a great friend and mentor.

I'm also very grateful to my cousin, Professor Daniel Dayan; writer and sociologist, Professor Philippe de Wailly; doctors Albert Castro and Claude Timsit, for their very judicious advice; Mady Mesplé, soprano and remarkable teacher; Francis Bardot, singing teacher; Sabine de la Brosse, medical journalist; Dr. Jean-Jacques Maimaran, a longstanding friend and colleague.

A very special thanks to my friends and awe-inspiring colleagues, Professors Robert. T. Sataloff and Michael. Benninger, for whom music, art, and science are intimately linked.

My observation of the voice's vibrations and of the harmony of words has helped me to understand better the hidden face of the artist.

Robert Hossein made me vibrate time and time again as I watched him direct his artists and mimic his characters. His ardor, his passion, is infectious. As for his voice, you know how it is! His charm seduces us.

James Conlon, a remarkable international conductor, doesn't read music, he lives it. He doesn't direct the orchestra, he uses it as a painting palette on which each color is a musical instrument. His wife, Jennifer Conlon, a soprano, contributed to my scientific research.

Cyprien Katzaris, a pianist, brings Chopin to life for us, identifies his fingers with his whole body. In his view, he doesn't play, he interprets; he makes the instrument his emotional vibration.

Thanks to these musicians, I was able to fathom the complexity of the loop between our vocal emission and our auditory reception—is the human voice not also an instrumental synthesizer? Is it not simply the meeting of the rational and the chaotic, from which harmony is created?

Charles Aznavour, singer and poet, invites us into his world of harmonics, texts, and suggestive words. Years meant nothing to him; the wrinkles of the voice never concerned him. Roberto Alagna is an exceptional tenor whose vocal print enthralls the public. Levon Sayan, so supportive of these artists, knows how to galvanize them.

Georges Mary invited me into the backstage of this universe in which the clown who laughs is sometimes especially sad, in which the artist remains fragile under the spotlights.

The ventriloquists Christian Gabriel and Valentine Vox helped me understand the mystery of these magicians of the voice.

What was remarkable in the writing of this book was the involvement not only of my professional circle, but also of my close friends. They stimulated me when necessary, they calmed my excessive ardor. I would like to express my loyal friendship and gratitude to Alain and Josette B., Bernard and Edith L., Alain and Roselyne C., Jean-Claude and Irène D., Sydney and Nicole O., Francis P., Franck H., David and Caroline C. and Nicholas B.

I also wish to thank Nicole Lattès at Editions Robert Laffont, as well as Malcy Ozannat, whose advice was of precious help in adapting my sometimes overly scientific language in order to make the *Odyssey of the Voice* an easier read.

My numerous travels led me to consider Man's voice within the context of his culture, his traditions, his social background, his climatic environment. Moreover, numerous scientific, anthropological, artistic, and musical works transported me in the space-time of the human voice, from its origins to this day.

To all who stood by me, and to all who inspired me, to these numerous artists, sculptors, painters, singers, actors and writers who allowed me into their emotional world that is so richly hued, in which science is an instrument and not an end, nor a beginning:

A big thank you!

Part 1

To the roots of the voice

Chapter 1

Back to the origins of the voice

Long before the advent of man,
long before that of the voice
there was the big bang that rocked
the universe out of its silence.

The human voice in its vibration reflects our own evolution. A complex alchemy between our DNA, our thought processes and our expression, our voice is particular to Man. Both master and tool of our thoughts, it is the articulation of language. Whether on a grand scale or on a minute scale, it expresses our imagination and is part and parcel of time and space. Man speaks. What multiple paths has Man's voice been down? Since when? What was there in the very beginning? What strategy did it adopt in order to evolve into the language of the 21st century?

How did life create the Word? Did the particles of DNA that engendered speech come from the cosmos?

Organized chaos

Picture the beginning of the universe, some 14.3 billion years ago, after the mighty Big Bang. The cosmic plasma is just unremitting chaos. Then the Sun takes shape. It begins to illuminate space

4.6 billion years ago. Today, it's halfway through its given lifetime. It's just another star among so many others in our galaxy: the Milky Way.

Our solar system was created from a central core of gases that generated its own gravity. Rocky microparticles called planetisimals and gaseous elements revolved around the star to be.

Under the influence of acceleration and gravity, the vertiginous merry-go-round causes these microparticles to concentrate into a central sphere—the Sun. Around it, the eight planets such as we know them take form. The ninth, Pluto, is more of an asteroid than a planet. Asteroids and comets coexisted with our planets in this interstellar maelstrom.

Fifty million years go by. The Sun is formed. The planetisimals solidify at varying distances from the Sun, forming the four rocky or telluric planets: Mercury, the closest to the Sun, Venus, Earth, and Mars. The gases are forced outward beyond the Sun, creating four gaseous planets: Jupiter, Saturn, Uranus, and Neptune. An incessant molecular waltz characterizes them. Their composition is 98% hydrogen and 2% helium. Saturn would float on the sea!

Another 50 million years go by to create our planetary ballet. 100 million years have elapsed since the Sun was created. Our solar system is in place. Planet Earth revolves around the solar star, outer space is empty or nearly so: 2% hydrogen, nearly 98% helium. The reverse of the composition of the gases that make up the gaseous planets. Outer space is silent, or almost silent: a secret melody animates it. The residual echo of the Big Bang still travels through space, measured at three degrees Kelvin. The ambient temperature is practically absolute zero.

The Earth basks in the Sun without burning

Planet Earth has found its place, 147 million kilometers from the Sun. An ideal distance: close enough not to be frozen like Mars, far enough not to be burned like Mercury. The solar rays reach the Earth in 8 minutes.

The Earth has a circumference of 12,700 km. It revolves around the Sun in 24 hours. That is its daily cycle. 500 million years ago, this same cycle took 18 hours. The Earth was then the densest planet in the solar system, with the strongest magnetic field. Today, the Earth is still subjected to volcanic activity; this makes it a living planet. Its central core is ferrous, burning at over 6,000 degrees Celsius. This molten core is the source of the Earth's gravitational energy. The Earth spins at a speed of 29.79 km per second. But the sun also revolves around something, and that something is the center of our galaxy, 30,000 light-years from the Sun. The diameter of the Milky Way is 90,000 light-years. The solar star spins at 230 km per second. Therefore, it takes the Sun 250 million years to do a full rotation around our galaxy. Since its creation, it has already completed 18 full rotations.

But to get back to our Blue Planet, which has not always been blue. We human beings are constituted, made up of, structured by inert atoms. This magical cohesion gives life when it's reproduced. It creates Man. Calcium, carbon, hydrogen, nitrogen, and oxygen make up our body and produce its energy. They are the indispensable particles of DNA, or deoxyribonucleic acid, the molecule of life. Thus, the infinitely great and the infinitely small come together. Order and disorder complete each other. It is the meeting of yin and yang. Harmony in the making. The Blue Planet emerges. The composition of its exceptional atmosphere allows procreation and the perpetuation of Life.

When we breathe, we breathe in oxygen. The air we breathe in is 22% oxygen, 0,1% helium, and nearly 79% nitrogen. This means that the air on Earth is dense enough to allow the propagation of vocal waves. No so on Venus, where the air is 100 times denser than on Earth. The concentration of CO_2 on Venus is 96%, which precludes any life such as we know it, and any form of voice. On Mars, the atmosphere is 100 times less dense than on Earth. The composition of its atmosphere is similar to that on Venus. No question of speaking on the Red Planet either. The timbre of our voice is directly related to the density of the air we breathe. When we breathe in pure helium, we quack like a duck. The helium affects the vibration of the vocal cords, producing a weird tonality. Their vibratory energy is modified by the density of the air. The less dense the air, the sharper the voice; the denser the air, the deeper the voice. It seems that the human voice is only possible on Earth.

The moon, faithful satellite, but since when?

The cycle of life on Earth depends not only on the rotation of the Earth around its axis and around the Sun, but also on our satellite, the Moon. The Moon's balancing act in space is astounding. The

Moon gives rhythm to our life cycles, to the female menses, to the tides. How was the Moon created? How did it come to be suspended in space, faithful companion to the Earth? Its mass is theoretically too important compared to the Earth's for it to remain our satellite. Earth is the only telluric planet with a satellite, though Mars does have tiny satellites, 16 to 28 km across. Let's pursue this line of inquiry.

The air on the Moon is less dense than on Earth. In fact, it has the same density as the Earth's crust. Recall that the core of the Earth is ferrous, while the core of the Moon is not. Could the Moon possibly be a chunk off our planet?

Our planet has finalized its form. The Moon doesn't yet exist. A certain tranquility reigns. The Earth is differentiating itself from the other planets and has distanced itself from the Sun. The time: 4.5 billion years ago. But the tranquility is about to be disrupted. A monstrous asteroid, one-tenth the size of Planet Earth, hurtles through space. It is almost as big as Mars. It smashes into our planet and amputates part of the Earth's crust. Thus was the Moon born. Gravitational fields were to make possible the impossible. Instead of drifting in space, the satellite gravitates around our planet. Apparently, the Earth's bachelor days were short-lived. It has nearly always lived alongside its old friend the Moon. But after the crash with the asteroid, the Earth is slightly off its axis, causing it to revolve forever around the Sun. The gravitational forces between the Earth and the Moon allow a harmonious balance to establish itself. This symbiosis plays a major role in the appearance of Life on Earth, as indeed it does in the moods of living beings on our planet.

The lunar cycle and the nautilus: a clock of the past

In the 21st century, the Moon revolves around the Earth in 29.5 days. But this hasn't always been the case! A beautiful spiral shell, the chambered nautilus, brings us a clock of the past. The shell is inhabited by a mollusk that creates a new transverse partition inside the shell every lunar cycle, carefully remaining in the portion of the shell nearest the exit. Each day, the mollusk also carves a new ridge inside the shell. Thus, the present-day nautilus has 29.5 ridges per partition. Nautilus fossils dating back 45 million years have 29.1 ridges per lunar cycle. 2.8 billion years ago, they had only 17 ridges.

In those distant times, the lunar cycle was, therefore, 17 days. The lengthening of the lunar cycle is a secondary manifestation of the progressively greater distance of the Moon from our planet. Each year, it's 3.5 cm farther from us, due no doubt to gravitational forces. So we are not about to lose our Moon! Thus was our world formed, such as we know it today.

Planet Earth becomes the Blue Planet

The Moon revolves around the Earth; the Earth revolves around the Sun; the Sun revolves around the center of the Milky Way; the actors of the Universe are in place. The Earth becomes blue thanks to our atmosphere. Life can appear. The only missing element is DNA.

In space, between the Earth and the Moon, a white light surges at vertiginous speed. A gigantic bolt of light illuminates several hundred kilometers of the surface of the Earth's crust. This unidentified flying object has a long plume behind it. It crashes. This UFO brings with it molecules from the living world: it is a comet, made up of snow and water. Mixed in with this dirty snow are other small, hard, strange elements. Silicates. And organic matter, amino acids, elements that are indispensable to life, as is water. That event marked the beginning of life on Earth.

Back then, thanks to this comet, one could drink interstellar water! Is it the same water that hydrates us today? Perhaps. This reminds us that we are all particles from the cosmos and that we owe the humidification of our vocal cords to these comets that came seeking our planet. The origin of life, particles of water, numerous organic molecules have just disembarked from the luminous spaceship that is the comet, itself interstellar dust, a flying object from our galaxy, vehicle for the transmission of life. But this only pushes further back the question of the origins of life: if it did not start on our planet, where did the first molecule of life come from? The comets brought us the missing link of the Blue Planet, the transition from the inert to the living.

Apparently, the impact between the comet and Planet Earth made possible the creation of the first living cell. Cells that would enrich the Earth's crust and its atmosphere. Is DNA a product of that crash between the comet, solar energy, and the Blue Planet? Such is the theory proposed by Whipple in 1950.

But how did *FOXP2* (Enard et al., 2002) develop, that amazing, incredible gene of the human voice, specific to the human language? What is the real story of DNA and of its mutation throughout those billions of years? Only Man has an articulated language. A language he forms with his mouth and larynx and controls with his brain. This gene is but one of the elements that make the human voice possible. For indeed, everything is complex. Experience shows us that the magic of life on Earth was made possible by the linkages and complementarity between molecules, cells, gravitational forces, and photons.

The first unit of life appears on Earth

The first cell to appear on Earth was not the determining factor in this story; for it was rather the cell's reproduction, billions and billions of times over, that produced the complexity of the human being.

But how did this cell first materialize?

Given the existence of billions of galaxies and billions of stars, does DNA exist only on Earth? The relative positions of the Earth and Moon relative to the Sun, the presence of Jupiter, which balances gravitational forces in our solar system, are almost unique ingredients that make life possible. Water is indispensable for the sustenance of life, but is not a sufficient element on its own. The temperate temperature means that proteins don't coagulate or freeze. Man is thus an exceptional multicellular harmony, a chaotic system, complex and regulated by a great variety of factors. And like the trajectory of a leaf falling from a tree, Man's breath, cardiac rhythm, thoughts, and voice are not governed by fixed, rational laws. Man is dependent on parameters of which the fundamental characteristic is an extreme sensibility to the initial conditions. He is chaos within perfection. Planet Earth allows evolution by virtue of its harmony within its galaxy and, above all, by virtue of the preservation of its atmosphere.

Charles Darwin published a revolutionary piece of work in 1859. Called *The Origin of Species*, it would provoke a paradigm shift in scientific and philosophical circles, shaking prevailing beliefs. Darwin put forward two theories: first, evolution is the fruit of natural selection; second, the origin of evolution was a cell. Today, we would say that the origin of evolution was a gene.

Darwin and evolution

This visionary had already proposed a scheme, which, though undoubtedly clear, was nevertheless reductionist. For it suggested that, over time, the cell had evolved to produce the medusa, the fish, the amphibian, the reptile, the bird, and the mammal, in that order.

Around the time that Darwin publishes his work, a different theory on spontaneous generation is also being hatched, a theory according to which inert matter can spawn living matter. Louis Pasteur emphatically disagrees. In 1864, he proves the theory's lack of validity. Inert matter can't spawn living matter. Only a living cell can reproduce a living cell, and this theory is still valid today, at the start of the 21st century. A living cell can't be reproduced synthetically. Man cannot play with the Golem!

The creation of DNA

If one gives credence to the belief that the universe has a beginning, then logically it must also come to an end one day. The search for the origin of the first amino acids, and therefore of DNA, leads Stanley Miller to attempt the following experiment in 1953: he mixes different gases, then produces a flash. He observes the creation in vitro of amino acids. A huge disappointment is in store, for later the gases now thought to have been present in the cosmos 4.6 billion years ago will be found to bear no similarity to those used in Miller's experiment. Thus the origins of the first living cell remain an enigma.

How far back to the origins of Life?

Why such focus on the cell? The cell is the basic unit of life of our organism, which has billions of cells. This unit has another constituent part: the genome. The genome appeared some 3.8 billion years ago, 800 millions years after the start of the solar system. First to appear were single-cell micro-organisms like the amoeba or ciliated protozoan. Their basic structure resembles that of our body's cells. We are a mass of ciliated protozoa. The ciliated protozoan shows a certain complexity. It requires nourishment, reproduces itself, and dies. This has been its pattern for billions of years. Thanks to the electron microscope, we now understand much better both the mystery of the cell and its harmony. It's like a ship with an imposing frame: the pilot's cabin is the nucleus with its chromosomes, the seat of our DNA. The nucleus is surrounded by cytoplasm. Embedded in the cytoplasm are power stations called mitochondria. These tiny organelles transform nutrients into life-sustaining energy. The mitochondrion organelle is the only element of the cell outside the nucleus to possess a DNA molecule. Why?

A bacteria invades the cell

The mitochondria are one of the only energy resources sustaining our survival and they are part and parcel of our cells. This wasn't always the case. In the early days of our planet, the mitochondrion was more than likely bacteria with its own DNA. When living matter appeared on our planet, the mitochondria invaded the cell. Living matter and, more specifically, the sexual cell resulted from this symbiosis. The mitochondria provide energy, the cell makes reproduction possible.

Interestingly, there are seven times more mitochondria in the cells of the vocal cords, the eye muscles, and the heart muscle than in the biceps muscle. The energy fueled by the mitochondria serves to synthesize proteins. These proteins, which are specific to each gene, impart the particular nature of each organ—the kidney, the heart, the brain—and of each function. The genome specific to the voice is among others *FOXP2*. Thus, the voice also has its origins in DNA. The chemical reactions necessary to the production of protein are in place. When protein is created, it is used for a precise purpose and for a specific function. It can also be stored for future use, or for an emergency. The cell derives its personality from protein. It has a membrane, a lining that protects it from the outside world. The lining is permeable. It allows in the messages addressed to the DNA, as well as energy resources intended for the mitochondria. It allows out toxins, as well as messages required by other cells. These messages concern, more specifically, glandular cells and brain cells such as neurons.

Survival is harmony

The survival of a cell depends upon the coexistence of all parameters, not only in that cell, but also in our body, and in harmony with all other cells. It becomes clearer why the synthesis of the living cell appears to be impossible. DNA, a giant, monstrous molecule, is in the shape of a double helix. Watson and Crick "discovered" DNA in 1953. They demonstrated its presence in every living cell, proving that it is essential to life and to reproduction. All living organelles contain DNA. Even better, this spiral molecule contains the secret of our evolution and the key to our personality. Coded, it can mutate. It's specific to each person, except in the case of real twins, called monozygotic twins. Here we are confronted with true clones. Born from the same ovum and the same spermatozoon, which give life to two distinct but identical living beings with exactly the same 30,000 genes and their molecular resonance; and paradoxically, affinities close to extrasensory perception as well as telepathic gifts that are difficult to apprehend in our rational world. This is in contrast to dizygotic twins, formed from one ovum and two spermatozoa. Thus, one can give birth to a girl and a boy who look alike, but have different DNA. Monozygotic twins look exactly alike. They also have identical voices to begin with, but the scars of life introduce perceptible differences over time.

DNA is formed from four basic elements called bases: adenine, cytosine, thymine, and guanine, or ACTG. This alphabet of life writes the story of our existence. Given DNA's length, a million pages would be required to write all the bases that make up the DNA molecule. It's stored in the cell nucleus, in a space no bigger than a few thousandths of a millimeter. In this sense, the "genetic" code is a true language, but one that is the mother language of all languages. The combination of these four essential molecular units dictates its law. One could almost say that it enables the creation of Man in its image, or that "it's a case of language creating Man rather than Man creating language," as was claimed dramatically by Jacques Monod on the 3rd of November 1967 at the Collège de France. It seems that a direct, almost filial, link exists between the genetic code and the human voice. Could the discovery of the *FOXP2* gene be the first stepping-stone toward this scientific and philosophical possibility?

DNA has been transmitted for over 3 billion years. It has suf-fered several mutations: mutations that have caused a physical, physiological, and morphological transformation of the species. The mutation acts directly on the chain of DNA bases and on the coded message. It can modify, break, transform, or alter the gene. It is both a distortion and a modification of the writing of our genetic heritage. If nowadays it is often considered an inauspicious disturbance, in the history of time and space it has enabled the evolution of the different species and, in particular, of the human race.

The DNA clock

How did we go back to our origins? It was thanks to the theory of "the DNA clock": it would appear that the influence of radioactive solar rays on our planet modifies and creates a regular mutation of DNA, in the order of 0.23% every million years. Thus, our DNA, which differs from that of the chimpanzee by 1.6%, suggests that 7 million years separate us from our common cousin. This remains in the realm of probability, given that the impact of solar photons on our planet may have changed due to climatic influences. But for all that the hypothesis is attractive, it probably requires further research. This regular mutation of our planet over time allows us to date var-ious species. We are indebted for this theory to Sibley and Ahlquist.

First, the clones: all cells are identical

As a fundamental constituent of the cell, DNA reproduces itself in a simple manner in the case of the unicellular organism. This was the first form of reproduction in the early days of life on Earth. It is known as mitosis and entails a division of the cell into two parts that are identical to the original cell. Thus, way back, no evolution was possible, as reproduction was purely a cloning process . . .

The cell has a sex: new cells are different

Then a revolution occurred. No one knows exactly why or how. The first cells to appear 3.8 billion years ago do not join up to produce multicellular organisms, they keep to themselves. They don't seduce. They don't couple, because in order to reproduce, they merely divide themselves. They draw their energy from the solar rays that flood our planet. These single-cell living organisms, called eubacters or prokaryotes, are cells that contain DNA, but have no nucleus. They still exist today. Back then, with the help of the photonic rays of the Sun, they enabled oxygen to be formed from the carbonate gases of our planet's atmosphere. This mechanism is called photosynthesis. Nearly 2 billion years go by. Our atmosphere changes. The density of the oxygen in the air becomes sustaining. Multicellular living organisms, or eukaryotes, are able to exist. From now on, DNA is concentrated in one part of the cell's nucleus and surrounded by a membrane. The cell has a sex: male or female. We no longer have cells dividing in two to produce clones, we have two cells coupling to produce a new cell. A cell that carries the characteristics of the parent cells, but differs from them both. Besides, in order for a gene to arise from a phenotype manifestation, such as blue or brown eyes, it must be activated and stimulated. A gene can also be present in the DNA chain and remain dormant—no one will know of its existence! These are the first manifestations of Man's evolution.

Earth is enveloped by the Big Blue

The sky exists. The ocean exists. Mountains and valleys give relief to the Earth's surface. Living organisms take up residence. The sexual cell appears. The meeting of male and female cells will allow the miracle of evolution to take place. The coupling of two sexual cells, or gametes, each of which possesses half the number of chromosomes of the cell to be, exists in every animal on Earth.

Every cell in a sexual living organism possesses 2N chromosomes, which make possible the birth of a gamete with N chromosomes, and so gives life to a new living organism that contains these 2N chromosomes. A man has 46 chromosomes: 44 autosomic chromosomes, plus 2 chromosomes called sex chromosomes: the X and Y chromosomes. A woman also has 44 autosomic chromosomes and two XX sex chromosomes. The gamete is the basic unit of procreation. The spermatozoon of a man contains 22 autosomes (numbered 1 to 22), plus a sex chromosome with two types of gametes: X or Y. A woman only has one type of gamete: the ovum.

The ovum also has 22 autosomes (numbered 1 to 22), plus an X-sex chromosome. The coupling of the two gametes will produce a male if the Y spermatozoon penetrates the ovum, a female if it's the X spermatozoon.

The mitochondrion is loyal to the mother

The spermatozoon only passes on its nucleic DNA. The ovum, on the other hand, passes on its nucleic DNA and keeps its mitochondria, and therefore its mitochondrial DNA. Whatever its sex, a child will have its mother's mitochondria and both parents' chromosomes. As soon as the spermatozoon penetrates the ovum, it loses its flagellum. Only the nucleus, which contains no mitochondria, passes through the ovum's membrane and, therefore, only the chromosomatic male information will be contained in the definitive egg. The theory that Eve had mitochondria stems from this observation and would tend to demonstrate that we all descend from the same African mother. We shall examine this in the next chapter.

The sexual organism is the key to evolution

What advantage accrued to Nature, over a billion years ago, from the complication implicit in reproducing by means of a sexual chromosomal mechanism rather than by means of a simple division? This complexity allows the living organism to go down an exceptional evolutionary path. Nothing will be cloned. Genes, the true masters of our ancestors and of our lineage, become subjected to multiple variations. Of course, these variations may be secondary to a mutation, but they may equally be secondary to a genetic compounding of the chromosomes of the parents' gametes when the embryo is formed. The resulting living being will be unique, but will bear the stamp of its past.

DNA is almost immortal. What changes is its envelope.

After this first revolution—the appearance of sexual organisms—comes the revolution of the food chain, of predator and quarry.

Natural selection is under way. Some are better armed than others. Astonishing but true: one species, namely the shark, has not evolved for the past 400 million years! The world of fossils tells us that multicellular marine living organisms appeared some 570 million years ago; trilobites and plants such as ferns appeared some 400 million years ago. The trilobites are already a very complex living being. Their eyes are formed by around a hundred facets, much like the eyes of flies today. These were probably the very first eyes on Earth, just as Man is probably the first living being to have spoken on the Blue Planet.

These trilobites, the first living organisms to see on Earth, passed on this faculty to numerous species. Who knows, the human race could be the starting point for other species with the gift of speech.

The shark has kept the same appearance throughout evolution. Its body is made of cartilage, because bony structures did not exist back then. It owes its survival to the fact that it is the master predator of the Ocean. It's at the top of the food chain. Together with the ray fish, it stalks the oceans devouring defenseless fish without fins or teeth, fish that appeared 530 million years ago. The first fish fed on plankton. But fish with a central bony skeleton appear on the scene relatively quickly. Calcium phosphate, an essential component of bone, survives the passing of time and provides us with proof of these animals' existence in the form of their fossils. Numerous species appear and disappear with the passing of time and the changes of climate. The diversity of the living world is astonishing. Slowly, it evolves toward the primate.

The living organism struggles against gravity

Fish now have a bony skeleton that forms their central structure. They live in the oceans. The respiratory system came on shore with the amphibians and reptiles. The missing link between the fish and the salamander is the acanthostega that lived 350 million years ago. The metamorphosis of the animal world that enabled the conquest of the continents started 330 million years ago. The skeleton evolves.

The locomotor system, until now separate from the pelvis, becomes welded to it to provide support for the body on land. Now gravity comes into play. Motion on shore requires a reasonably stable and solid bony structure. The respiratory system also has to adapt to the atmosphere on land. As the seas gradually recess, giving way to dry land, and lakes gradually disappear, the animals that lived in those waters have to adapt themselves to life on land. The reptile progressively becomes master of the land. Plants develop. Seas and rivers share this watery universe. The shark conserves its supremacy. The reptile will slowly but surely evolve toward the mammal. The intermediary species between the shark and the reptile is the ornithorhynchus (the duck-billed platypus), still with us today. A strange, indeed, very strange animal. It is warm-blooded. It breast-feeds its offspring. Yet it lays eggs.

Evolution undergoes a catastrophic change 250 million years ago. For reasons still to be explained, over half of the then-living marine organisms disappear.

Here come the dinosaurs!

The magnificent epic of the dinosaurs started around 220 million years ago. These exceptional reptiles are kings of the planet. A tropical climate reigns. It promotes gigantism, not only in plants, but also in animals. The Earth becomes a palette of colors, flowers grow. A new species of tiny animals appears: mammals.

Communication through sounds arises. At this stage, it is only embryonic, but it exists. It's made possible by the presence of ears on these tiny mammals and primitive ears on the dinosaur. For the ear is a prerequisite for acoustic communication. The mammal already has small auditory ossicles, a tympanic membrane and the beginnings of an internal ear. *The chain for integrating the human voice has seen the light.* The receiving organ for our language has made its appearance. The ear of the dinosaur is much more primitive. So now noises can be picked up and grunts can be emitted. The voice isn't yet formed, but it's on its way. How will the mammal forge a place for itself on a planet dominated by the dinosaur?

Catastrophe or miracle?

The time is 65 million years ago. The sky is clear. The sun is shining on the horizon. Suddenly, an asteroid streaks through space at a speed of 16 km per second. A ball of fire lights up the skies of the Blue Planet. It approaches fast. It picks up speed as it penetrates the stratosphere. It heads straight for the Gulf of Mexico, in the Yucatan peninsula. The asteroid has a diameter of 12 km. It crashes straight into the peninsula. The angle of attack is 30 degrees. The impact of the crash is terrible. A 300-km-wide crater is formed, testimony to the monstrous cataclysm, without precedent, that Planet Earth has just suffered. A cloud of smoke, dust, and rocky debris rise into space. In a matter of a few hours, a few days, it covers North America, then the entire planet. At the moment of impact, fires propagate. All is burned to a cinder over hundreds of kilometers. The shock wave destroys the animal and plant worlds within a radius of thousands of kilometers. Worse still, the brutal and intense warming of the atmosphere releases nitrogen into the air. A chemical reaction takes place, resulting in devastating acid rain. The landscape on Earth is one of desolation. These fatal downpours are accompanied by impressive thermal energy released by the impact, causing radiant heat on Earth.

At the site of the crash, iridium, deformed quartz and microdiamonds are found both in and around the crater of the Yucatan. These discoveries back up the theory put forward by Luis Álvarez, according to which the dinosaurs were wiped out by an asteroid.

Thus, the collision causes a deluge, considerable thermal energy, and chemical chain reactions and plunges Earth into darkness for a period of several months, if not years.

The Sun can no longer warm the planet. The dust screen neutralizes the effect of the solar photons. The Earth enters an Ice Age. Photosynthesis is practically nonexistent. No photosynthesis, no oxygen. Thousands of species—90% of plants and 70% of animals—disappear forever. The reign of the dinosaur meets its end. Catastrophe or miracle? The reign of mammals could open out: the human race is not far off.

Life reclaims its stake. The thick cloud of smoke thins. Blue skies reappear. Photosynthesis reconquers the planet. Mammals continue their evolution, leading them inexorably toward *Homo vocalis*.

To admire the bird winging its way across the ocean is to behold the ancestor of the dinosaur . . .

The mammal comes knocking at the door

The climate becomes more temperate. The evolution of mammals accelerates impressively. The evolution toward mankind is underway.

We witness the appearance of the first marsupials, with an external ventral pouch in which the fetus matures. Next to appear, and directly in line with Man, are placental mammals, mammals whose fetus develops inside their body, in the uterus. The space-time path continues its unstoppable journey. Communication means between mammals improve and diversify spectacularly. Bats, which first appeared 55 million years ago, use echolocation to find their bearings via ultrasound. Dolphins also communicate thanks to sonic location and emit other peculiar sounds that we shall come back to.

The launching gene for speech in Man seems to be *FOXP2*. It is about to be activated and stimulated. (Unless it did not exist before, and its appearance is due to a mutation.)

However, evolution is evolving, not only thanks to DNA mutations, but also thanks to the food chain. All grass-eating animals depend on the plants that they ingest. Plants are themselves the end result of the transformation of solar energy into biological energy, are they not?

During its embryological life, the mammal will live through a speeded up version of what mankind went through over several hundred million years. Namely, the meeting of two cells called gametes, followed by the appearance of metazoans, small living organisms with two layers of cells. Followed by living organisms with three layers of cells. In the human embryo, these layers are known as the ectoderm, the mesoderm, and the endoderm, the very essence of Man's structure. The endoderm, basically a mass of cells, is none other than the internal layer from which our digestive system evolves. The ectoderm serves as an external casing and the mesoderm is the bit in the middle that forms our viscera. And there we have the makings of the human embryo! Such is Hoertl's theory, at the end of the last century. The nine-month-long intrauterine life of man's offspring bears a curious resemblance to the evolution we have mapped out from the amoeba to Man.

Life has a universal master plan

I was very impressed by the following experiment. The development of the eye is determined by a group of genes. Researchers removed this group of genes from the embryo of the *Drosophila* fly. At birth, the baby fly was blind, it had no genes of the eyes.

Then they destroyed the same group of eye genes (located in the same place on the DNA chain) in the embryo of the immune mouse and replace it with the genes removed from the *Drosophila* fly. A baby mouse is born with the eye genes of the *Drosophila* fly in its DNA, and it sees! This experiment suggests that the location of genes is universal, that their location on the DNA chain is precise, and that it is practically identical for all animal species. Thus, one group of genes "creates, builds, and develops" the eyes; another group creates the organs of the trunk, then the pelvis, and last of all, the brain. They don't have to be activated to appear. This understanding of the genome tends to support the view that animals have the same master plan as do insects, fish, birds, or humans. In this case, the genetic information to create the eyes exists, it imposes itself. To prevent its transmission, it has to be removed.

Elsewhere, for other functions, the gene exists, but needs to be activated if the function is to materialize. Is that true for the human voice? We will explore that later with Frederic II from Prussia. A function may also be nonexistent because the genes for it do not exist, it will then depend on a new mutation of the DNA.

The genetic heritage of Man and ape is very similar. Only 1.3% distinguishes us. Therefore, 98.7% of the ape's DNA is identical to Man's, even though the ape has 48 chromosomes against Man's 46. This may seem like a minute difference, but in fact, it's considerable. For example, we know that in Man, if a single amino acid is missing from the hemoglobin molecule, which has around 574 amino acids, survival is impossible. In other words, here a 0.017% variation spells the difference between life and death.

The ape's brain is much smaller than Man's. Yet it seems that the ape's genes, if not identical to Man's, are extremely comparable. Analysis of the proteins destined for the brain reveals much greater molecular diversity in Man than in the ape. In a matter of a few million years, the maturation of the brain evolved astonishingly fast to produce *Homo vocalis*.

The DNA in our chromosomes contains our full story, from the origins of Man on our planet until now. Could it be that DNA is none other than Life itself and that only its carnal envelope changes?

Chapter 2

The evolution of
the human voice

*The evolution of the species, the evolution of mankind
is like a notched wheel that can only turn in one
direction. The reverse motion does not exist.*

Numerous paleontologists present the odyssey of evolution as a logical progression from the four-legged ape down to two-legged *Homo sapiens*. They are convinced that the ape's erect position on two legs resulted from his having come down from the trees to take up permanent residence on the ground. Others, like Sir Arthur Keith, argue that the ape became a biped before he came down from the trees. Whichever way it happened, it enabled encephalonization, articulated speech and, therefore, the creation of the voice.

The newborn baby of the 21st century resembles our ancestor *Homo erectus*

The different theories put forward concerning the language of *Homo erectus* agree on one point: his laryngeal system resembled that of a newborn baby's. His cortex will become the site of areas specific to language: Broca's area and Wernicke's area. Such individualization is only sketchy in the chimpanzee, with its highly developed limbic system. But in Man, stimulation of the limbic system doesn't bring on articulated speech; it provokes only cries and noises.

Thus, *Homo erectus* was probably capable of some sort of highly succinct form of verbal expression. Judging from the size of his skull and the "brain print" found inside the various fossil skulls found in Africa, he was slow to conceptualize and slow in his speech. For the "brain print" ridges left by the areas of speech on these fossils—he spoke: he is *Homo vocalis*!

Another element must be taken into account. *Homo erectus* was adult by the age of twelve and died around the age of thirty. Specimens of an older age are rare. Specimens of women with osteoporosis are even rarer. Thus, the apprenticeship is short-lived, but sufficient already. Thanks to his voice, he forms predictive and abstract thoughts. He uses his own experience to invent new words and new concepts and to discover a more elaborate language. In 1912, Korbinian Brodmann demonstrated in a comparative study that in the cat, 3.5% of the brain is devoted to language, as against 17% in the chimpanzee and 30% in Man. This frontal lobe, let us not forget, is the master brain. But the acquisition of language co-opts the whole brain in, and is different from the acquisition of, the voice.

Man, a survivor of evolution

Through living longer, he developed his voice

Along the millenniums, Man's longer life span allowed him to develop his voice and brain to an exceptional degree. Indeed, if we are able today to refer to scientists of the past millennium, it's because their oral communications were written down; this passing down of knowledge fueled progress. Most researchers make noteworthy discoveries after the age of thirty. The experience they have acquired enables them to share their knowledge with younger students. These younger students, by the time they are twenty, already possess the same theoretical knowledge as their masters, themselves in their forties and fifties. This tuition or transmission was at first oral, which underlines the importance of this precious gift that is the voice.

The pen of our intellect has been writing our voice for several millennia. First, the voice enables thinking, and the mind then makes use of the voice to express itself through the voice. Both contribute to the acquisition and discovery of our scientific, artistic, and intellectual heritage. In a snowball action, they are both active participants in their own progress and evolution.

Charles Darwin's findings in 1859 on the comparative anatomy of the great apes classify Man as a direct descendant of the primates and not as a singular phenomenon. Man has been unseated from his throne. He is the last link in the chain of evolution. In the same way, Nicolaus Copernicus, man of the cloth and Polish canon, in 1543 dislodged the Earth from its central position in our universe. He published *De la révolution des sphères célestes* (The revolution of the celestial spheres) in which he expounds his heliocentric model of the universe, going counter to the age-old theory that the Earth is the center of the universe. A geocentric model that was oh-so-comforting and perfectly in tune with our pyramidal way of thinking. The convictions of two millennia are shaken; yet Copernicus was wrong, because he believed the Sun to be the celestial center of the Universe, the Earth being just another planet among others.

Thus, within a gap of three centuries, two revolutions shake prevailing ideas. Nicolaus Copernicus, mathematician and astrophysicist of the 16th century, dislodges the geocentric model of the Universe with his heliocentric model. Three centuries later, Charles Darwin, anthropologist of the mid 19th century, provides proof that Man is a species of mammal.

A direct lineage between the ape and Man doesn't seem very likely. It would be more correct to say that they are cousins with a common ancestor, as demonstrated by the arguments provided by the recent theory of the clock of nuclear DNA. In 1927, Henry Fairfield Osborn, Director of the American Museum of Natural History, opted unequivocally for two distinct phylogenic trees. He had foreseen the existence of DNA and its mutations.

The bottleneck of evolution

Natural selection allows Man to survive because his ability to escape predators effectively guarantees his descent. Articulated speech was probably one of the most appropriate of acquisitions for this permanently upright creature from the savanna.

The lion, the jaguar, and the zebra are four-legged: not only because this particular anatomy imparts excellent stability and remarkable speed when in movement, but also because these animals fit into the scheme of evolution. A scheme that began with the fish, with its four fins, and continued with the amphibians, salamanders or frogs, reptiles, crocodiles or lizards, and finally mammals, with their four legs (see Plate 1). Cetaceans, whales, or dolphins all have, as does *Homo sapiens*, five fingers on their upper or anterior limbs. However, Man is the only permanently biped mammal and his brainpower is exceptional.

Natural selection brings us *Homo sapiens*. Nevertheless, we must introduce another concept here: the concept of "the bottleneck of evolution," which will attempt to elucidate for us why all men on our planet speak. This scientific enterprise is essential if we are to understand how the human voice, articulated speech, and the five thousand languages recorded on our planet, came about.

The planet of the primates

A species, through a mutation of its DNA, produces a genetic variation. Its genetic identity card, or genotype, changes; therefore, its physical aspect or phenotype also changes. For example, the original population resembles the mutant, much like the chimpanzee resembles Man. Inasmuch as this mutation has created a new species, this species can become a "superpredator," a predator that imposes himself, colonizes, invades the planet, and may even at times exterminate the species that bred him. Such is the bottleneck theory.

This theory can itself be secondary to climatic influences, the climate then taking on the role of "supreme predator." Men survived the Ice Age because they built shelters, learned to make fire, to clothe themselves. This adaptability of Man's explains the diversity of his geographic distribution. Of the 185 primates in existence today, from the lemur that weighs 80 grams, no bigger than your thumb, to the gorilla, that weighs 150 kilos and stands nearly 1.80 meters, Man is the only primate able to live under all latitudes. All other primates require richly treed forests or tropical forests or the savannas of Africa, Madagascar, or India. Man owes his survival not only to the fact of being a biped, which freed up his hands, but also to the frontal positioning of his eyes, which gives depth to things; to the verticalization of his thorax, neck, and head, which enabled the development of his encephalon; and to the adaptation of his articulate mandible and maxillary dentition, which gave him the means for articulated language. Primates are not the only species to enjoy the advantages of frontal vision. The cat, the owl, and the eagle also do.

As we know, nearly 65 million years ago, the dinosaur disappeared from our planet. During this same period, the appearance of primates was to turn our planet into "the planet of the apes." Primates, a word invented by Carl von Linné, means "first" in Latin. This 18th century scientist classifies Man as the first living creature on Earth, which is not exactly true. The Tertiary Age allows a particularly exuberant development of monkey and ape species. First were the prosimians, with the tarsier and the lemur, then the simians, with the proconsul, the baboon, the orangutan, and then the gorilla. Nearly 23 million years ago, the evolution of mammals slows considerably. The planet cools down. These climatic bottlenecks favor certain primates and disadvantage others.

Some time later, 17 million years ago, the climate becomes temperate, the Earth heats up. The diversity of mammals now is impressive. At the top of the ranking we find the monkey, the ape and, soon, Man. Thousands of different species roam his savanna. Dry land is gaining ground due to the migration of the continents and decreasing sea levels. Lakes form. The plant world is luxuriant. Animals, fish, reptiles, amphibians, birds, terrestrial or marine mammals are legion. *Homo sapiens* is not far off.

Different cold periods arrest the evolution of primates. 15 to 16 million years ago, then 5.3 million years ago, and finally, 4.5 million years ago, we encounter Ice Ages. These eras are most propitious to the appearance of grass-eaters, hominids, and certain families of primates.

The common denominator of this new race, the primate, is the development of the cranium and, ipso facto, the brain. We see the primates evolving into different groups. The first will give us, amongst others, the gibbon (hylobatides), the second, the orangutan (pongides), the third, the family of the gorilla, the chimpanzee, the bonobo (panines), and finally, *Homo sapiens* (hominids), the only permanent biped.

The mutation of monkey into Man: when and how?

The fundamental transition from the big apes to Man appears to have taken place 5 to 10 million years ago. Back then, we had a common ancestor. If DNA and the study of DNA have enabled us to delve into this prehistoric period, let's not forget how much we have learned from fossils. The proconsul, which appeared 20 million years ago, evolves progressively toward the hominid. The first irrefutable trace of a biped was found in a print left in the volcanic ashes of Tanzania nearly 3.7 million years ago. How did permanent uprightness come about? The enigma is still unsolved. But, as we shall see again in the development of the brain, bipedalism was a key factor in Man's evolution. In the eighties, Yves Coppens puts forward a climatic and geographical theory of evolution in "East Side Story," on the origins of Man and the great apes. Nearly 7 million years ago, the tropical and equatorial forests of Africa suffered an earthquake that was to change the face of the world: it produced the Rift, a mountain range that creates a geographic and climatic cleavage. The clouds are now unable to cross over the mountainous ridge. To the East of the ridge, Africa dries up. In contrast, West Africa experiences a milder, seasonal climate and is subject to a rainy season with monsoons. The first hominids adapt to this change. Man experiences his own evolution from the *Australopithecus* to *Homo sapiens*.

Man carries with him the story of the evolution of his voice: his jaw originates from the first fish, which had teeth, 350 million years ago. You'll recall that the shark already existed back then. Man's middle and inner ear originate from the reptiles, which lacked an outer ear. His pilosity and complete ear (outer, middle, and inner ear) go back only as far as the first mammals. Finally, his erect stance came about progressively, allowing the development of his brain, the descent of the larynx, and the beginning of the voice, apparently some 5 million years ago.

Weight for weight, Man's brain today is five times bigger than that of the apes. But this wasn't always the case, as the following numbers and comparisons illustrate.

The brain of *Australopithecus* (5.5-2.5 million years ago), the man of the savannas, weighed 400 g; that of *Homo habilis* (2.5-1.5 million years ago) 600 g; of *Homo ergaster* (2-1 million years ago) 800 g; of *Homo erectus* (1-0.4 million years ago) 900 g; of *Homo sapiens* (0.3 million years ago to the present day) 1,400 g. This cerebral hypertrophy resulting from evolution endows Man with speech; indeed, his neocortex, the part of the brain that regulates speech, develops to an extraordinary degree.

We know from molds taken from his skull, which show the negative of "the brain print" on this bony cavity, that *Australopithecus* had a projection of language in his brain. Astonishingly, the molds reveal an important asymmetry between the right and the left lobe, more marked in *Homo sapiens* than in *Australopithecus*. The right brain enables the analysis of spatial structures, recognition of objects, and the management of information such as musical harmonies. The left brain is Cartesian, mathematical, and analytic. The blood flow carried by the meningeal veins, whose trajectory is also imprinted on the skull, is more important in *Homo habilis* than in *Australopithecus*, especially at the level of the frontal, temporal, and parietal lobes, testimony to the particularly important development of language—its function, conception, production and comprehension—and of words registered only in the dominant lobe, in areas of the brain called Broca's area and Wernicke's area. Therefore, one can reasonably deduce that 5 million years ago, the premises of the voice already existed.

By the time *Homo habilis* appeared, Man was speaking

How did Man speak? How many words were part of his vocabulary? A strong assumption authorizes the following hypothesis, based on the tribes of New Guinea who are still in the Stone Age and for whom fire is still an essential element of their faith. These tribes use 6,000 words and often address each other through intelligible stomach rumblings, in which the sacred has its place and the abstract conscience, characteristic of Man, replaces behavioral consciousness. Speech sets the foundations for the first human civilizations. But first, the full expression of speech requires a syntax and the semantic construction of words and sentences. The erect stance means that a fundamental element is now vertical: the articulation between the spine and the base of the skull, or occipitus. This is also particular to the human race. It brings about the development of specific areas of the brain that predispose the development of

Man as we know him today, and more particularly, the development of speech. In the monkey, the spine and the occipitus form a 45° angle. In Man, and this is a capital element, the angle formed is 90° (see Plate 2). The cranium is as if resting on the spine. This being the case, it becomes easy for the larynx to drop lower down inside the neck and take up its perfect position for articulated speech, at the level of the fifth cervical vertebra. Thus, the development of sympathetic resonance chambers at the level of the head and the neck becomes possible.

Through having articulated speech, Man emits vowels

The molding of the chimpanzee's voice box, owing to its small size, makes it impossible for chimpanzees to articulate our five vowels. The difference in the distance from the vocal cords to the teeth, the difference in volume and surface, not only of the vocal passage, but also of the resonance chambers, indicates that only Man, primate of primates, is capable of articulated language. Apparently, according to research by Jeffrey Laitman, Neanderthal man can pronounce the vowels *a - i - e - o - u* only to a limited degree. The base of his skull is flat, and the mandible is protracted, features that suggest that the Neanderthal man had very scant speech and a larynx that was still perched very high. Yet, a tiny little bone lost in the neck is of capital importance. Called the hyoid bone, it holds fast the powerful muscles of the tongue. First found in Neanderthal man in 1983, in Kebara, near Mount Carmel in Israel, it testifies to an already evolved language. Tombs and symbols nearby suggest that prayers were customary. Was the voice then already in the service of the abstract, of religion? Thus, the evolution of the human voice inscribes itself in a dynamic process and a mutation that engages not only the brain, but also our phonatory mechanics.

The man from Tautavel

In *Homo habilis*, the larynx remains perched high up in the neck, the expression of speech is basic. Yet it does exist, as shown by the cerebral imprint of Broca's area on the bony surface of the cranium.

No doubt we must wait for *Homo erectus*, nearly 450,000 years ago, before the human voice becomes satisfactory. The base of the skull rests on the spine at a 90° angle. The larynx is level with the middle cervical vertebra. The oral and pharyngeal cavity is adapting to the spoken language. It was in 1971, in the Caune area of Tautavel, in the Oriental Pyrenees, that the Tautavel man was discovered: flat forehead, broad face, and a 1,200 cm^3 brain. His mandibles were also recovered. They show a lesser prominence of the very powerful internal padding on the bone structure that limited the range of movement of the tongue in *Homo habilis*. There's more room for the tongue; consequently it can move around the mouth more easily. It can now arch backward better to create the different vowels that form the backbone of our spoken language.

Yet, a question arises. Before we spoke, before our voice became our privileged means of communication, how did we manage? This was an era of signals, of indices, as pointed out by Boris Cyrulnik. For example, for a small ant, a simple olfactory molecule is a key signal for communicating with its colony. One that is key to the ants' survival, inscribed in their genetic heritage. In the case of Man, we can go so far as to say that his voice, indeed, his language, is indispensable to his survival. His mind turned him into *Homo sapiens*, whose ineluctable evolution on our planet requires of him constant creativity. For unlike the salmon that returns to its breeding grounds, Man by nature constantly seeks out new territories.

Man crossed over the threshold of the articulated voice: he spoke

But, for all that, our voice boxes play a fundamental role in setting the pitch of the voice, in determining the beauty of its timbre, and its harmonics and in defining our vocal print. In Man their essential role is to enable articulated speech.

First, room has to be made for this resonance chamber. It requires a structure that is both hard in certain places, so that we have fixed reference points, and soft in others, enabling us to modify our resonators. If Man can speak and not the primate, from a strictly mechanical viewpoint it's simply because the larynx dropped down inside the neck. This extraordinary downward migration of the larynx, by 7 to 8 cm, consequent to the verticality of *Homo sapiens*, is the indispensable cofactor of the human voice; the other cofactor being, of course, his brain.

A larynx level with the fifth cervical vertebra—has this always been the case for us? As it happens, no! The newborn baby can suckle and breathe at the same time up until the age of eighteen months without any mishaps. Radioscopy has revealed that the newborn baby breathes, swallows, and vocalizes just like the chimpanzee. In that, he is no different from the big apes and all mammals, able to drink, and breathe simultaneously throughout their lives. Thus, the lion, the gazelle, or the panther quenches its thirst as quickly as possible while continuing to breathe, and can thus in a matter of minutes be ready to remove itself from the path of predators.

Between the ages of one to eighteen months, the newborn's larynx drops, as we have seen, from level with the second cervical vertebra, to level with the fifth cervical vertebra (see Plates 3 and 4). Hence onward, he can drink or breathe, but cannot do both at the same time. He forms his voice box, which will enable him to form his articulated language. The monkey, on the other hand, is deprived of the benefit of this evolutionary arrow from time, for its larynx is still placed high (see Plate 5). This is what distinguishes Man from so many primates.

Of course, the size of our brain is a key factor. But it is the multiplicity of factors, the magic of this perfect symbiotic evolution throughout our body, this genetic concatenation caused by progressive DNA mutations that made possible our articulated language: the human voice. Thus, one day, Man crossed the threshold of the spoken language.

In the fascinating delvings carried out during the 20th century in the gorges of Olduvai in Tanzania, a corner of Africa that holds a privileged place in the quest for our roots, Louis Leakey and Yves Coppens, among others, provided us with a glimpse of the first signs of the human voice. Judging by the shape of the cranium, the imprints of the brain on the bone, the skull's angle with the cervical spine, and the presence of a resonance chamber allowing for speech and the emission of vowels, it would seem that this "ancestor man" was also able to speak over 3 million years ago. As remarkably described by Jeffrey T. Laitman, the most important evolution in *Homo erectus*, aside from his brain, was the forming of the resonators.

A machine for exploring the time dimension of the voice

If we could send out a machine for exploring time, we would see that about 15 million years ago, the very first primates communicated through stomach rumblings, shrieks, and shouts. The chimpanzee's vocal cords are also shapely, but less so than Man's. Its larynx mostly serves for breathing, but also for communicating. As evolution ran its course, this phonatory communication sharpened the structure of the vocal instrument. The evolution of laryngeal elements peaks with Man. His vocal cords are long and well-rounded, with precise, delicate vibratory edges, their friction reminiscent of a bow on a violin string. Man's vocal cord is the only vocal cord with three layers of epithelium cells on its surface, in all other mammals it has only two layers. It's also the only one with such a wide vocal register, up to three octaves. The expansion of the thoracic cage and the elasticity of the costal apparatus provide Man with the ability to control his exhalation and with a great capacity for withholding air in order to bring forth a powerful voice.

In this prehistorical world, men hunt for food, run on firm ground, and perfect their language. The tribal chiefs impose themselves through their voice. The men have dominating voices. I cannot say for sure which of the larynx and the brain came first, but it seems reasonable to assume that this evolution was synchronous in all the anatomic elements previously described. Several elements are specific to Man: be it the descent of the larynx, the forming of fleshy lips with external padding existing only in humans, the original epithelial structure of the vocal cords, or localized cerebral specificity, such as Broca's or Wernicke's areas. Within this evolution, Man is only a link in this species of mammals endowed with speech. Intellectual faculties, the faculty to adapt, and vocalization are three essential ingredients for the evolution of language.

Will tomorrow's language call upon other forms of communication still conveyed by the voice? Will telepathy be a new means of communication? Is Man the first link in the species *Homo vocalis*?

Chapter 3

The fossil voice

The human voice is immaterial and leaves no trace.
To go back to its origins therefore seems impossible.
Yet the intangible wind leaves its signature
on the mountainside.

Language, the human voice, phonemes, vowels, and consonants—these are all impalpable elements that leave no tangible trace behind them. Yet indirect witnesses of a fossil voice do exist.

A couple walks side by side in the savanna, in the Olduvai Valley, in Tanzania. This walk takes place 3.6 million years ago. Time will preserve a record of it, discovered in 1978 by Mary Leakey. The couple left imprints of their footfalls in the clay soil. Volcanic ash deposits enable researchers to date them. The analysis of those footprints provides us with a measure of the rhythm of their gait, the amount of downward pressure exerted, the regularity of their stride, even the degree of spring in their pace. Not far from there, fossils of skulls with narrow auditive canals were also found.

Small furrows on the inside of these ancient skulls tell us that the couple was probably chatting companiably of this and that. The molds of the skulls reveal to us the whorls of the cerebral cortex, an indelible record of the evolution of our voice, of our speech, and of our thought processes. These same molds mirror back to us how the brain was organized: one can but wonder, on the one hand, at the extraordinary resemblance between *Homo sapiens* and the big apes and, on the other, at worrying differences between them.

Man is born unfinished: the fossil skull

The development of the brain of *Homo sapiens*, compared with that of the big apes, is awesome. We seem to be confronted with a real quantum leap, with no evident intermediate evolution, an abrupt metamorphosis along the path of evolution. A link is missing in this evolution: why does Man's brain continue to grow so much after birth?

Man is the only mammal with such cerebral growth; a growth that takes place up until the moment of birth, of course, but the brain also continues to grow rapidly and efficiently after birth. At birth, the newborn's skull presents an impressive likeness with that of the chimpanzee. Yet a few years later, the difference between them is spectacular. Man develops in a way that is specific to the human race and this enables him to develop his most precious trump card: his brain. The human adult's brain is three and a half times greater than a newborn's. It seems that he is born "unfinished." It is as if the true gestation period were nine months inside the uterus and twelve months outside it. The elements that are indispensable to *Homo sapiens* only take shape around the age of eighteen months: the ability to prattle, to conceive words, to begin to stand on two feet, the descent of the larynx, standing upright.

The growth of the human brain such as we know it today is not what it was 3 million years ago. Today, a baby is born with a brain of around 400 cm³, which by adulthood will have grown to 1005 cm³. A few million years ago, the skull of *Homo habilis* was much smaller, as indeed was his baby's. This much we know, because the birth canal of "Mrs. *Homo habilis*" was much narrower than the birth canal of women today. However, in those foregone days a baby's brain continued to grow ex utero to the same relative degree as today.

Comparatively, the human brain is ten times larger than that of reptiles and one hundred times larger than that of amphibians. Whales, dolphins, and certain primates have bigger brains in absolute terms. However, Man owes his supremacy to the size of his brain relative to his body mass. For the brain represents only around 2% of our body mass, but it is very greedy: it consumes 20% of our body's metabolic energy. In order to be fully operational and efficient, the brain requires that the body's temperature, arterial pressure, and glycemic level remain constant. A change in any one of these elements can upset our whole organism. Headaches, dizziness, torpor, and convulsions are the early warning signals of such changes. The brain consumes a considerable amount of energy, which is why regular balanced nutrition is so important, at any age, to provide the energy that the brain requires.

The fossil larynx: key to our evolution

Like the cerebral imprints found on fossilized skulls or ancient footprints preserved in clay, the discovery of a larynx, a mandible, or a hyoid bone provides us with indirect evidence of the articulated language of our distant ancestors.

The larynx, indispensable instrument of our voice, also "speaks" of our past. It consists mainly of muscles, cartilages, and joints. Surprisingly, the smallest elements of the larynx, only a bare few millimeters in size, give us remarkable insights into the evolution of the voice box from ape to Man. Called the arytenoid cartilages, these elements are symmetrical, one for each vocal cord. They allow the vocal cords, which are also symmetrical, to open, close, shorten, or lengthen. The study of these small bones by Dr. Lampert, in 1926, enabled us to better understand the evolution of the larynx. The articulation of each vocal cord, left and right, is formed between the arytenoid and the cricoid, a small, unique cartilage perched at the top of the trachea. Lampert analyzed the facets of this joint in both apes and Man. He found that the slope of the joint between the cricoid and the arytenoids increases with respect to the horizontal as a function of a species' closeness to the human species. The slope is 25° in lemurs or mycetes, 45° in cebus monkeys or barking monkeys, 55° in chimpanzees. In Man, the slope is 60°. Thanks to this degree of tilt, the joint has a wider range of motion, from 0 to 60°. The larynx is able to lift up and rock more quickly and efficiently. The movement of the laryngeal instrument in all three dimensions is thereby greatly improved. The slope began its evolution with the mycete monkey, some 15 million years ago. By the time *Homo sapiens* enters on stage, he can play his voice like an instrument.

Because of this angle, our laryngeal space has a most unusual shape. Due to the considerable individuation of the cricoarytenoid joints, it has five distinct sides. This feature is specific to Man. In other mammals, the laryngeal space is four-sided. This gives them more breathing space, thus ensuring excellent airflow, essential when giving chase or fleeing. They thus dispose of a sufficient reserve of oxygen when they breathe in, taking in a maximum volume of air in a minimum lapse of time. These small arytenoid cartilages aren't the only mechanical elements that come into play in phonation.

The other anatomic element that is specific to Man, but only from the age of ten, is the way the surface of the vocal cords is structured. As in the case of skin, this surface is called the epithelium. In all mammals, the epithelium is made up of only two layers, and so it is in Man until puberty. But then a third layer forms, and this imparts impressive precision to the projection, pitch, and timbre of his voice.

The corrugations of the hidden face of the skull

The imprints of cerebral circumvolutions and whorls left by the cortical areas of the meningeal venous network on the inside of fossilized skulls allowed us to map the brain of the ancestors of *Homo vocalis*.

Let us look at this in more detail. For the last several million years, a noticeable asymmetry of the left brain is obvious, more often than not at the expense of the right brain. These developments correspond to the specialization of each cerebral region, linked, for example, to the lateralization of the projection of the hand, of capital importance for making tools and for emphasizing vocal expression. The density of the meningeal venous network in the anterior areas of the brain reflects intense local cerebral activity. This part of the brain manages the complex relationships between the physical and the social environment. The molds reveal an expansion of the parietal area, which plays an essential role in the analysis of information collected by the receptors of our sense organs, and, consequently, in the brain's response to this information. As regards the projection of language and the human voice, in *Homo habilis* one notes for the first time the imprint of a swelling on the left temporal lobe corresponding to Broca's area, the area involved with the *production* of speech. Just behind lies Wernicke's area, the area concerned with *understanding* the spoken word. These molds are the irrefutable testimony that a vocal brain already existed back then. The projection of the motor area of the hand is contiguous with that of the motor area of the voice. That may be why "we speak with our hands."

From the bivouac the voice is born

The development of a cultural environment greatly boosts the evolution of the brain. The men regroup in tribes. They fashion tools and weapons. They make figurative drawings. During the preglacial periods, they are forced to gather in shelters to protect themselves from the cold. These huts, or caves, become a center for cultural exchange and social interaction, and this stimulates the creation of new words. Fire is a central feature, meals are a social affair. But when the climate warms up, it is no longer necessary to take shelter. Now the tribes congregate essentially for nourishment reasons, to hunt and gather food. In Ethiopia, camp fires or bivouacs as old as 1.3 million years and even 2.4 million years have been found. The conquest of fire can be dated unequivocally to 1.4 million years ago. Archeological remains of burnt clay were uncovered in Olduvai. Darwin seems to be right when he claims that Africa was the cradle of mankind. But the classification of animals must be credited to the Swede Carl von Linné, in the mid 18th century. He was the first to identify *Homo sapiens* by name, alongside the chimpanzee.

Man and chimpanzee: a common ancestor
8 million years ago

The discovery of the first human bones provided a solid basis for the theory of evolution. The infinitely small was to be a precious ally in helping us understand the process of evolution. Already, in 1954, researchers had analyzed different immune systems, notably hemoglobin chains. This protein chain, made up of amino acids, consists of 574 amino acids organized into 4 different chains. These form a three-dimensional globular structure (two alpha chains of 141 amino acids and two beta chains of 146 amino acids) that is repeated invariably in all our red blood corpuscles, 6,000 million, million, million times. If even a single amino acid out of the 574 were to change, the hemoglobin molecule would become unreliable. Our body could no longer be oxygenated. The outcome would be fatal.

Molecular anthropology was born from this approach. The molecular clock is an impressive concept. Mutations, if they can ever be accidental, seem to be regulated by chronological biology, a predictable space-time cycle: a 0.26% mutation of DNA apparently occurs every million years.

A comparison of Man's chromosomal or nuclear DNA with that of the chimpanzee allows us to place our common ancestor 8 million years ago. That was when the occasionally erect chimpanzee bowed out to the exclusively upright Man. Being permanently upright brought about a specific positioning of the vertebrae and, moreover, different curves. The curve just under the base of the cranium frees the cranial cavity beautifully and enables a better development of the cortex and the descent of the larynx and the hyoid bone. Additionally, a new curve forms in the sacrum, between the pelvic wings. This means that during childbirth, the newborn's head is forced to turn and exit toward the front of the pelvis rather than toward the back of the pelvis, as is the case in all other mammals.

The gene of speech: a revolutionary concept

Could there exist a gene for speech that would account for the short time frame between *Homo habilis*, our ancestor adapted to living in the trees, and *Homo ergaster*, hyperspecialized for walking and running, and in whom the development of the left brain was probably the single most important development? The study of fossil skulls underscores the massive progress of his brain in relation to language as compared with *Homo sapiens*.

The research team of Wolfgang Enard and Swante Paabo discovered a gene purportedly specific to language, *FOXP2*. This gene is apparently located on the two alleles of chromosome 7. In other words, a binary copy of *FOXP2* is necessary for normal speech. The great apes lack this feature. This gene is seemingly indispensable for the development of the voice, and thus of articulated speech, with its required control over the larynx, the mouth, and the other elements of the voice box. These studies by the Max Planck Institute in Leipzig and by Oxford University provide the missing link in evolution, which is none other than the mutation of a gene that became essential for human speech. The importance of this gene had already been recognized in the case of certain anomalies of the voice, such as dyslexia.

This mutation would seem to have been one of the starting points for speech for the entire human race on our planet.

A common African mother gave us our voice

The blame is on the mitochondria

Once again our DNA, in this instance mitochondrial DNA rather than nuclear DNA, enables us to track down our original mother. The bottleneck in the evolution of the species is addressed in a theory developed by Alan Wilson and his collaborators at the University of California at Berkeley in 1987: the theory of "mitochondrial Eve." These researchers examined the mitochondrial DNA of 147 women deemed to be representative of the female specimen on our planet.

We know that during fertilization, the spermatozoon penetrates the ovum and only its head, with its 23 chromosomes, fertilizes the ovum, which also has 23 chromosomes. The tail of the spermatozoon remains outside the ovum.. Consequently, the big difference between these two distinct entities, soon to become one, is that the ovum and the spermatozoon bring different components into the new cell. One of them—the ovum—still has a nucleus, a cytoplasm, and mitochondria. The other—the spermatozoon—leaves its flagellum "at the door" and procreates only with its nucleus, with no cytoplasm nor mitochondria. The spermatozoon provides only nuclear DNA, which determines the sex of the child to come. Within the cell, the only organelle, apart from the nucleus, that has DNA is the mitochondrion. Therefore, any mitochondria in the body of the child resulting from this fertilization can only be a legacy from the mother. If the human race goes back to a single original mother, we must all have the same mitochondria. And indeed, this is what the theory of the mitochondrial Eve demonstrated; for humans taken from five different continents all turned out to have similar mitochondrial DNA, taking into account DNA's clock. It is worth noting here that mitochondrial DNA only has

37 genes distributed over 16,569 nucleotides; this is meager compared with nuclear DNA, which contains 3 billion nucleotides and some 25,000 to 30,000 genes!

Several scenarios unfold from this study

First scenario: we all descend from the same original mother, who herself had no ancestors. Her existence was due to a DNA mutation. However, this doesn't explain the existence of human fossils that are 200,000 years older, according to the DNA clock. Thus, this first hypothesis hardly seems credible.

The second scenario is worthy of a science fiction movie. The human race was wiped out—except for one couple, that survived. We are all survivors from the same continent, the same region, the same village, indeed the same hut, in central Africa. And we had ancestors prior to this tragedy. This woman, our Eve, belonged to an important population of *Homo sapiens* and was the only woman to survive, along with one or more males. This tragic episode of our history took place 200,000 years ago.

The teacher from Cheddar

In the 1990s, a skeleton some 9,000 years old was found in the small English town of Cheddar. According to the writings of Bryan Sykes, a mitochondrial analysis of the skeleton was possible. The same analysis carried out on a history professor teaching at the local school revealed a mitochondrial DNA profile that was almost identical. The mind boggles at such a close hereditary match, nearly 9,000 years apart!

Genetics and languages

Trying to attribute the origins of our voice to a single genome seems reductionist. Some 5,000 languages are spoken on our planet. Some classification attempt is possible. Roots of words appear in different populations, just as roots of genes do.

We know today that if Africa appears to be the mother continent of the human voice, it is also the mother continent of 400 Bantu languages, among others. We also know that some languages have disappeared. Thus, a genetic origin can't be found for languages. Besides, if an English or French family adopts a Vietnamese child, the child ends up speaking the adoptive parents' language without accent. Equally, if a Masai family in the plains of Tanzania or Kenya adopts an occidental child and teaches the child Swahili, the child will also one day speak Swahili without any accent (plus he will understand the language of the lion, the panther, or the eagle). Therefore, the complexity of our voice is such that it cannot be purely genetic.

Chapter 4

The voice: a learning experience

The voice, pathway between the real and the virtual worlds, is something we learn, build and are characterized by. Voice is the very characteristic of Man.

"Man is a naked biped," Plato proclaims.
To which Diogenus retorts:
"This plucked chicken is Plato's Man."

*O*nly Man has a proper voice. He doesn't just mimick. His voice isn't an object. It lives: it evolves, it becomes richer as the millennia go by. Creator of thoughts, the voice also creates a connection between the individual and the collective.

How was Man one day suddenly able to speak? At what point did he differentiate himself from other mammals in this 4.5 billion years old world? Is Man the only creature on earth with this faculty? True, the mechanism for speech is already in place in the two-year-old child. The cerebral commander stores, learns, and perfects itself. But which came first, the voice or thinking? Was the voice the result of a chance genetic mutation? Is it necessary to our survival on this planet?

The articulated language of our ancestors is taking shape. The mechanics of speech fall into place. They enable the construction of thoughts and thoughts in turn express themselves through the same mechanics. The creation of our abstract world is underway. Words enable us to give names to things and thus to conjure them into existence.

Listening fathered today's voice

From the embryo to the fetus

For the first two years of the newborn's life, its apprenticeship by its mother is a key element for its still incomplete brain. Education, intelligence, but especially, initiation to the spoken word, enable the little one to share in the cultural world of its species. A fundamental aspect of evolution, acoustic communication, is at the origins of the human voice. Thanks to the ear, the fossil aspect of the verbal expression of our thinking yields its secrets already in the early stages of pregnancy. The ear is composed of three parts: the external ear, with its external auditory canal; the middle ear, with its three little ossicles nestled behind a membrane called the eardrum; and finally, the internal ear, with its two distinct structures, the cochlea, which regulates sound and appreciates frequencies, and the three semicircular canals that manage our sense of balance. In the early fetus, the cochlea at first resembles that of a fish, recognizing only low-pitched sounds, then that of a bird, and, finally, that of a mammal, capable of hearing relatively high-pitched sounds. From the sixth month of intrauterine life, the cochlea of the inner ear of the unborn child can only benefit from hearing a wide range of frequencies, different musical instruments, varied types of music, or superb voices. The vibrations will stimulate its cerebral circuits, activate the auditory area of the brain and its connections within other regions or areas of the brain.

The unborn baby perceives two types of sounds: the mother's internal noises, and speech or singing outside the womb. But, in order for external noises to be heard, they have to pass through the abdominal wall, the uterine wall, and the amniotic fluid. This means some of the vibrations will be absorbed along the way as they travel from the outside world to the ear of the unborn child. The fetus is more sensitive to its mother's voice, which it hears both internally and "out there," than to other voices. The unborn baby is also more sensitive to high-pitched voices. This seems to be innate rather than acquired. Thus, even completely deaf parents will find their newborn highly receptive to voices with highly pitched harmonics.

From the eighth month, the fetus can recognize an octave. The earlier the baby's musical education, the better the baby will be able to sing and charm with its speaking voice. One week after its birth, the baby begins to turn its head in response to being spoken to.

Communication in Man and animals

A baby communicates first and foremost with its mother. A dialogue normally entails talking to someone else, but it can also entail talking to oneself.

Long before our advent, the singing bird colonized our planet, followed later by the marine mammal. But acoustic communication is not present throughout the animal world. It presupposes a transmitting organ and a receiving organ. Only vertebrates and arthropods have this privilege. In the early stages of evolution, arthropods' transmitters and receivers were on their feet, body, thorax, and abdomen, instead of on their head. In this species, the basis of communication is a coded rhythm. Mosquitoes, crickets, and cicadas emit sounds that are recognizable to us: the "zzzzz" so typical of the mosquito is the sound produced by the vibration of its wings. When a cricket chirrs, it rubs its wings together. When the cicada chirps, it uses a complex percussion system in which transmitter and receiver are one and the same organ, drumsticks, cymbals, and percussion all lodged in its upper body. Tens of millions of years will go by before the transmitter and the receiver emigrate to different parts of the body and specialize. The transmitter is the phonatory organ and the receiver is the acoustic organ. Amphibians were the first animals to acquire this characteristic.

Where arthropods, such as the cicada, possess a percussion instrument, amphibians possess a wind instrument. Man has both a string instrument and a wind instrument: his larynx. Acoustic communication isn't something you can palpate. Its existence begins and ends every time a sound is emitted. It requires a transmitter as well as a vibratory receiver specific to each species' environment. This acoustic communication evolves in all four spatial dimensions. The receiver, or ear, develops as it evolves. The human voice, fruit of our vocalizing, creates an impalpable, fleeting vibratory imprint in our atmospheric environment. The human voice is the imprint of the breath of life.

In the 21st century, nearly two hundred species of primates exist. From the smallest, which can fit into your hand, to the gorilla, the initial melting pot seems to have undoubtedly had a common origin. We certainly manifest specific characteristics. Over more than 60 million years, despite climatic changes, Ice Ages, and other such vicissitudes of our solar system, the mammal slowly but surely progresses toward the evolutionary outcome that is the human race. Many species become extinct after only a furtive appearance on our planet. Man and his powerful voice survive because of his exceptional adaptability in the face of climatic changes, and this after nearly 7 million years.

The voice: an apprenticeship with a time limit after birth

Will Man, now in possession of all the required elements for articulating sounds, vowels and consonants, finally speak, just as he is going to breathe, walk, or run? If he were not to learn how to speak, would he understand language? Is his genetic heritage sufficient now for his voice to be an innate utterance?

To the quest of the primal voice and the King of Prussia

"I, Frederic II the Great, King of Prussia, want to know the primitive voice used by the very first man. Staff at my palace shall bring up several infants born by my peasants. My servants shall not address them. They shall be disguised as wolves and shall remain silent before them. The infants shall be well nourished and well looked after." Thus it probably came to pass that centuries ago, this sovereign, open-minded and a philosopher at heart, decides to understand how the voice comes about. Is there a "natural voice"? He tries to solve the riddle of language. Frederic II the Great persists in trying to determine which of Latin, Greek, or Hebrew the original language was. Which language would a child spontaneously use without any prior coaching?

These infants are raised by people who never speak to them. They are isolated Their eyes see no facial expressions during three to four years. Their ears receive no acoustic input. They are immersed in a strange and secluded world. The result is impressive. They wriggle. They don't speak. They grunt.

Yet the mechanical structure for speech exists. Yet the brain is Man's brain. Yet they can walk. Yet they are permanent bipeds, the upright is present. But the voice as it should be simply doesn't exist.

They are put back into the real human world between the ages of three and four. Toward the age of five, they are in an age group in which they should be speaking, expressing themselves, not just eating and drinking. But these young children still aren't talking. They were not introduced to the world of speech nor to the world of the voice. Neither were they taught how to communicate with others, in any word or sign languages. Consequently, the apprenticeship and ontogeny of the voice were not possible. It was easy to draw a conclusion: Man's offspring isn't born with a primitive voice, and more than that, this capability seems indispensable for his continued existence. These infants' fate was a sad one: all became severely mentally retarded and died by the age of puberty. Therefore, the voice must be learned within a certain time limit after birth.

Is the voice indispensable to our survival? Ontogeny apparently is indispensable if *Homo sapiens* is to become *Homo vocalis*.

Man no doubt owes his survival over all these millions of years to communication, to the exchanges he was able to create with his own species in order to survive. His creativity is in part fueled by his own voice, but mostly by other people's voices.

Kamala and Amala in India

A few thousand kilometers from Prussia, centuries later, two little girls called Kamala and Amala live in a den deep in the forest, practically since their birth. Huddled at the back of the den, normally occupied by wolves, they cling together for warmth through the icy winter. The year is 1920. On a November day, Dr. Sing approaches the den. No wolf is nearby. Two living creatures grunt, squeal, and emit plaintive cries. Their hands are rough, their knees and feet covered in calluses. They crawl on all fours despite being capable of standing. Sing observes them. Rooted to the spot, they stare at him open mouthed, tongues hanging out. They reek of wolf. A few minutes go by. They begin to drink water, more accurately, they lap it up.

Amala and Kamala, wolf-children, only eat raw meat. They can't speak. They must be three to four years old. Sing adopts them. He brings them back into Man's world, to the world of spoken language. Months go by. The two little girls don't adapt. They waste away. Amala dies a year later, having learned only a few words. The return to civilization proved fatal for her. Kamala is stronger. She has better adaptive capacities. Yet eight years later, just as she reaches puberty, she too passes away. Despite Dr. Sing's efforts, her vocabulary stagnated below fifty words during those eight years. She could barely communicate. Her apprenticeship of the "civilized" world had come too late in her life.

The wild boy from the Tam valley

In France, in the dense forest of Tam, in the heart of the Aveyron, farmers and shepherds discover a small mute child. He walks like a man. He's almost naked. He roams the forests of Lacaune and runs off as soon as anyone approaches. He emits only grunts and animal cries. Unlike Kamala and Amala, he eats no meat; he is a vegetarian. On the 8th of January 1800, the wild boy, aged about 10 and soon to be known as Victor of Aveyron, leaves the world of forests for that of men. He takes shelter in the house of Vidal, a dyer, at Saint-Sernin. Two days later, taken into the village, he is handed over into the care of Dr. Jean Itard, a physician, who takes him in. The challenge of educating the boy, of changing the imprint of those early years in the wild, is enormous. The challenge of introducing him to Paris is almost superhuman. Yet Dr. Itard travels up to Paris with him by coach and takes up residence in his house in Batignolles. They arrive in the capital on the 6th of August and remain there until 1803. The scientific community is eager to see the boy, and he is handed over to satisfy their curiosity. His apprenticeship proves long and arduous. He learns a primitive, basic vocabulary, but will never adapt to this new world of Man's. He is entrusted to Mrs. Guerin, who looks after him for the next seventeen years, from 1811 until his death in 1928. During all those years, he never acquired more than a rudimentary language. This raises the question: what is normality? To which Dr. Itard will later respond: "Man isn't born Man, but is coached to become Man," in his book *Memoire et Rapport sur Victor de l'Aveyron* (Essay and Report on Victor of Aveyron).

Young Victor, Amala, Kamala, these wild children, these wolf-children, walk on two legs. The shape of their cranium and the size of their brain are human. But their spoken language is nonexistent: fewer than 200 words in Amala's and Kamala's case and 500 words in Victor's case. One can understand their asocial, even violent, behavior, behavior conditioned by fear of people and of the unknown. Animals among men and men among animals, they couldn't integrate. We're far from the legend of Tarzan the ape-man "Me Tarzan, you Jane"!

We see here the important role the human voice plays in our entire body, in our appearance, in our identity. It is part and parcel of our survival and of the human species. As the millennia went by, the voice continued to improve. While it's true that a man raised among wild animals can barely speak, the chimpanzee when raised by Man doesn't develop an articulated language; it only develops sign language and, even then, only within a very specific context. It can transmit this language to fellow chimpanzees. Its capabilities are comparable to those of a two- to three-year-old child. But let us be wary of not drifting too complacently into anthropomorphism. Already in 1623, Jobson, the Captain of a British ship, was to exclaim with astonishment, when faced with a strange man: "He lives in the forest and doesn't want to speak with us." The strange man was an orangutan. In order to become fully human, we have to undergo the apprenticeship of articulated language.

The road of the voice

Does it lead us to Lucy?

The most ancient bipedal woman in history is Lucy, discovered in 1974 by Yves Coppens and Donald Johanson. She owes her name to the Beatles' song "Lucy in the Sky with Diamonds," which by chance was being played over and over on the radio that day. Her bones, recovered from a dig in Hadar in Ethiopia, form a 105-cm-high skeleton when reassembled. It is 3 million years old. Researchers were able to establish her profile by analyzing her fossil. She was two-legged. She stood almost upright, as evident by the curved lumbar spine, the basin-shaped pelvis with its forward-curving iliac wings, the smooth head of the femur, found also in the big apes, and the straight shaft of the femur, proper to Man. Yet she lacked something, something the voice requires if it is to develop normally. This something is the position of the larynx, the uprightness of the cervical vertebrae and the 90° angle between the first cervical vertebra, or atlas, and the cranium, found in *Homo vocalis*. In Lucy's case, the head is bent and juts forward. The cranium doesn't rest on the atlas and forms an angle much greater than 90°. There's no real verticality. Lucy didn't speak like we do! She couldn't pronounce all the phonemes we dispose of today.

The key organ of the human voice, the larynx, is also found in many animals. The "vocal larynx" may be the appendage of Man, but its primary structure in the animal kingdom allows two other functions: it is used as a sphincter and for breathing. From fish to amphibians, from reptiles to dinosaurs, from birds to mammals, the larynx is present.

The larynx: the morphing of evolution

In certain animals, the larynx allows a vibration, the creation of a fundamental sound associated with harmonics. In others, like the reptile, there is no creation of harmonious vibrations. Only the emission of what we call noises, in other words anarchical vibrations, irregular, aperiodic, similar to the noise made when clearing one's throat, or like the hiss of a snake. In 1921, V. U. Negus, professor at the Royal Academy of England, published a remarkable piece of work on the development of the larynx in the animal world, from fish down to Man. If we are to understand the larynx, we need to understand the role it plays in the respiratory tree and as a framework for bringing oxygen into the animal's organism. Oxygen is indispensable to life and breathing is an indispensable link in the complex world of the living on Planet Earth. Whether from the atmosphere or from water, whether in gills or in the lungs, oxygen is brought from outside the animal into the animal.

Nature has concocted different stratagems for accomplishing the dynamics of this inspiration. The gills are a simple organ. Fish don't have lungs. The water flowing past them caresses the branchiae. These capture the oxygen in the water and expel carbon dioxide. The branchia were probably the very first larynx on our planet, and its function was purely for breathing.

Evolution then makes its inroads and a fish discovered in the Nile, called *Polypterus* or *bichir*, displays not only branchiae, but also the beginnings of lungs. This imposes the existence of an orifice that canalizes the air into the depths of the body. This early blueprint of a lung also creates the blueprint for the larynx. The *Polypterus* was able to breathe both in and out of the water. This evolution can be attributed to the drying out of rivers and lakes, it allowed these marine creatures to survive. Being able to breathe on dry land was the only chance these species had of surviving. The "lung fish," or *Geratodus*, was discovered in 1931 in Australia. It has not only a larynx, but also a pharynx and the beginnings of an upper respiratory and digestive tract. The larynx now has two functions: breathing and constriction. Breathing and swallowing are accomplished via the same tract in the neck. When a bolus is ingested, it passes through to the esophagus. The closure of the glottis prevents its descent into the lungs. The glottis is the space at the base of the larynx, between the vocal cords. This glottal space is structured by muscle fibers, which enable it to act as a sphincter; in other words it's able to close, thus isolating the lung cavity from the pharyngeal cavity. These elements remain relatively supple, devoid of any cartilage. They open passively during inspiration. In Man, the 5-mm embryo possesses this type of pharynx. We are now at the dawn of the age of the vocal larynx.

Fish become amphibian

The laryngeal odyssey continues. The larynx and the pharynx are now equipped with specialized muscle fibers that are better suited to the laryngeal function. They cross over, giving additional power to the larynx. The beginnings of a cartilage makes its first appearance in tritons and salamanders. The cricoid cartilage and the two arytenoid cartilages are outlined. The larynx now has both breathing and sphincter functions and has a sketchy vibratory mechanism that enables frogs to croak.

Amphibians turn into reptiles

The larynx is still a small organ, with a minor vibratory role. Now the cricoid ring appears at the base of the larynx and at the top of the trachea. As mentioned before, the little arytenoid cartilages allow the vocal cords to open and close and articulate with the cricoid. Again, similar structures are found in the eight-week-old human fetus. The thyroid cartilage, essential for the protection of the larynx, will make its appearance only later, providing a shield-like structure in front of the laryngeal muscles. In the crocodile, this cartilage is tied to and fuses with the cricoid cartilage; in effect, it forms a single cricothyroid cartilage. This cartilaginous mass allows for the insertion of muscles used mainly to close the larynx and use it as an efficient air sphincter.

Reptiles turn into birds or mammals

The laryngeal sound instrument is developing in reptiles and birds. Where breathing, in amphibians, is limited to swallowing air, in birds, mammals, and a few evolved reptiles, breathing requires a few thoracic movements. They breathe in actively and breathe out passively. If rigid cartilaginous rings didn't form the trachea, it would quite simply collapse during inspiration, as when an endo-tracheal suction is performed, or when you suck out the air in an almost empty ball, the walls of which are practically touching. The consequence of such a collapse would be asphyxia. This is what happens in a newborn suffering from tracheomalacia.

The mammal evolves

Evolution continues its work. The larynx becomes fully formed. The angle between the axis of the mouth and the axis of the laryn-geal tracheal tube starts to change in species.

In the crocodile, the angle between the larynx and the mouth is 0°, they practically form a straight line. In dogs and cats, the angle between these two axes is relatively small, 20 to 30°; in the chim-panzee, it's 60°. The ideal angle is almost reached. In Man, the angle enables the larynx to become a structure that's quite distinct from the oral and pharyngeal structures and creates a resonance chamber that is the key to articulated language. It is the result of the perfect angle of 90° between the axes of the mouth and the larynx.

The cartilages of the larynx (arytenoids, cricoid, and thyroid) are now very distinct in the mammal. A joint is evolving, the cricoarytenoid joint. Another is forming: the cricothyroid joint. They will be of major importance to the spoken word. The muscles between the cricoid and the arytenoids also begin to play a crucial role. They allow the larynx to open and therefore enable respiration. Other specific muscles will allow the larynx to close, protecting the lungs from something going down the wrong tract. The vocal cord inserts itself at the back of the throat on the arytenoids and at the front on the thyroid cartilage, where it almost touches the other vocal cord. Thus, the larynx now has two vocal cords forming a V. Joined at the front, they open and close at the back. The larynx is both a wind instrument and a string instrument. During phonation, the vocal cords close and create vibrations in their mucous membrane. The membrane, but not the cord itself, undulates and vibrates against its partner. When a singer produces the *A* note, it vibrates four hundred and forty times a second. Thus, vibrations are formed on the vocal cords and vowels and consonants are formed in the resonance chambers. Is this what happens in animals?

The larynx can sometimes be strange: from the bird to the dolphin

In birds, the larynx is called "syrinx." Located where the trachea splits into two, at the point where the bronchi end, the syrinx is used only for singing. In marine mammals such as dolphins or whales, the closure of the larynx is replaced by closure of the blowhole. That's how these mammals breathe, through a vent on the top of the head, not through the mouth. This enables cetaceans to keep their mouths open under water, their home habitat, without fear of inhaling seawater and choking.

From monkey to Man: the resonator chambers

From fish to reptiles, from dinosaurs to birds, from cetaceans to Man, the larynx is the organ that best represents evolution. Its ultimate vocation in this third millennium seems to be the human voice. But this is probably also just a stage in the long history of evolution, and others will follow.

Only primates have a space between the soft palate and the epiglottis. In monkeys, it is very short, in Man, it is very long. This will enable him to speak. Man's palate is shorter than any other mammal's. He's one of the only mammals with a uvula right at the back of the soft palate, in its center. It's a relic from the very long soft palates of the animal kingdom. The epiglottis prevents choking and extends practically to the base of the cranium in all mammals, cats, cheetahs, antelopes, and dogs; whereas in Man, it stops under the tongue.

As for the positioning of the larynx inside the neck, only Man has the lower portion of his larynx ending level with the fifth cervical vertebra. In the human embryo, the larynx is only 14 mm long and level with the cranium, as it is in bears and dogs. When the fetus is two-and-a-half months old, the larynx migrates down to the second cervical vertebra, more or less where it is in chimpanzees and gorillas. Now the epiglottis is no longer in contact with the soft palate. Only in the seventh month of the life of the fetus will the larynx reach the third cervical vertebra. This frees up more space between the soft palate and the epiglottis, making it comparable with the space found in chimpanzees. Then, up until the twenty-fourth month, the larynx will continue on its downward path until it reaches its final destination.

The whys and wherefores of this descent have many explanations: our upright posture, the flexibility of our spinal column, the angle between our first cervical vertebra and our cranium. Our vocal cords become parallel with the ground. They are in a horizontal plane, perpendicular to the trachea.

Our approach to the mechanics of the voice would not be complete without some insight into the evolution of the jaw. Man's jaw is clearly less developed than that of other primates. We have no prognathism, our chin doesn't stand out. Our oral cavity is practically vertically beneath our cranium. Our tongue also plays a major role when we speak: it has maintained an imposing muscular mass. It has partly lost its flatness and is level with the oral and pharyngeal cavities. It has helped push the larynx farther down the throat. When at rest, the larynx is level with the fifth cervical vertebra, but when you sing or talk, it can rise up to the fourth cervical vertebra or drop down to the sixth cervical vertebra.

From antelopes to cheetahs

As regards the internal structure of the larynx, in Man the small ary-tenoid cartilages are separate, which can't be said of the kangaroo, for example. Thus, Man's phonatory agility is maximal thanks to the independence of the laryngeal cartilages. The joint between the cricoid and the arytenoids (cartilages of the larynx) has a small meniscus, just like the knee, which can suffer from inflammation or arthritis.

The glottal space, or the space between the vocal cords, has a very specific triangular shape, proper to humans, with its apex at the front of the throat and its base at the back.

But our evolutionary path continues to surprise us as we fol-low the progress of the larynx. The importance of the arytenoids isn't immediately apparent. Their shape and length, the angle they form with the cricoid cartilage, are specific to each species. In horses and antelopes, the length of these arytenoid cartilages is seven-tenths the diameter of the glottis, but in Man, with his rela-tively slow speed, their length is four-tenths the diameter of the glottis. The explanation is simple. The arytenoids allow the glottal space to open wide. They allow a maximum of air to be taken in very quickly, as the glottis controls its passage. Man has no need to run very fast to escape from or catch a predator. For example, a gazelle can cover 500 m at a speed of 60 miles per hour, a cheetah covers 100 meters at a speed close to 70 miles per hour. The glot-tal surface of the gazelle is 30% greater than that of the cheetah. It's a case of the function "creating" the organ.

Gripping branches with false vocal cords?

Overhanging the vocal cords in the larynx are two ventricular folds, also known as false vocal cords. In Man, their phonatory contribu-tion is limited. In the salamander, the frog, and the crocodile, they play an essential role. These laryngeal pseudovalves enable the larynx to resist the pressure of water and prevent the lungs from being inundated. In mammals, and especially in primates, the false vocal cords allow better use of the upper limbs: strange, is it not? These ventricular folds are more developed in the gibbon, the ban-dar, and the chimpanzee, but less so in the gorilla, because gorillas are more land bound and spend little time swinging from branch to branch. What causes this?

The upper limbs are used to hang onto branches and swing from tree to tree. The abdominal pressure exerted by the additional pressure on the larynx gives much greater muscular strength. The false vocal cords reinforce the strength that is exerted, as happens if you push when constipated, or when lifting weights and dumbbells. Breathing stops, the thoracic cage is immobilized, abdominal strength is maximal, the contraction of the upper limbs is maximal and gives great strength. Thanks to evolution, Man no longer needs to hang by his arms and swing from branch to branch like the great apes. Highly developed false vocal cords are no longer justified in his case. But when he moves his arms, it causes a contraction of the muscles that insert into the rib cage, and the thoracic cage needs to be immobilized for an effective and powerful contraction of the pectoral muscles. This is readily observed in athletes lifting weights. When a weightlifter is about to lift a weight, he contracts his larynx, blocks his breathing, and contracts the false vocal cords to better isolate the lungs from the pharyngeal cavity and thus improve the muscular efficacy of the upper limbs and of the abdominal and pelvic muscles. He uses his larynx as a sphincter that prevents air from passing through the glottis and provides added force with which to contract the diaphragm completely and effectively.

Man is the mammal with the least developed ventricular folds, because he doesn't swing from branch to branch and is earthbound. When he needs to apply pressure, as would a singer, the diaphragm is perfectly controlled. The inhalation is blocked when it is two-thirds complete, and this ensures excellent precision for the diaphragmatic muscle. This control is key to controlling a vocal exhalation. Thus, should these ventricular folds be removed, there would be a very slight reduction in the strength of our upper limbs, in the blowing power of the wind-instrument player, or in the performance of the weightlifter. Phonation would be practically unchanged, but there would be a slight reduction in the lubrication of the vocal cords.

In the first days after birth, a newborn baby can support its weight by grasping with its hands. It can hang holding onto its mother's finger or the pediatrician's. This grasping test is done in the nursing ward. It is an archaic reflex. If the reflex is lacking, it means the baby was born prematurely or that it suffers from a psychomotor dysfunction. From the twenty-eighth day, the baby can maintain this grasping reflex for two minutes. This aptitude persists until the third month. During this period, an examination of the larynx shows important ventricular folds, which later diminish in size.

The deer has no need to grasp and has no ventricular folds. Vestiges of ventricular folds are observable in dogs, but in amphibians, reptiles, birds, and cetaceans, they have practically disappeared.

Man will speak or sing

Where balance is perpetually lacking, a new balance emerges. Thus, complex sciences such as biology, physiology, or physics have a common denominator: DNA, our genetic heritage. One can hardly refute the anatomical continuity of the cerebral area between the great apes and Man. The beginning of the human voice marks a violent discontinuity, a profound mutation, one that *FOXP2*, the gene of the voice, can't totally explain. This discontinuity reveals a multiplicity of associated factors and dissociating them seems impossible. Audition and the larynx are intimately tied in with language. These two transmitting and receiving poles are the alchemy of the human voice.

One nerve controlling voice and emotions

As we delve into the mystery of articulated language, we come across an astounding discovery: a single nerve controls the muscles of the vocal cords: cranial nerve 10.

Thanks to this nerve, we are able to modulate our vocal cords, to separate them in order to breathe, to close them in order to speak. It creates our voice, it can slow down our cardiac rhythm and increase the acidity level of our stomach. It conjugates our emotion and our verbal expression. Small wonder then, that our voice betrays our deepest feelings and our inner self.

And so the human voice, mirror of our thoughts, is still, in the early stages of its evolution. Only 10% of our brain is exploited. Our articulated language, the essence of communication between six billion human beings on our planet, allows us to assimilate and memorize an impressive amount of data. If Man didn't speak, would he be like his cousin, the great ape? This is indeed what the lives of those wild children suggest to us.

The breath of the primate and the singing voice

In Man and in the great apes, the ribs in the upper part of the thorax enjoy a certain degree of mobility, whereas in other mammals, they are fixed. This is a crucial observation for singers and teachers, because herein lies the secret for the optimal control of the "head voice" and the "chest voice." This mobility of the ribs, when associated with the muscular synergy of the entire body, gives the professional singer the option of two vocal registers. Controlling the amount of air pressure is indispensable, the more so when singing. Perfect control of the power and pitch of the voice requires mastering the exhalation. It also requires suppleness and elasticity, not only of the laryngeal apparatus, but also of the pulmonary, muscular, and abdominal breathing apparatus. If you strain too hard, what can happen is that the false vocal cords may be brought into play, as well as the vocal cords. In that case, you'll sound like Louis Armstrong.

In Man, we can consider the pulmonary capacity, or the thoracic cage itself, as an amplifier, as it is in the bird. Whatever the opinion of certain scientists, the pulmonary resonance chamber does exist, everyone has one, it's specific to each of us. It's like the wood of a violin, you don't play on the wood, you play with the wood! It acts as an amplifier. A singer's silhouette is often a good indication of vocal tessitura. A baritone or a contralto is normally tall and slim or slender, with powerful vocal cords and a relatively stretched larynx. A tenor or soprano will tend to be solid and compact, with shorter, well-shaped vocal cords. The high-pitched voice of a child is due not only to a lack of hormonal influence, but also to the smallness of the larynx, the shortness of the vocal cords, and their extremely fine edges, due to the epithelium having only two layers of cells.

Whistling and whispering: yet another expression of the virtuoso vocal cords

The spoken voice and the sung voice both require the vibration of both vocal cords. The strident, very high-pitched voice produced when you scream, known as the "whistle voice," is an exception: in this case the vocal cords don't vibrate. They're very close to each other, very taut. Expelling the air under very strong pressure produces this sound, as when you breathe on to a blade of grass held between your hands. Moreover, spectrographic analysis of the sound produced by "the whistle voice," or by a real whistle, shows the single trace of a basic sound, with no harmonics. The same occurs when you whistle through your lips. Do it now: the vocal cords are still working to control exactly the force of the air you exhale. They separate and get closer without ever touching, enabling you to control the strength and pitch of the whistling, helped by constant movements of the tongue. Conversely, an *A* sung in a maintained vibrato voice is rich in harmonics, the entire edge of the vocal cords vibrates and this creates the pitch and the origins of the harmonics. To be more precise, the vibration of the falsetto voice is quite different. Here, during the vibration, only the middle third of the vibrating cord remains half open, with very sharp vibrations. This technique is only possible for very high-pitched frequencies.

Digitalized laryngeal fibroscopy shows that when you whisper softly, without straining, the vocal cords remain open. They may move in slightly, but they never touch. There's no vibration involved. The whispered voice is created by an exhalation passing through the glottal space and into the pharynx. It's modulated by the voice box, which produces the various phonemes heard by the other person, or persons.

Straining while you whisper is very bad for the vocal cords, as it provokes an aperiodic noise in the larynx. The vocal cords partially move in toward each other, they brush together lightly, but don't vibrate. The friction between the edges of the two vocal cords can cause microtraumas.

The voice is the DNA of our thoughts, and the word is its gene

DNA alone cannot give us a voice

The concept of genes in our DNA is now well established. The gene is the indispensable unit that allows a species to hand down information from one generation to the next. We owe our survival to the stability of our genetic heritage and to mutations that favored Man's evolution. Our genes are both architect and master builder, but also, paradoxically, message captors. Some of them are active, others passive. They enable the synthesis of the proteins that will provide energy for our muscles or for activating our brain circuits, seemingly in just a few milliseconds. This genetic baggage transforms itself, according to the species, in a survival instinct. We have seen that sheep can drink and breathe simultaneously. Indeed, they drink as quickly as possible in order to avoid predators. Man no longer needs this protection as he's at the top of the food chain. His behavior is different. He's going to activate and stimulate other genetic aspects of his DNA, better adapted to his survival.

When words behave as genes

Man's evolution apparently is owed to our sex genes. For it is the male/female alliance that allows our genetic heritage to become richer. I believe that the evolution and apprenticeship of *Homo vocalis* down all these millions of years was also kindled by another concept: words are the genes of the voice and, consequently, of our thinking.

The voice constructs itself, becomes richer, is kept alive thanks to our verbal past. The transmission of the intangible word is the secret power of our knowledge base. Pregnant words, words rich in meaning, are the genetic units of our intelligence.

The ethologist Richard Dawkins has put forward a seductive theory whereby certain words rich in meaning are the equivalent of a "gene." The "meme" would be the genetic unit of our vocal language. In his book *The Selfish Gene*, he makes the point that Man's culture stems not only from our DNA heritage, but also from our heritage of the human language. Something Jared Diamond seems to corroborate in his book *The Third Chimpanzee*, in which he claims that Man is none other than the third chimpanzee that dresses and talks.

The voice is hereditary and is fed by our past

The voice has developed only in Man. Whereas so many mechanical, chemical, and neural factors are handed down genetically through our DNA to create the "voice organ," words have to be learned. The living voice transmits this knowledge to Man's offspring. The learning of the voice and of words is the key for his evolution and survival.

Each word that is understood means that another can be understood. Little by little, a suite of words takes form, and combinations of these words enable us to form, nurture, and express our ideas. As it grows, this language also allows us to interact with others, to form relationships, and only between two people of the same generation, but also between generations. Thus was the flame handed down from Aristotle, over two millennia ago, to Leonardo da Vinci, some five hundred years ago, to Einstein, less than a century ago, and finally to us today. A kindred spirit moves us when we keep the Olympic flame burning on its travels. But language represents much more, it is the flame of our emotions, of our thinking, of our survival. In the Western world, many philosophers or scientists know over 250,000 words.

At the dawn of the third millennium, we are still inventing new words to convey new ideas, such as to "digitalize" an image: these new words could be conceived as a major mutation. They appear out of nowhere, unlike words that are transformations of an earlier word, such as "admin" instead of "administration." The progression of our cultures over the past two thousand years, but more so over the past century and a half, has been fueled by our spoken and written word, by the interchange between religion and science, between the farmer, the poet, the researcher, and the philosopher.

When Man encounters the power of the word

The scientist teaching a class communicates an idea, which is seized upon by his pupils. The human voice is the medium that propagates this cerebral and intellectual evolution. The spoken word demands the attention of the other person, or persons. There must be some cerebral interactivity. But, and this is remarkable, the spoken word never dies. The idea behind it can pass from one person to another, it can be added to or deformed, but it will always be present to some degree, just like our genetic heritage. Is the vocal, auditory, or cerebral stimulation of "the other" indispensable?

The Word is a double-edged sword. Words enabled the transmission of culture through the millennia. They made possible the development of the various monotheist religions over four thousand years. They allowed the creation of scientific works and the development of philosophical concepts. They can cause a chain reaction of wars and intolerance. For example, the word "nazi" alone means atrocities. Half a century ago, this word did not exist. It should have never existed.

In another domain, the Big Bang theory of the origins of our Universe ferries exceptionally rich mental imagery, which we owe to Stephen Hawking. The expression "Big Bang" now evokes questions about the origins of life, the stars, the Milky Way, our planet, and outer space that require us to reconcile our rational mind and the dreamer in each of us!

A word invested with strong meaning becomes part of our existence and enables each of us to form other words. It survives only through communication with others. Selfish and isolated, it dies with us. Words reflect the level of culture of a person.

The path taken by the voice is a long one, shared not only with DNA, but also with the apprenticeship of words since millions of years. This same path has built up Man's strength into what it is today and made possible all his discoveries. The voice has memorized Man's energy. Its territory is Man, its future is tomorrow's Language, its present is Life.

Chapter 5

Cerebropolis at the controls of the voice

The brain, housing of our emotions and thoughts,
creates the jewel of our voice.

The Voice, the Word, Pronunciation, Understanding live in Cerebropolis

On the 12th of April, 1861, Mr. Le Borgne is referred to Dr. Paul Broca's clinic with a gangrenous infection of the leg. The surgeon is less interested in the infection than in the language dysfunctions Mr. Le Borgne presents. It seems he can only pronounce one syllable: "tan." There is no evidence of any buccopharyngeal paralysis, no facial anomaly, no other deficiency. Yet all he can say is this one syllable. It is his only mode of oral expression. All his other functions are working. His comprehension of language, his cognitive functions are unaffected. He becomes known as "Mr. Tan." He succumbs to the gangrene on April 17th, 1861, a few days following his admission to hospital. His autopsy reveals a lesion of the left brain, specifically in the third gyrus of the frontal lobe. The region of the brain dealing with language has just been discovered. The next day, Paul Broca presents his findings to the Anthropological Society, of which he is Secretary. His deduction is that the lesion of the frontal lobe caused the loss of speech. The location of the human voice in the brain has been pinpointed for the first time. Neurosurgeon at the Kremlin-Bicêtre Hospital, Professor at the School of Medicine of Paris, Paul Broca was the first to demonstrate that the brain presents distinct areas that are specialized by function. The link is now well established. Language dysfunctions are associated with a cerebral lesion. The area involved, for "area" is the name used from here on to describe the different regions of the brain, becomes known as Broca's area of speech. It is specific to Man. It carries the essence of the human voice. This approach marks the beginning of the associations since made between "function and cerebral projection." Neuroanatomy is born. Since the 19th century, it has never ceased to enthrall scientists investigating the mysteries of our brain.

These findings will spark numerous vocations. Carl Wernicke completes Paul Broca's findings. This German neurosurgeon, after studying medicine in Breslau, studies neuropsychiatry in Vienna under Heinrich Neumann. He was very influenced by H. Meynert, with whom he worked for six months. His doctoral thesis, *Der aphasische Symptomenkomplex*—The symptomatic complex of aphasia—(1874), describes a form of sensorial aphasia caused by a lesion affecting the reception and comprehension of language. The cerebral territory concerned with the comprehension of language, rather than with its pronunciation, bears his name: Wernicke's area. He thus introduces the concept of an auditory image of the word that leaves an imprint on the cerebral cortex after it has been heard. He describes the existence of an internal lexicon stored by the brain. He associates the dysfunctional comprehension of language with a lesion located very precisely in the posterior part of the first temporal gyrus. The premises for researching the brain, control center of the voice, are being put in place.

The learning of the voice requires audition. The cerebral projection of audition is located in the left and right cortex. Surprisingly, a unilateral lesion of the auditory area provokes a slight decrease in one's ability to perceive and locate sounds, but does not lead to deafness. This is because audition has a bilateral projection. The left ear inputs information of one type to the left brain, and information of a different type to the right brain. The right ear functions in the same way. Strangely, when the auditory area of your brain is stimulated, you hear only high or low musical frequencies, never words. Toward the middle of the 20th century, Norman

Gershwin, an American neuropsychologist, consecrated and further clarified the importance of the different cerebral projections of the human voice. Broca's area and Wernicke's area work hand-in-hand in the comprehension and emission of articulated language with the indispensable help of the temporal planum, which connects these two "actors."

A lesion of these areas does not have the same consequences. Each area of the brain plays a highly specific role.

Wernicke "writes the word," Broca "reads it out loud"

Broca's district

Broca's aphasia arises from a lesion of Broca's area, for example after a stroke. More precisely, it is the production of language that's affected the ability to form words. Speech is now slow, chopped up, punctuated: just a succession of syllables. The victim of a stroke manages a few phonemes, stops, then starts again, but in an anarchical fashion, with no rhythm. The word "sun" is pronounced "sss . . . su . . . n." There is no grammatical composition. Verbs are often used in the infinitive: "He try." There is no construction of sentences. The victim can understand everything, but struggles to make himself understood.

Wernicke's district

A lesion to Wernicke's area is different. Production of language is unimpaired. What is impaired is the internal lexicon, our inner dictionary of all the words memorized over the years. The victim of this type of lesion has "verbal diarrhea." Sentences appear to be correct, phonation is satisfactory, but he talks on and on and on. His logorrhea is uncontrollable and incomprehensible. The proper sequencing within sentences is respected, but the words thus strung together make no sense. Words are distorted, phonemes modified: "sleep" becomes "seep," "dolphin" becomes "dopin." The phonological treatment of language is impaired here.

The Ancient World tracks the voice to the brain

Such dysfunctions were already well understood in the Ancient World. From hieroglyphs written on papyrus paper under the Pharaohs in Egypt, we learn that nearly three thousand years ago, they were operating on the brain: "If you examine someone with a staved-in temple, and get no answer when you speak to the person, it means the use of language has gone." These writings show that at the time of the pyramids, the cerebral projection of the voice had already been identified. In Psalm 137, verses 5 through 6, of the Bible we can read: "If I forget you, oh Jerusalem, let my right hand wither, let my face become paralyzed, let my tongue stay stuck to my palate and may I lose all memory of you." Is this not a clinical profile of the consequences of a stroke in the left brain? For it is the left brain that enables speech and that controls the right side of the body. It enables the integration of the spoken word, of language. Wernicke's area, where our private lexicon is stored, is at the cross-roads of the cerebral circuits involved with vision, hearing and motion of the left side of the body. The hind portion of this area receives visual information, the lower portion receives sonorous information and the lateral portions control physical motion.

Wernicke's area is the brain's "scribe" for language. Broca's area "reads language out loud." It acts as spokesman for language.

Voice spasms—yet the larynx is normal

Mr. Paul, fifty-four years old, professor in a provincial university, consults me in great distress. When he speaks, he is intelligible, logical, his syntax is normal, but highly punctuated. "Whhhen . . . I sssspeak, my vvvoice is chhhhoppy, spppastic. My lll . . . arynx was examined. They fffound nothing wrong. I dddon't understand." And indeed, upon examination, his larynx is normal anatomically. Yet the vocal cords stutter, they jerk, even at rest. He adds: "If the phone rings when my secretary is out of the room, I prefer not to answer. Answering the phone panics me, but I have to answer, it could be urgent. I pick up the phone awkwardly, with difficulty. I put it to my left ear and say 'Helllo?' I'm nervous, anxious. My hands are moist. My throat is tight, I choke on my words. Yet I know that my vocal cords are normal, all the brain tests have come up negative. I have been told that a control center may have got scrambled somehow, it can't control things as it did. Doctor, how come this complex brain of mine can't control my voice properly? I don't even have proper control of my hands when I want to emphasize something during my lecturing at university! Quite simply, I can't speak properly, whether with my voice or with my hands!"

His muscular mechanics, his larynx, his breathing are all normal. Further neurological tests don't reveal anything new. In fact, Mr. Paul suffers from spasmodic dysphonia, which affects the command controls. In people afflicted with Parkinson's disease, or who suffer from uncontrollable, involuntary facial spasms, the voice is perturbed, sometimes unrecognizable, shaky, deformed, the control only partial. Yet the larynx shows no abnormality. But if we are to understand this speech problem better, we need to enter into the private world of the brain, inside *Cerebropolis*.

A Journey to the center of the brain: to Cerebropolis

Voice and thinking: the comings and goings of our Self

Communication is based on phonemes, which feed the intellect. Words stimulate our brain, improve our vocabulary, our voice. Our thoughts also use words to express themselves. The voice establishes itself, its language closely connected to the hand, whose cerebral projection is very close to the brain's area of language. The lateralization of the hand and of language is "handled" by the dominant hemisphere. One must differentiate the left and the right hemispheres, which are asymmetrical. Is Man's brain, such as we know it, the outcome of a single, brutal mutation, or of several progressive evolutionary mutations?

Three brains in the center of Cerebropolis

We don't have one brain, we have three. Their story begins several hundred million years ago. The fish, the reptile, the bird, the primitive mammal, and the evolved mammal, each has left its mark. What an extraordinary machine our central nervous system is, with its billions of cells and connections!

1. "Cerebropolis First district"

This is the safeguarding brain, the brain we share with fish, reptiles and birds. It will take care of the basics such as hunger, temperature control, fear response, territorial defense, and crucial reflexes. Our survival is in the care of this reptilian brain: it controls all our vital functions. It also controls some hormones, with the thalamus. The thalamus has two lobes. Sitting in the center of the brain, it constitutes the largest nuclear mass (a mass that contains the nuclei of our neurons) of the brain. A small appendix at the base of brain, the pineal body is a gland that controls the secretion of melatonin and the third ventricle This district of Cerebropolis houses the sections on mood, memory, and hormone control.

2. "Cerebropolis Second District"

This is the limbic system, *limbus* being the Latin word for arc or girdle. We share this brain with mammals like mice, gazelles, dogs, cats, or cheetahs. At the base of the brain, the hypothalamus is located medially, below the limbic system. This "Second District" controls our strategy for survival. It is the seat of our emotions, of our affective world, of nostalgia, but also of our memory and memories. Here we find several peculiar structures. The hippocampus, highly developed in birds, is the seat, among other things, of the biological compass that ensures our sense of orientation. The cerebral tonsil, so called because of its almond shape, is symmetrical. It allows primitive instinctive reactions. This structure is essential for decoding emotions and, in particular, any stimuli that threaten the organism. It regulates aggression, fear, our biological rhythms, our primitive behaviors. The medially located pituitary gland and hypothalamus orchestrate our hormonal world, highly sensitive to stress and emotions.

3. "Cerebropolis Third District"

This is the third fundamental building block of our nervous system. The evolved brain, the commander of the voice: the Cortex. The most sophisticated, also the most superficial, it sits right on top, under the cranium. We share this noble brain with the other primates. The areas of Broca, of Wernicke, and others that we will discover later, live there. The brain is capped by what is known as the "noble" brain, the cerebral cortex. It has six layers of cells that will tell us, later on, the story of our species' evolution (see Plate 6).

The network of Cerebropolis

What a confusion of neural cabling governs us, yet all is perfectly orchestrated, managed, and classified! Our nervous system is composed of the spinal cord, which runs down inside our spine. Thirty-one pairs of spinal nerves radiate from it. The brainstem at the base of the brain gives rise to the cranial nerves.

What is striking in the assembly of the cerebral hemispheres is how all the controls have been concentrated into a really compact volume. Everything is centralized. The totality of the information relating to all our functions is accounted for here, both by afferent nerve fibers and by efferent nerve fibers.

We have reviewed the different parts of the brain. But note that all is not separated into a left and a right brain. If you look at the inferior part of the brain, just above the brainstem and just below the base of the brain, you will find the intermediary brain. It sits medially, and we only have one. It is the seat of the limbic system. The superior part of the brain, which is paired and asymmetric, consists of our two cerebral hemispheres, the striate body with its cortex, the white matter and lateral ventricles, and the interhemispherical commissurae with the corpus callosum sitting between the left and right hemispheres.

The little Cerebropolis, also called the cerebellum

The cerebellum—our little brain—consists of two hemispheres joined together posteriorly by the vermis, the most ancient part of our brain in evolutionary terms. These cerebellar hemispheres present a few gyri (hills). Fish present similar structures.

The cranium, safety belt for our thoughts

A surprising fact: our body has a central frame, the skeleton, protected by muscles draped over it, also skin, mucous membranes.

Our only anomaly: the brain. It has its own bodyguard: the cranial box or cranium.

When you suffer a cranial trauma, for example in a road accident, is a fracture of the cranium really bad news? Not always, on the contrary. Let's take an analogy. Imagine you delicately drop an egg on the floor, and the shell doesn't break. The egg must absorb the shock. Pry open the shell carefully in one spot and look inside. The yolk and the white are all mixed together. Now drop an egg so that it breaks on to the floor. Behold: the shell has absorbed the shock this time, but the yolk and the white haven't mixed together. We can draw a parallel with the brain and the cranium now. If the skull absorbs the shock, leading it to fracture, chances are there will be little wrong with the brain. When the shock is first largely absorbed by the cranium, and then by the brain's protective padding or cushions, called the meninges, it doesn't usually cause any major internal lesions. When the cranium doesn't fracture, it is the brain itself that registers the shock and in this case neurological alterations are likely. The shockwave will have perturbed the inner structure. Of course, a violent cranial trauma alters everything.

The cranial box is extremely solid. Like the eggshell, it protects the noblest fruit of Man's evolution: his brain. But the brain is not in direct contact with the skull. The meninges, a sort of cushion made of liquid and fibrous tissues, serve as an interface between the hard bony structure and the very soft brain. It is no surprise that the protective membrane in contact with the inside of the skull is called the *dura mater* and the one in contact with the brain is called the *pia mater*. For indeed, as their names suggest, they nourish the brain with indispensable energetic nutrients. Between these two protective membranes is a liquid, known as the meningeal liquid or cephalorachidian liquid, itself associated with a webbing called the arachnoidea, because of its resemblance to a spider's web.

A paradox: the role and the volume of the brain

The brain of an African elephant weighs 6 kg. Man's weighs 1.5 kg, is 16 cm long, 14 cm wide, and 12 cm high. Its relative mass is the greatest in the entire animal kingdom. In Man, the brain reveals multiple gyri on the neocortex. Only Man has such a highly developed structure. The precision of the cerebral projection of the various functions is impressive. If you stimulate a precise spot on the left temporal lobe, the right hand moves. This stimulation is accompanied by articulated language learned at two or three years of age. Stimulate the same region in a chimpanzee, and he will lift his right arm and cry out. Thus, the response to a specific cerebral stimulation is much more selective in Man than in the chimpanzee. We owe this to the considerable increase in brain surface provided for all the areas of the neocortex by the abundant gyri, which allowed each area of the brain to become ultraspecialized. In the reptile, the neocortex is practically nonexistent.

Our paleocortex, or reptilian brain, is similar to that of the dog, the panther, or the deer. Its volume is also similar. The brain's evolution is specific to each species and specific to subgroups within the species. Thus, a parrot's brain can vary in size by up to 300% across subspecies of parrots, as well as present differences in the way the areas of the brain are assembled. But all men have the same brain. What we do with it is another story!

Each species has its own cerebral imprint

The dolphin has an acoustic lobe that is particularly developed. It masters ultrasounds that are more readily perceived under water. The elephant, because of its environment, needs to perceive low-pitched sounds and infrasound. These propagate better in a savanna-type landscape. Does the migrating bird not have an innate compass to guide it? The dog has exceptional flair, as does the salmon trout—it remembers smells in the water that guide it back upstream to its breeding grounds. But at what age does this type of cerebral projection appear in Man? Medical imaging techniques used to explore the brain led to an exceptional discovery. Just after birth, vocal development gets under way, and neuroimaging unveils its mysteries and its progress to us.

The human voice is a "team sport":
neurons talk to each other

The voice is the indispensable stimulus for its own evolution. Take the case of a child born deaf. The deafness is bilateral and complete from birth. Soon after, atrophy is noticed in the area of speech.

Since he cannot hear, he doesn't communicate verbally. Then an atrophy of the left and limbic lobes is detected, although these lobes were in place before the baby's birth, ready to ensure the development of his voice. Thus, the human voice, with its potential for development not only in communication with others, but also with oneself, preserves, activates, and generates the circuits of the areas of the brain concerned with language. It is the indispensable stimulus for this function. If the voice doesn't stimulate the first neuronal connections between the three brains, these areas of the brain will switch off.

So the voice activates, develops, builds, forms, and initiates new neuronal circuits. The acquisition of speech, of music, of the abstract will conquer new ground in the brain. It stimulates information recall. It accelerates the assembly of a word lexicon and the apprenticeship of foreign languages. The voice stimulates its own development. In the same way as the activity and training of an athlete sculpts his muscles, cerebral stimulation in the first months of life shapes the vocal intelligence of the child. Stimulation through voice and music activate the cerebral structure of the human language and the faculty of anticipation.

Our vocal development is tied to our behavioral development. Our psychological, social, and cultural environment has a definitive impact on the development of the human voice.

The voice by nature is a social mechanism. The word "social" stems from the Latin *socius*, which means "companion living in an environment shared with the same species, with like people." Man can't live isolated from his own kind without it affecting the way he develops, without it impacting his very essence. These interactions with his own kind provide him with the opportunity to construct his identity, to respond to statements, to cut others short, to learn words that feed his linguistic universe. Feedback from our fellow men is indispensable. Otherwise, it would be like trying to play a game of tennis alone! Man's offspring, from a tender age, puts together the tools of language. From apprentice of the voice, he will soon progress to being its master. The presence of others, interacting with others, confronting opinions, brings about the metamorphosis of this vocal animal into *Homo vocalis*.

The learning of the voice is facilitated by Broca's area (for speech), Wernicke's area (for a lexicon of words), and the temporal planum (for the communication of language). These three privileged sites are all located in the left brain for all right-handed people and for most left-handed people. It is undoubtedly the dominant hemisphere. This asymmetry is hormonally determined under the influence of testosterone. Two thirds of left-handed people are men. But over four fifths of people on Earth are right-handed.

The awakening of our brain

Identifying things by name, mastering this concept—is this not the first and foremost fundamental step of vocal ontogeny? Now we enter the newborn's psychological and affective world and its cognitive and motor development. Jean Piaget has identified six stages of development, occurring at one, four, nine, twelve, eighteen, and twenty-four months. The first mumblings of the baby enable it to request food, an object, a toy. Later, these mumblings evolve so that the baby can communicate its feelings, share its sadness or joy. Thus, the human voice progressively becomes the ideal vehicle for symbolizing the world it represents. Actions said to be "pre-intelligent" occur in the first to fourth months (Stages 1 and 2) and prolong the development of reflex activities. They build up solid ties between mother and child. Between the ninth and the twenty-fourth months (Stages 4 to 6), intelligent behavior is established, the most important, in Man's case, being articulated language. His transitional period is between the ages of nine and twenty-four months.

An anthropomorphic approach with respect for the animal world

Sue Taylor Parker, an anthropologist at Sonoma State University in California, decided to apply Piaget's observations of his own children to the bandar monkey. Her conclusions are impressive. The monkeys were observed to go through the same stages, but in a much shorter lapse of time (three to five times shorter). However, from the ninth to the twelve month onward, the learning process stops. The monkey's voice can't go down this particular evolutionary path, because the road was never traced to begin with. Articulated language doesn't exist. Vocal communication is poor and the monkeys show little interest in the various objects brought to their

attention. Their sign language remains succinct. For all that Man
has an authentic language, D. Listel stipulates, he is only able to
teach a symbolic form of communication to animals, even to specimens such as Washoe and Kanzi, the well-known chimpanzees
whose story we are about to discover.

In the sixties, Allan and Beatrice Gardner teach sign language
to Washoe, the chimp. He knows one hundred and fifty sign-words.
His teachers produce a scientific film on him that goes around the
planet. Yet very quickly, limitations in his apprenticeship become
obvious. There is no syntax. In other words, Washoe can't build
sentences or fathom the correct sequencing of words. Each sign
corresponds to a specific object, an expression of hunger, a concrete action. But present Washoe with a new object, and he is incapable of describing it by creating a new sign for it. Conceptual
learning is just not possible.

In 1986, Savage and Rumbaugh "educated" Kanzi, a bonobo,
the chimpanzee thought to be closest to Man. True, having learned
graphic symbols, he was able to combine them in a certain order
and establish links between hand signs and a lexicon. But, as in the
previous case, he was incapable of creating a new concept, and his
slowness showed just how limited he was. We are very far from the
human voice, which has led to the creation of over two hundred
thousand words and made possible conceptualizing and storytelling.

Washoe's or Kanzi's use of language is exclusively on demand,
following a specific stimulus. The abstract does not exist for them.
It is not unlike a Pavlovian reflex. A child, on the other hand, resorts
to language to inform, communicate an idea, declare an opinion,
foresee a situation, share an emotion, create something he has
imagined. The chimpanzee manages to master a few hundred signs
only by virtue of an arduous apprenticeship and a gift for mimicking, which is impressive, but limited basically to replicating.

Yet the chimpanzee has its own language. It is astute, it has
some form of intelligence. An anthropomorphic approach is interesting, but it should not make us forget our respect for the animal,
nor its nobility. In 1997, De Wall was to witness a highly interesting
scene amongst monkeys. A female chimpanzee finds a fruit. She
emits a specific sound that means "alarm, watch out, we're under
attack." All the chimpanzees scamper off, which allows her to finish her meal undisturbed, nobody being around to steal the fruit
from her. So even among animals, "faking it" happens. But the basis

of the fake is behavioral. Many such feints have been recorded amongst female chimpanzees. I. Pepperberg also tested the apprenticeship of language in Alex, a gray Gabonese parrot. In this case we are dealing with true articulated language, but the language that these parrots learn is created by Man for Man. These experiments therefore have limited validity and applicability.

So we are confronted again by the question of the secret of the human voice. Does cerebral genetic programming exist? Already in 1968, Noam Chomsky had dared to consider such a hypothesis. Is the mystery of the human voice in part contained by our DNA? We reviewed earlier the inner structure of this molecule and saw that the *FOXP2* gene is most likely one of the elements of the human language.

Asymmetry of the cerebral hemispheres in primates

Just like Man, the great apes, in other words, tailless monkeys such as the chimpanzee, the gorilla, or the orangutan, present an asymmetry of the cerebral hemispheres. Therefore, they have one hemisphere that dominates. For all that they lack a Broca's area, they do have a temporal planum, that superior region of the temporal lobe concerned with the treatment of communication and language. It is significantly more developed on the left than on the right. Indeed, research carried out by W. Hopkins, of the Yerbust Regional Primate Research Center, revealed that nearly 67% of chimpanzees have a dominant left hemisphere. But this species also has a dominant ear, and that's the right ear. So the question posed here was: does the chimpanzee lack only articulated language? This analysis seems a little simplistic. Of course, the anatomical position of the larynx is essential for speech. But vocal intelligence is also an operative factor.

The dominant hemisphere talks, but both hemispheres control the muscles that do so

We are told that the voice is under the control of the dominant hemisphere. Yet the muscles used for phonation contract on both sides. Our vocal cords also contract on both sides, which produces a symmetrical vibration. How can this voice structure claim to be controlled by one hemisphere? Neurons and callous fibers of the brain cross over from the dominant hemisphere to the other hemisphere, calling into play the muscles of phonation on both the left and the right side simultaneously, synchronously, and harmoniously as soon as they are needed for speech. Control of the body's muscle mechanics and of the muscles used for speaking is bilateral. The noble areas of the brain used for language are unilateral. The creation of language requires the motor capacity to organize the phonatory mechanics, already conceived and thought through, in the areas of the brain concerned with language. You can see how complex this organizational blueprint is.

Machinery and function of the voice

If I want to say a word,

1. Wernicke's area finds that word.

2. The temporal planum then puts it into context.

3. Broca's area enables its pronunciation and passes instructions to the motor areas of the right and left hemispheres for these to activate symmetrically the muscular mechanics of phonation. I now pronounce the word.

Pathologies have made possible this type of observation. When the left brain is affected, the right side of the body stops functioning. Each cerebral location has a specific function. A lesion of the front right lobe causes dysfunctional articulation: the mechanics of articulation are affected. It comes through as a motor aphasia that can be accompanied by hemiplegia. It is hard to understand the person, but he can express himself. When the left lobe is affected in a right-handed person or in a majority of left-handers, this affects not only the motor functions, but also the central speech center. Earlier, we saw the consequences of an expressive aphasia caused by a lesion of Broca's area: slow, labored speech, in telegraphic style. The worst part for the victims is that they can understand everything that is said to them. They are conscious of their pathology, but they're also conscious that they are incapable of speaking intelligently and fluidly. This verbal incapacity is often accompanied by problems with writing.

It can also be accompanied by a quite different aphasia, caused by a lesion to Wernicke's area. If this area alone is affected, it is like being verbally blind and deaf. One can understand neither the written word nor the spoken word. The speech dysfunction is accompanied by a problem in understanding. The victims can't control their own conversation. The fluidity of speech is correct, but there are errors in the words and phonemes. In this case, the victims aren't conscious of their errors nor of their aphasia, which is caused purely by dysfunctional thought processes, not by a mechanical dysfunction of the larynx.

In another register, we have dyslexia, which affects some 3% of the population; also stuttering and mumbling. Stuttering normally develops between the ages of 3 and 5 years. It existed in the days of Hippocrates, Aristotle, or Demosthenes, of whom we know that he put pebbles in his mouth to learn to speak properly. This affliction, more frequent in men, is called by some "the neurosis of speech," described by Jean Tarneaud in 1934. Others claim it is hereditary. Research carried out in the mid 20th century revealed that out of five pairs of monozygotic twins, all stuttered. Stuttering can be caused by several factors, be it an emotional shock, a trauma, or a fright. Heredity facilitates its occurrence, but need not be involved. There are as many types of stuttering as there are stutterers. There is no value in trying to coerce this form of verbal dysfunction into a straightjacket. It affects only the spoken word, which is why singing is not affected by it. Over 70% of stutterers stop stuttering after puberty. In fact, a speech therapist is essential to a favorable outcome for these verbal dysfunctions.

But our brain also creates our laughter and our tears. Laughter is a complex, emotional reaction, bringing into play motor phenomena related to our face, our phonation, and our breathing, phenomena that are rarely controlled and that can cause laryngeal spasms. Expression through laughter is very freeing. Some Chinese medicines use it therapeutically.

Our brain map: an astounding workstation

Let's go back to settle the map of *Cerebropolis*. We humans of the 21st century possess our ancestral brain (*Cerebropolis First District*), also called the archeocortex, seat of control centers vital to our organism; the paleocortex (*Cerebropolis Second District*), seat of the unconscious and involuntary personality, that expresses itself in our moods and spontaneous reactions; and the neocortex (*Cerebropolis Third District*), important seat of our conscious personality and will power. This seat is also the only control center for Man's articulated language.

The brainstem, or archeocortex

Composed of the medulla oblongata and two cerebral peduncles or mesencephalons, the brainstem sits above the spinal cord. Where a lesion of the brain hemispheres causes dysfunctional behavior, a lesion of the spinal cord is irredeemably fatal. Even a partial lesion brings on a vegetative state that requires permanent medical assistance. The spinal cord assists vision and hearing. Hearing, we saw, is indispensable to the creation of the voice. The noble nerves of our body, called the cranial nerves, come off the brainstem (except the first cranial nerve, which controls our sense of smell and is joined to the brain by nerve fibers located on top of the ethmoidal sinus, also known as the olfactory plate, a relic from our reptilian life). We have twelve cranial nerves, these are paired and symmetrical.

The cerebellum: motion and voice

This smaller brain, like its bigger brother, is made up of layered cells showing the three phylogenic periods: arche-, paleo-, and menocells. It is joined to the brainstem anteriorly. The cerebellum plays a major role in coordinating movement and balance. But unlike the brainstem, it is not essential to our vital functions. Here sits the memorization of language, work, and apprenticeship. Whereas the left cortical hemisphere is the seat of language, for these activities the right hemisphere of the cerebellum is dominant. It plays a major role in acting, since it combines memory, language, and motion in space.

The encephalon: two continents of our life moored together by three bridges

It comprises a left brain, a right brain, and a base. These are not independent. Three sets of cabling, or nerve sheaths, form bridges, the major one being the corpus callosum. Thus, information is able to cross over from one side to the other, and from back to front, or front to back.

The limbic system or paleocortex: the crossing district of our emotional brain

As we have seen, the limbic system is the behavioral and emotional brain. It sits at the base of the left and right brain hemispheres, inside and contiguous with the temporal lobes. It is at the junction of the efferent and afferent neuronal paths of the neocortex.

The neocortex: a cerebral projection proportionate to its usage

This came later in the evolutionary timetable. It overlaps the hemispheres and its convoulted topography reveals hills (gyri) and valleys (sulci) or brain circumvolutions. In the present state of our knowledge, six layers are recognized on the surface of the neocortex. Each manages cellular circuits.

In 1909, Cajal was to ask himself the following highly pertinent question: given that we use our hands intensively, is their cerebral projection proportionate to their usage? The answer is yes. The cerebral projection of functions that involve using the hand is greater, no doubt because that area of the brain is frequently stimulated. Conversely, a function that is rarely used will have a corresponding cortical projection that is smaller and thinner.

The greater the cerebral stimulation, the more frequently the projection controlling a function is solicited, the more the projection will develop in the cortex, taking up more space and becoming thicker. In a blind person, the vision area atrophies, but the others become more finely honed. The same happens with regard to the voice, as we saw in the case of wild children.

Broca's area and Wernicke's area are the epicenters of our language center

If Broca's area and Wernicke's area are the epicenters of our language center, the voice has multiple cerebral projections, notably as regards our memory function (without which we would be incapable of assimilating words), our auditory function (without which we would not be able to learn to use the voice), the area of the temporal planum (with which we construct our voice), and the motor area (mechanical assistant of the spoken word).

Without doubt, the most crucial projections are located in Broca's area, level with the lower left frontal sulcus or groove concerned with speech, and in Wernicke's area, level with the first and second temporal gyri in the left hemisphere, concerned with the perception of words and linguistic symbolism. But adjoining these territories are areas concerned with the motor aspects of language sounds or phonology, word storage, comprehension, sentence construction, and the rhythm and musical quality of speech. These words first have to have been memorized and therefore heard: that's the job of, among others, the parietal lobe, which plays a part in the perceptual brain. The occipital lobe has a major role to play in vision; it enables you to read words. Thanks to multiple and complex cerebral connections, the voice develops and establishes itself with apparent ease (see Plate 7).

The higher functions of Man: the circumvolutions of the brain at the origin of language

Functions such as hand movements, language, vision, memory, the apprenticeship of foreign languages, and many others, stimulate and allow the development of the brain. Throughout the evolution of mammals, from the cat to the mouse, from monkey to Man, the cerebral cortex displays a similar cellular structure: a cellular structure identical in Man and other mammals and consisting of six layers. In 1984, Meynert demonstrated that the cortex doesn't have the same thickness all over, although the six layers are encountered all over. This difference in thickness is due to the variable frequency of stimulation of different areas of the brain. More recently, in 1980, Rockel removed a sample of neurons from the cortex and found that for a comparable volume, the bandar monkey and Man have the same density (146,000 neurons per mm^2). The human cerebral cortex, with a surface of around 22 dm^2, contains around 30 billion neurons; the chimpanzee's, with a surface of 4.9 dm^2, contains 7 billion; the gorilla's, with a surface of 5.4 dm^2, contains 8 billion.

The mouse is down at 65 million neurons. Apart from cephalopods (the octopus and squid family) endowed with several million neurons, invertebrates such as the sea squirt only have 2,000. Here, Darwin was well inspired when he said that "Man's body structure bears the indelible imprint of an inferior origin." Did the sea squirt not endow us with neurons?

The billions of neurons of the human cerebral cortex are, of course, supported by an awesome number of interneuronal connections. The adaptation of the neocortex to the voice has been hugely boosted by stimulations to this part of our brain, firstly, over millions of years, and secondly, during our own lifetime. The fact of wanting to speak and create words to materialize our thoughts stimulates the creation of new cerebral circuits and extends the cerebral space dedicated to this function. The wherewithal is there, it just needs to be activated to become functional. A function can activate a cortical area that was inactive. It will keep the new circuit on record and use it to build other circuits. Thus, the brain autostimulates itself to grow, provided it receives sufficient external stimulation. The cerebral hemispheres are asymmetric, favoring the left hemisphere, and, more specifically, the temporal planum.

The brain of the fetus is formed between the tenth and the twenty-seventh weeks. Broca's area is in place: the voice is therefore innate! But if it is not stimulated, it can't manifest itself and won't exist, or rather, it will remain dormant.

The cerebral landscape:

We all have two hemispheres, each comprising five lobes. Four of them are well known: they contain nearly 70% of our neurons.

1. The *frontal lobe*, anteriorly located, seat of Broca's area, is just behind the forehead. This lobe is concerned with voluntary movement and the coordination of movement. This motor cortex is also responsible for our sense of touch, as it has a sensory portion. Thinking, certain memory functions, reasoning faculties, and our manners belong to this lobe.

2. The *temporal lobe* above the ear houses Wernicke's area, the auditory function, our sense of taste, and other memory functions.

3. The *parietal lobe* sits in the median part of the cortical hemisphere. It is concerned with body sensory awareness, involuntary movement, and spatial orientation. It also provides feedback on touch sensations.

4. The *occipital lobe* located at the back of the brain is the seat of vision.

5. The *insula*, the fifth lobe nestled in the interior face of the hemispheres, intervenes when we yawn and controls the vestibular complex.

Our lobes are marked by fissures which subdivide into gyri. Each hemisphere shows two or three fissures and grooves. These fissures or grooves allow the brain to significantly increase its surface. You only find such developed fissures and grooves in Man. The central fissure, called Rolando's fissure, appears around the twenty-eighth week of gestation. It forms a slightly vertical line on the lateral face of the hemisphere. Anteriorly is the frontal lobe, posteriorly the parietal lobe. There is a second important fissure known as the Sylvian fissure (see Plate 8). It appears in the tenth week of gestation and forms an almost horizontal line, perpendicular to Rorlando's fissure. The frontal lobe is also anterior to the Sylvian fissure. The frontal lobe is the seat of voluntary movement, controlled by means of efferent fibers that run from our brain to our muscles. Behind the Sylvian fissure lies the projection for sensory awareness of these same body parts: it is the afferent fibers that bring the information to the brain. The Sylvian fissure is horizontal and forms a boundary with the parietal lobe above, and the temporal lobe below. It separates the frontal lobe at the front, from the temporal lobe at the back.

Our brain map: a mystery to be revealed?

Penfield undertook several experiments in the 1950s. Voluntary subjects presenting a brain tumor agreed to electric stimulations around the tumor, while conscious, but under local anesthesia. The stimulations either activated or inhibited the zones treated. Thus, stimulating a sensory area provoked a sensation, stimulating a motor area provoked a motor reaction that was coherent with the specific zone treated.

But, and this comes as no surprise, no zone specific to the human voice was found. No stimulation provoked speech. It is the teamwork between different areas that makes speech possible.

Stimulating Broca's area provokes the utterance of a few vowels, but never sentences. These experiments gave us a better understanding of the multicenter projection of the human voice; it also taught us to undertake only minimal ablation of tissues surrounding a brain tumor, in order to avoid touching the area concerned with language. In 1989, G. Ojeman observed from a sample of 117 patients that, even though the cerebral projections are always located in the same place, they vary very slightly from one person to another.

The neocortex is the seat of the higher functions of the primates: the hand, the pharynx, the larynx. Neurosurgical exploration backed by microelectrodes enabled the neuromotor and neurosensory mapping of our body. The projection for the head is low, near the base of the skull; the projection of the feet is on the top of the head. What about this left brain dominance? It also exists in mammals, as well as in birds, notably so in parrots. Since the days of invertebrates, with their grossly primitive nervous system, mammals have developed a complex nervous system. This has enabled Man to develop the motor coordination and sensory functions necessary for human speech.

Memory and voice

The human voice can't exist without prior memorization of words. Memory recall operates on two levels: short-term memory and long-term memory.

Short-term memory enables us to store for a few hours or a few days, sentences, words, or melodies heard here and there. It is an extension of our immediate hearing faculty. But what an extension! A ray of sunlight is retained on our retina for a few tens of seconds. But words or a melody are perceived by the brain in 50 milliseconds, by the ear in 2 to 5 milliseconds, and can be retained for several days. The information is stored in the brain for some time before it is obliterated. Amnesia can wipe out long-term memories or short-term memories, depending on which neuronal circuits are affected. Interesting experiments have been carried out on short-term memory. They revealed that our capacity for immediate retention is limited to seven items. We are not able to memorize more than seven items in our short-term memory, whether the information is visual, vocal, or sensory. If we add an eighth item to our short-term memory, it will wipe out the first item and we are back on track with seven items.

Our short-term memory is backed up by our long-term memory, which enables us to have memories and to conceive of time. This long-term memory is the melting pot that will enable the creation of new words, new sentences, and original thoughts. We are taught at school early on to recite poetry and to retain formulas such as $E = mc^2$. This knowledge apprenticeship enables us to store dozens of thousands of words in our brain. It is indispensable to human evolution. As Richard Dawkins explains, the "meme" is the gene of the word on which the structure of language is built. Auditory information, the stimulus of our voice, enters the brainstem, is conveyed to its cerebral projection, then, through multiple connections, interacts with the language areas and recognizes the musical instrument—the violin, the piano, the harp. The projection for auditory input is only millimeters from the projection for Wernicke's area. In professional singers and musicians, these areas are highly developed. Their corpus callosum, the bridge that brings cabling to the two hemispheres, is also enlarged. Indeed, families that are great music-lovers develop these areas from early childhood. Each hemisphere does its share of listening. The auditory area of the right hemisphere integrates one-third of the input from the right ear and two-thirds from the left ear. Conversely, the left hemisphere integrates one-third of the input from left ear and two-thirds from the right ear.

Within the audiophonatory loop, this mode of functioning plays an important role. It is this feedback that makes the difference between having a good ear or not, that explains why a person with a hearing deficiency can't become a tenor, a baritone, or a soprano, a pianist, or a guitar-player. You need that audiophonatory loop. Take the example of older people whose hearing becomes progressively worse. Their voice changes, it becomes monotonal. The timbre of their voice loses its warmth and its harmonics.

Communicating through gestures: even in one's head

"Free hands"

Once we were able to stand upright, thus freeing the upper body, we freed up our hands. As described by André Leroi-Gourhan, our stance went through four evolutionary periods.

The first period was that of the walking quadrupeds. Their brain shows the first traces, along Rolando's groove, of a finer motor organization of the anterior face muscles, with, at the front, the center of sensibility.

The second period is that of the prehensile quadrupeds, who began to sit. This sitting position temporarily frees the upper limbs. The hand is also freed episodically. But there is no alteration to the way the head is carried. Their neocortex shows a precise motor organization that's particularly well-developed and specialized as regards the hands.

The third period is that of the monkey. Again we encounter the sitting position, but this time, the head is carried differently, creating an angle that approaches the vertical. The facial and manual projections of the neocortex are highly developed, especially those of the hand and thumb.

The fourth period is that of the upright stance so characteristic of Man. The major change here, of course, is the complete freedom given to the upper body, with free use of the hands, but especially, the cranial suspension that gives more room to the brain and provides the opportunity to develop afferent and efferent connections in relation to articulated language.

Throughout his evolution, from invertebrates to reptiles through to *Homo sapiens*, Man appears to be the only species that escaped anatomical hyperspecialization. Consider the mammoth's tusks, the horse's legs, the brain of singing birds, the highly developed acoustic signals of the bat. Man is able to adapt to all situations. His hands, his sight, his hearing, his uprightness, his ability to express himself, his speech make him unique and independent. The main key to all this was the mechanical liberation of the back of the head brought about by his upright stance!

The quantum of the brain: the neuron the citizen of Cerebropolis

Numbers that makes me feel dizzy!

Our voice is created through the synthesis of information by the whole brain. Billions of cables and connections between our neurons make possible the very existence of vocal expression. Our vocal mystery resides, among others, in "Cerebropolis."

For experienced detectives like us, the key exhibit is without doubt the cerebral quantum: the neuron. What are the characteristics of this cell?

The word "neuron" was invented in 1890 by Waldeyer (who also coined the word "chromosome") to design a cell that is unique in its ability to form a giant communication network. This marvel comes to us from the animal world. Our nervous system contains 300 billion cells, forming two large families: the first, that of our neurons, carries information; the second, that of our glial cells, props and supports the brain's structure. "Mysterious butterflies of the soul, whose fluttering wings may one day, who knows, provide us with the answer to the secret of our mental life." Thus did Santiago Ramon y Cajal, Nobel prize-winner in 1906, describe these noble elements of our brain that are steeped in a nutritious fluid known as the cerebrospinal fluid. The image of fluttering butterfly wings was revisited much later to support the theory of chaos.

Our neurons, close to 100 billion in number, have the body of their cell in the gray matter of our brain. This gray matter is only a few millimeters thick. In order to ensure its expansion, it folds over itself, forming fissures and grooves on the brain's surface in the cerebral cortex. In Man, the cerebral cortex occupies 50% of the volume of our brain. As we saw earlier, our neurons are organized into six parallel layers, except in the visual cortex, which has seven layers of neurons.

Some 100 billion synaptic junctions connect these nerve cells to each other. Each neuron receives 10,000 different signals from other neurons through its dendrites. A single neuron then sends 10,000 new signals to 10,000 other neurons via its axon. This information is propagated at a speed of 200 to 360 kilometers per hour. These numbers are mind-boggling!

Where the cell bodies of neurons form the gray matter of the brain, their axons (think of them as wires down which the neuron sends information) form its white matter and entwine to form thick cabling, which in its thickest part forms the corpus callosum. A bridge formed of several hundred million fibers, it is the only element that connects the left and the right hemispheres.

Right bank, left bank: a bridge uniting them

This bridge, the corpus callosum, between the right and the left hemispheres—how indispensable is it? Can it be obliterated, can it be sectioned? Its role is better understood thanks to a case of severe epilepsy.

A certain Mr. Pierre, an epileptic, at the start of the 1960s considers his condition to be intolerable. He can no longer bear the repeated fits that are invalidating and painful, both physically and psychologically. He hears of a possible treatment that may, if not cure him, at least make life tolerable. He decides to volunteer for an experimental procedure that consists in severing the corpus callosum. He is anxious when admitted to hospital. The neurosurgeon informs him that he'll be operated on the next day, and that he may not survive. He goes ahead nevertheless, he can't bear to live on like this. The operation goes well and the outcome is extraordinary. No motor deficit, he walks normally, is able to feed himself normally, apparently talks normally. The epilepsy has practically disappeared. Both Pierre and the neurosurgical team are euphoric. A few days go by, then Pierre and the surgeon notice some anomalies. The harmony between the two hemispheres is gone. Each is now an island unto itself. Reason and emotion can no longer intermingle. Pierre is right-handed. His left brain was dominant, his language center resident there. Now, when asked to read the word "knight" with his right eye covered, he finds he can't understand the signs before him. Normally, the visual information carried by the written word is integrated by the visual area of the right occipital lobe, then transmitted to the left frontal and temporal lobes, seat of the brain's language center.

But the connection between the two hemispheres has been interrupted; the cabling of the corpus callosum has been severed. The right occipital lobe can no longer pass on the information corresponding to the word "knight" to the left hemisphere, to be integrated by Broca's and Wernicke's areas. Pierre no longer sees words. He sees geometric shapes. For him, words and letters no longer form a language; all he sees is a string of curved and straight lines. The visual stimulus is still there, but its translation, its representation, and its concept are now lost somewhere in Cerebropolis. The afferent message exists, but the verbal response no longer exists, and neither does the efferent message. This illustrates aptly the complementarity of these two hemispheres that work together to facilitate the integration of the world of language and voice.

Cables, cells, electricity, and junctions

All those billions and billions of synapses have three fundamental roles to play in this meeting of neurons. The neuron is a one-way highway: the cell body is the departure point, the axon is the road and it ends at the synapse. If the axon heads for a muscle, its direction is "centrifugal": it is going to deliver a motor message from the brain to the muscle via the synapse. Another type of axon runs sensory information from the periphery back to the brain: its direction is said to be "centripetal." Thus, the brain has efferent (centrifugal) fibers exporting motor information and afferent (centripetal) fibers importing sensory information.

In Cerebropolis, three steps are required to activate a neuron. For example, if you decide to contract your biceps, the first step is the information that runs from your brain to the biceps via the efferent fibers. This will order the muscle fibers to contract. The second step involves another neuron, which informs the brain that the biceps has indeed contracted. This information goes from the muscle up to the brain via the spinal cord; this is sensory information. Some 14 million neurons allow this type of sensory message to be delivered to the brain. The third and final step is one of integration. The information has been delivered to the brain. Now it will be translated, interpreted, decoded by other neurons to establish its meaning. We know how important this step is from Mr. Pierre's case.

Above, the simple contraction of a muscle was illustrated. Things become hugely more complex in the case of a vocalization exercise. You decide to sing the *A* note. The efferent neurons bring about the contraction of numerous laryngeal muscles. The afferent neurons inform the nervous system: "Job done." This information is integrated by the third group of neurons.

But that's not all: you need to adjust the musical note. Now the return of sound comes into play. You modulate, correct, perfect the tonality you are aiming for. All this is done in a few hundredths of a second. Our brain, the virtuoso *Homo vocalis*, is able to recognize, adapt, and repeat a musical note in one-fifteenth of a second. An orchestra conductor can distinguish fifteen different notes or fifteen instruments in a second. Repetition of the exercise helps to memorize the techniques, the movements of the laryngeal muscles, and the vibratory patterns of the exercise as the sounds will be produced, but the emotional content has to be created afresh every second. Either it's there, or it isn't, but it can't be repeated! The interpretation given harmonizes the exercise. The apprenticeship, based here on repetition of this process, calls on the left brain for the solfeggio and on the right brain for the harmonics. The vocalization exercise thus memorized is ready for recall. The next time you rehearse the same verses, you adjust your voice much faster, and more efficiently, than the first time around. Training one's muscles and brain is as important for professional singers as it is for athletes.

The neuron: the chatterbox citizen of Cerebropolis

The mastermind behind this exploit is the neuron. It's a unique feature of our organism, from all points of view. It can't divide. Nothing else achieves this degree of complexity, which makes it very difficult to replace. When it dies, it's final. While alive, it never stops communicating with its kind. It is a great chatterbox, as well as being a one-way messenger. It can create new connections on command. Its shape is very characteristic: reminiscent of a tall tree with shallow roots and a long, slender trunk, capped by a crown of leaves and branches. The branches are dendrites 2 microns in diameter, which capture information from other neurons. The center of the apex of branches is the cell's body, with its nucleus and numerous mitochondria. The trunk is the axon, which can be a few millimeters to over a meter long. The roots are the synapses, 50 microns in diameter, the endings of the neuron.

The information is received by the dendrites, gets transmitted to the cell body, runs down the axon to the synapses, and crosses over to another neuron or to a receptor organ. The reverse flow never happens. Let's take a concrete example: I'm going to pronounce a few words, then fall silent. The silence will diminish the activity of the different language areas of my brain. The neurons are switched off. Now, I want to pronounce the sentence: "What a beautiful sunset!" The cerebral stimulus of the language center has been activated. The neurons get busy. The excitatory synapses transfer the information toward the motor zones of my larynx. The expression levers of my articulated language and larynx are activated. Several dozen million interneuronal connections have been put to work and guarantee the harmony of the sentence I pronounce.

Through medical imaging, we have been able to observe that certain areas of the brain consume more oxygen than others when we speak. Functional magnetic resonance imaging, or f-MRI, confirms this information in real time and underscores the amazing speed at which information is transferred, as well as the importance of the dominant lobe.

The speed at which orders are transmitted

Even more surprising, whereas auditory information is conveyed by the ear at a speed of 40 m/s (144 km/h), phonatory information is carried by the nerve controlling it (the vagus nerve) at a speed of 100 m/s (360 km/h). The axon's nervous electric signal is insulated: it is surrounded by a sheath called the myelin sheath, which prevents any leakage of the signal. There is no dispersion during the transmission of the electrical information, which is, in fact, an exchange between the calcium and potassium ions of the axon's membrane. Even more extraordinary, this exchange of calcium and potassium ions, called the membrane's potential, takes place in successive bursts that are perfectly methodical, rhythmic, and synchronous. The energy that stimulates this electric current is itself generated by ATP, a molecule that is exclusive to our internal energy; without respite, it spontaneously recharges our nervous cells. This nervous impulse is universal across species. From the squid to Man, its structure is identical. Cellular respiration and the oxygenation of the lungs produce the energetic molecule for our whole organism, ATP, and create a nervous impulse which is none other than an electrochemical signal. Now we understand better why our brain consumes up to 20% of our energy. Rhythm is central to this nervous transmission. The message is not transmitted continuously, but sequentially, via thousands of small stimuli. The information is passed on to the end of the nerve. The junction between the two neurons works much like a plug. Neurotransmitters facilitate the transmission. There are several types of plugs, and thus several types of neurotransmitters.

Neurotransmitters: coordinating agents

Neurotransmitters, our hormonal molecular messengers, depend on and are influenced by our limbic system, our emotional brain.

They enable muscular activity, glandular secretion, a sense of pleasure, seduction, and the libido.

Acetylcholine: master of muscular contractions

One of the major neurotransmitters activates the musculature, including the muscles around the vocal cords: it is the cholinergic transmitter that controls muscle contraction. The junction "motor nerve/striated muscle" ensures an elementary "cybernetic" operation. Its law is "all or nothing." Either the muscle contracts—or it doesn't. But the strength of the contraction depends on the efferent and additional stimuli that set off successive microdischarges of acetylcholine. A minimum threshold has to be reached for the contraction to be set off. Then, an additional stimulus is required to achieve a certain degree of contraction and to control it with precision. The long vocal cord will seek its sharp, the short vocal cord its low. Thus, the striated muscle of the vocal cord will be solicited to stretch more and more. The brain, through its nervous impulse, determines the length, curve, and duration of the contraction. Can the vocal cord contract in the absence of a voluntary command from above? It seems not. Yet when you swallow the wrong way, a muscle reflex kicks in immediately, within a hundredth of a second, to let you cough. It is a loop reflex, and its neurotransmitter is still acetylcholine.

Adrenaline: activated by stress

This neurotransmitter, called noradrenergic, allows the secretion of adrenaline. Stress causes its secretion. It brings about an increase in vigilance, attention and cardiac rhythm. It increases our energetic consumption and stimulates our dynamic reserves. It activates our memory, comprehension, creativity, thinking, and speech.

Other neurotransmitters

The dopaminergic neurotransmitter (allowing the secretion of dopamine) has a different action. It confers the ability to feel pleasure and desire. A third group of neurotransmitters under research are the derivates of serotonin. They influence disposition, perception and levels of pain, relating to others, sleep, mood, and aggression.

The endorphins we secrete are auto-euphorizing drugs appreciated by endurance athletes such as marathon runners. They mask pain and make you feel good. They are also secreted when you listen to a voice you find seductive.

How do neurotransmitters pass on information?

In its structure, the neuron is no different from other cells. What characterizes the neuron is its vocation as message highway. It is our organism's "messenger-boy," delivering the latest news from the dendrite via the axon to the synapse, and never the other way around. How is the information passed on? The messages are both electrical and chemical. Within the cell, the message is electrical, then it becomes chemical at the synapses for an exchange either with the dendrites of another neuron, or with the receptor organ of a muscle or skin. Each electrical impulse delivers a base molecular unit. The number of impulsions determines the quality and amplitude of the message. The amount of chemical substance that passes through is perfectly proportionate to the information conveyed. A minimal threshold must be reached to set off the stimulus, otherwise the information can't be delivered. But the remarkable gradation of the possible response by these chemical microparticles allows for a dosage that's adapted to the musical sound we want to produce when the vocal cord contracts, to within one-eighth of a tone, from the *vibrato* to the *pianissimo* note we are after. This is comparable to the precision delivered to astronauts in space, who have to navigate their spaceship to within one-thousandth of a degree of the selected path!

Each impulse is precisely quantified. It delivers the message, setting up an action potential, a sort of electrical message with a goal—in this case a vocal sound. The dendrites can have 1,000 to 10,000 connections. Let's suppose we have 10,000 connections. If 6,000 of these are excitatory and 4,000 are inhibitory, only 2,000 excitatory impulses will be taken into account. In this case, it gives us a degree of precision of two ten-thousandths.

Experiencing one's voice: the afferent information returns to the brain

Until now, we insisted on the motor aspects of this neuronal chain of command. But there is also a sensory dimension, in that the brain is informed both of the muscle's response and of the quality of this response. For example, if I pick up a sculpture, I am able to pick it up because my brain orders the muscles of my shoulder, arm, and hand to do so. But I also know if the sculpture is hot or cold, dry or humid, if it is made of wood or of bronze—the brain receives this information: this is known as proprioceptive sensory information. This same sensory dimension operates when we use our vocal apparatus. It's essential. Thanks to this dimension you can experience your voice, its vibration. All the elements that enter into this sensory proprioceptivity help to regulate phonation. Sensory feedback from the muscles enables you to dose the laryngeal and breathing elements and control the vibration of the vocal cords in two ways: by regulating the muscular tone of the vocal cord and the power of the exhalation. It harmonizes the voice box and balances the breathing effort.

Every muscle has its own dedicated neuron that regulates the muscle's contraction. This is one of the elements ensuring harmony of coordination. But this motor control is centralized and controls several muscles at a time. It is centralized by the cerebellum, the reticular body, and the thalamostriated layer. A tumor of the cerebellum produces speech that's slow, laborious, choppy, punctuated, and even explosive. The thalamus plays an active part in speech delivery, in how we form words, in the control of elocution, in syntax. Moreover, it is responsible for our short-term memory. The cerebral cortex plays a key role in our voluntary and emotional language.

The integrity of the neuron is indispensable to the survival of the muscle it controls, to the reliability of the receptor it informs, to our proprioceptive sensations. Its impairment, traumatism, or degeneration spell the end for the organ or receptor it controls. Thus, a muscle can atrophy or become paralyzed if the nerve commanding it is severed or traumatized. For an organ to survive, it must be stimulated. If the nerve controlling the vocal cord were to be severed, the cord would atrophy and rigidify. It would lose all function.

Right brain versus left brain: the key to their harmony is in their symbiosis

This detailed review of the brain provided an outline of the role each hemisphere plays. The left brain plays a greater role in the treatment of language, in reasoning, mathematical analysis; the right brain is more involved in spatial relationships, musical harmony, and our emotional world. Are they completely independent? Absolutely not. Connections link them. They confront somewhat crudely the logical brain and the emotional brain. In left-handers, the projection of language is spread between the two hemispheres. This is known to some as lambilaterality. In 96% of right-handers and 70% of lefthanders, the seat of language is in the left brain. Only 15% of people are left-handed and 15% are ambidextrous. There are fewer left-handers among women than among men. Yet women have better verbal skills than men. Magnetic image resonance has highlighted the greater prominence of the language areas in the left brain in relation to concrete words. But when the brain is dealing with abstract words, it is the right hemisphere that is activated.

The projection of the human voice is different in men and in women. Sally and Bennett Shaywitz carried out functional cerebral imaging on a sample of male and female patients. They were asked to pronounce a few sentences, identical for all of them. The result was unexpected. In men, the projection of "phonological" language, in other words the detection of rhymes, occurred strictly in the left brain. In women, the left brain was also activated, but the corresponding area was also activated in the right brain. From this, one can conclude that in the West, language is a predominantly Cartesian function in men, whereas it is both Cartesian and emotional in women (see Plate 9). These findings led to more research. The differences in cerebral response between men and women listening to a text again highlighted the greater involvement of the right brain in women.

Neuroimaging has shown us that our brain evolves, of course, from birth to adulthood, but its evolution in men and in women is different. In our Western civilization, man is a soldier. He has to be decisive. His language must not betray any emotion. He is a warrior. It is no surprise, therefore, that his language center should be primarily in the left hemisphere, in his mathematical brain. Do we not encounter some men in the West with an apparently atrophied right brain? On the other hand, women's emotionality is obvious. Women have the right to cry. They let their right brain speak.

Jean-Paul Sartre liked to say "All is in all, and reciprocally." This probably holds true for our brain. For despite the specific role played by each portion of the brain, our voice finds its expression through the harmonious association of our left and right brain. We saw the importance of the apprenticeship of words through the example of young Victor, or of the little girls Kamala and Amala.

We have visited the impressive cerebral galaxy furrowed by neuronal highways. Reality is greater than fiction in this world in which the controller is apparently the Master of his destiny, thanks to the stimulations he himself unleashes. Yet is Cerebropolis really at the service of *Homo vocalis*, or of evolution?

Chapter 6

The receiver of the human voice

The human voice is the privileged receiver of our knowledge, subjected since our early childhood to our hearing and to our reception of the world of vibrations.

Philippe always puts the phone to his right ear: Why?

Philippe, age nine, enters my office, accompanied by his parents. He is wearing a blue and white checked shirt; he looks sporty and on the ball, perky. He questions me before I even have time to ask him the reason for his visit. "Doctor, can you tell me why my friends can listen to the phone with either ear?" An unexpected question. He continues: "I always put the phone to my right ear with my right hand. If I need to write, I then hold the phone with my left hand, but I still hold it to my right ear, never to my left ear. You can't hear anything on the left side!" The child is precocious. His parents confirm that he has never had any problems. I detect no anatomic anomaly when I examine his eardrums. He is in good health. But his auditory tests reveal that he is deaf on the left side. In fact, Philippe has never been able to hear on that side. As far as he is concerned, this is normal. His parents never realized that he has a problem; he never complained about it. Occasionally he mishears notes when playing the piano, but he speaks normally. The receiver of his voice has been unilateral since his early infancy. He had compensated for his left anacusis (total deafness) remarkably well with his right ear. The diagnostic was easy: a unilateral deafness that had had no impact on young Philippe's social life.

This contrasts with bilateral deafness from birth, which causes mutism. But the brain has extraordinary capacities: a child born of two parents who were born deaf will speak normally. Proof that the voice is alchemy of multifactorial elements we are still far from having fully understood. More than that, from the research of Kuniyoshi et al. (and it is amazing!), the f-NMR projection of sign language is in the same area: Broca's and Wernicke's area. So the deaf mutes "vocalize" with their sign language.

The ear is the exclusive receiver of the voice

The ear: an acoustical pathway

Man's ear is organized into three parts (see Plate 10):

1. The *external auditory canal*, which conveys the vibration down to the eardrum. A fine layer of skin that can sometimes be the seat of eczema protects it.

2. The *middle ear*, linked to the nasopharynx by the eustachian tube, begins after the eardrum or tympanic membrane and houses successively three tiny bones, the auditory ossicles: the malleus (tied up to the eardrum), the incus, and the stapes. The stapes footplate is linked to the internal ear by the oval window. It is the door of the cochlea to receive the vibrations that strike the tympanic membrane.

3. The *inner ear*, divided into two distinct sections:
   a. the one, with its three semicircular canals, is responsible for our sense of balance;
   b. the other, with its cochlea, is responsible for our ability to hear.

These elements develop in the embryo and are the building blocks for our voice receiver. The cochlea, shaped like a shell with its two and a half spirals, is the structure in the inner ear that enables us to perceive frequencies. For the singing voice, this "cochlear keyboard," as nicknamed by Professor Chouard, is an indispensable go-between bridging our brain and the world of sound. Only 2 mm in diameter and 35-mm high, it enables us to integrate at least three octaves. The cochlea of the lizard, only 0.04-mm high, can only distinguish low-pitched frequencies. The pigeon's cochlea is only 0.06-mm high. The guinea pig, with its 2.5-mm high cochlea, can hear up to 15,000 Hz, that is, very high frequencies. The human fetus hears: the cochlea and the stapes, are fully developed in the four-month-old fetus. In girls, the activity of the frequency keyboard is greater than in boys. These frequencies are notably more developed in the higher harmonics and are better perceived by the right ear (if the left brain is dominant).

A hearing receiver is essential for us to learn to speak. Our voice echoes inside of us. Hearing our own voice reassures us that we exist socially; if we can't hear it, we are isolated not only from others, but also from ourselves.

The embryo, then the fetus bathed in its amniotic fluids, perceives not only the mother's vibrations and internal noises, but also vibrations from the outside world, muffled and filtered by its protective cocoon. These sonorous vibrations influence the intrauterine development of the fetus. Its auditory sense is already stimulated, preparing the ground for the verbal apprenticeship still to come.

From the age of two or three, children stimulate and construct their own vocal stamp. One of the first elements to develop in the embryo, the ear is one of the last to be fully developed. Hearing educates a child. Hearing his own voice builds up his cultural edifice. Our voice enables us to communicate, to get our bearings; it can be authoritative or soothing, angry or emotional; it often betrays us, but it is always empowered by our sense of hearing. Our hearing consolidates our perception of what is "external" and what is "internal." Did Françoise Dolto not often say: "To speak is to live"?

Man's hearing

The newborn baby and high-pitched frequencies

At birth, the newborn experiences the equivalent of a seismic shock. After nine months of being "fed, lodged, and heated," he leaves his aquatic world for dry land. He produces his first cry, his first breath of life in our atmosphere. His world of sound is acquiring color. His voice is embryologic. A considerable flow of new information rushes to his brain. He was in a world without vision; now his eyelids open, and the luminosity is brutal. It blinds him. His left and right brains are experiencing photonic light for the first time. When his eyes finally adapt to daylight, his inner ear is ready to detect high-pitched sounds. Light and daylight are firmly associated with high-pitched sounds by this infant of ours. The acoustic keyboard and the photonic spectrum now coexist. This could explain why high frequencies are the realm of religion and sacred chants. The newborn prefers his mother's voice to all other voices. He recognizes its timbre, its melody, its rhythm. A few weeks later, he is able to detect the voice of other women. Yet a few more weeks must pass by before he recognizes his father's voice.

The discovery of our voice: it is through hearing

He screams, he cries: such is his vocal expression for now. He tenses his exhalation muscles and "screams" for all he is worth. This shrill scream of his has a frequency range of 400 to 450 hertz. Yet his voice doesn't break. Lullabies and sweet words don't calm him. He is hungry. Around the fourth to sixth week, his mother's tender voice now soothes him, he manages a few gurgles. At ten weeks, when spoken to, he looks toward the speaker, listens to him, tracks him down with his eyes; the body responds, concentrates. Toward the age of three to five months, he begins to babble. Language is making its first inroads. His larynx is still highly perched; he drinks and breathes at the same time. His vocal apprenticeship is beginning. His voice takes shape, is formed and constructed. His screams are no longer his only laryngeal expression.

At six to eight months, he listens to and recognizes different vocal timbres, he moves to rhythmic music. He perceives an octave, he can listen to music. From this privileged moment onward, he is given a name and is addressed by his name; the baby has now earned a new status in the family. He laughs, makes vocal noises, and manipulates objects. He acquires new language, his voice begins to establish itself. He seems surprised when he comes out with vowels and syllables that are chopped up, because he hasn't yet adapted his breathing to phonation. Pneumophonatory harmony appears around the ninth month. When he is spoken to, he is expected to answer within a specific vocal context. He eliminates certain vocal sounds and replaces them with a more expressive repertoire. Harmonics make their appearance and become lower pitched. He hums, repeats sounds and words that he has heard: "daddy," "mummy."

From his second year onward, he sings melodies, memorizes words, creates his own inner vocal dictionary. Prosody, the vocal rhythm of one's maternal tongue, begins to encrust itself in his cerebral cortex thanks to the voice's receiver, the ear. By the time he is two years old, his phonatory apparatus is in place, the central nervous system is being finalized, the multifactorial elements of the human voice are ready to interact. The suckling infant has become a child who is being taught to speak; he also learns to sing, he can use the major third intervals, and an adequate rhythm.

Then, from the age of three, he enters the universe of the "adult child" with his famous "Why?" or "Another story!"

The language-thought becomes the thought-language

The child learns to play a musical instrument. He fine-tunes his hearing—some will acquire the perfect ear. He builds the foundations of his vocal edifice. He improves, enriches, learns, and manages this new tool that serves his thinking. He invents new words, or rather reinvents them by pronouncing them his way. His left brain is absorbing words like a sponge: he has caught the "word mania" bug. Wernicke's area is still empty. It is ready to swallow up words, sounds, and phonemes. The area of the temporal planum facilitates the apprenticeship of grammar and he begins to form sentences. His right brain brings these elements together to form a harmonious and musical whole. Man's offspring is at the dawn of his voice. He is just starting to become aware of it. He listens to it, as he listens to other voices. By the age of seven, he is able to imitate, modulate, and play with his voice. His fundamental frequency becomes lower. He has "the voice of an angel." It will become sexual at puberty.

The sex hormones haven't yet made an impact on his larynx. The years between the ages of seven and nine are auspicious for the integration of music. "Absorbed" before the age of five, music is then "digested" at this age. It is not by chance that children's choirs are formed around children of this age.

Mathematics and the solfeggio are stored in the left brain, along with language. Harmonics reside in the right brain, our imaginative brain. Given the emotionality of the artistic world, one would think that a musical bent would overdevelop the right brain, swamping it with emotion. This is not the case. Learning the solfeggio and mastering musical techniques are such rigorous exercises that it behooves the left brain to take charge of this. Research carried out by Agnes Chan and Mei Chun Cheung using cerebral imaging shows that not only do musicians have a more developed left brain, but moreover, their left brain is more developed than is the norm. This is because music is unusually demanding on our cognitive functions. Our brain must be stimulated for our functions to develop, notably in the vocal and musical spheres, and this stimulation increases the capacities of the cortex.

The voice, the ear, and the mirror

The voice, support for our speech, can only exist once the child has gone past the stage of seeing himself as a reflection in a mirror and recognizes his separateness: when he says "mummy," he acknowledges her existence and the fact that *he* is not "mummy." Talking is a form of recognition that "things" have names and that the outside world is not just about tastes and food. Talking enables us to put in place a symbolic, verbal form of expression that evolves and creates milestones along the road of the voice, providing us with comforting reference marks. This vocal symbolism distinguishes us from other animals. One can always support the hypothesis that some language structure and communication system exists between a dog or a cat and its master, even more so between a parrot, a tiger, or a lion and its trainer, but be it as may, conversing about the latest fad, la commedia dell'arte, or our existential condition is strictly man to man. As Bergson points out, animals develop an internal connivance with their day-to-day world that allows them to adapt it, but they lack the capacity to reflect upon their fate. When a six-year-old child tirelessly asks the question: "Why?" it underscores the importance of the answers that feed the knowledge-base on which his future will depend. The concept of the word, symbol of our faculty of expression, is the basic unit of our knowledge of language, in the same way that the gene is the basic unit of our genetic heritage, DNA.

Animal behavior integrates the time dimension, as we can see from the migration of birds at certain periods of the year, or the peregrinations of whales in the oceans. Our voice, however, seems to be little influenced by the time dimension and its punctuation by days, nights, seasons, and climates. On the other hand, our emotional and auditory behavior is very pertinent to our voice.

The crucial point is not what I say, but what you understand

Hearing what the other person says doesn't mean that he'll be understood. "He didn't understand what I was trying to say, he was not listening." We often say this. The message is not just the words spoken, for these are modulated by how the other person listens to them. It is not what you say that is important, it is what the listener understands. That is the essence of verbal communication. You have different ways of saying the same thing, according to whom you're speaking. Speaking and listening both require some form of cultural, personal, and emotional apprenticeship that's a function of personal vibrations. The perceptual intuition of the vibratory wave perceives words. The symbolism of the word that the infant is going to have to learn, and in turn recreate, imposes a remarkable vocal ontogeny, especially in the bilingual child (refer to chapter 7 on Voice and language). Affect is built on harmonics. That's why a child always recognizes its mother's voice.

The filter of our voice is our ear

Speech is dependent on the previous acquisition of coordinated motor and intellectual activity. This imposes a rigorous learning process that inevitably involves using the ear to filter the voice.

What about the autistic child who hears everything, yet remains mute? He can make himself understood if he really wishes to. He speaks to himself, but others do not exist for him. According to Linda and René Gandolfi, "the dead-end street of language" in the autistic child is at the frontier between physiology and psychism, between the body and the psyche, between the coordination of expression and the coordination of thought processes. These children behave as if their vocal apparatus is paralyzed. Their hearing is functional and they react when spoken to. Genes specific to autism have been identified on chromosome 15. But a gene can't explain away all that is involved in such a complex behavioral symptomatology. It's just one of the elements contributing to this behavior.

Listen to yourself, and you will learn to speak and sing accurately

Louis Jouvet and Roger Blin, well-known comedians who were stutterers, mastered their voices brilliantly on stage. In another register, Enrico Caruso, Ruggero Raimondi, Mario del Monaco, Mady Mesplé, or La Callas offered their voices to opera. Opera requires an excellent ear, a total dedication to building one's voice; it provides the perfect example of the multifactorial alchemy between the tool (the vocal conduit), the receiver (the ear), and the master (the thinking brain).

When our voice takes its first steps down the road of evolution, it enables us to name things and to think abstract thoughts. Farther down the road, our thinking becomes master of our voice: the master that was the tool now becomes the master. Just as Michelangelo could see the sculpture waiting to be revealed in a block of marble, the poet, when he captures words, already knows how he will harmonize them to enable the actor or the singer to express their emotional universe.

Reproducing a melody or singing in tune depends on the vocal apparatus, but also on the ability to listen well. Our ear is the tuner of our voice. If we sing out of tune, it is not because our vocal cords are working improperly, but because our tuner, namely our ear, is "off." Why? For sure, a genetic component is at work. But above all, it is the education of the auditory organ from early infancy that makes the difference. The ear must recognize the note, perceive the harmonics and the melody if we're to reproduce them. Defective listening causes vocal distortions.

The first attempts of the human voice

We have seen that, historically, the evolution of the ear has gone hand in hand with the evolution of the larynx. Man expresses his past, his present, his future. He projects his identity not only on Planet Earth, but also in the intergalactic universe. The vocal filter, the ear, is part and parcel of the evolution of the species, or phylogeny, and of our presence on the Blue Planet. Animals can't envisage their future. They resort to language to defend themselves, to warn of an immediate danger, to seduce before mating. And yet, there are exceptions. When I began this research, I was greatly surprised to encounter in the animal world languages, tenors, lyrical singers—songbirds, dolphins, and other cetaceans, engaging in musical activity apparently for the sheer pleasure and beauty of it.

The bird and its music

Certain songbirds reproduce up to 50 different monosyllables in less than a minute. These are perfectly recognizable to their family, and especially to their partner. From the first day of life, the baby bird starts to twitter. It can almost sing. It must have learned this language in the egg. Its left hemisphere is dominant. The song it produces requires a particular cerebral structure and some form of learning, because the song is structured. Is it a language with its own syntax? J. P. Hailman and his team carried out remarkable research on titmice in this respect. Out of 3,500 different birdsongs produced by titmice, they isolated 362 different "sentences." The musical language encountered used not only sentences and silences, but also melodic curbs influenced by the speed of the song. This species of bird is very different from birds that merely cry out in relation to food or when in distress, in danger, or on the defensive. Thus, out of the 8,500 species of bird known to Man, less than 40% are songbirds. Among birds, singing is the prerogative of the male. They resort to song, as we find among mammals, on the one hand, to defend their territories and seduce the opposite sex and, on the other hand, to impose themselves as masters of their part of the woods.

From dolphin to Man

The pirate has turned into a dolphin

The language of dolphins is remarkable. The word dolphin comes from the Greek *delphis*, meaning "spirit of the seas." For the Greeks, the dolphin was a man, as the legend said. One fine summer's day, Dionysus travels from the island of Icaria to the island of Naxos. The sea is calm. The boat is out at sea. The crew, composed of pirates disguised as honest sailors, overcomes the rest of the men and passengers on board, intending to sell them as slaves. But they hadn't bargained for Dionysus. Guessing their intentions, in his rage he transforms the guy stays of the boat into snakes, covers the boat with creepers, and plays the flute. The terrified pirates jump overboard. Dionysius turns them into inoffensive creatures: dolphins, whose fate it is to patrol the deep waters.

The dolphin has two systems of sonorous communication

Its mouth is strictly for eating. It breathes through a blowhole on the top of its head. The dolphin is a marvel of nature. Its trachea passes through the esophagus and arrives directly at the vent via a duct. The dolphin can communicate in two ways: via ultrasounds and via sounds that are audible (to us humans).

Ultrasound makes echolocation possible. This enables dolphins to localize a prey very precisely to within a hundred meters, by night or by day, in clear waters or murky waters. Under the blowhole are six little bags stacked up symmetrically in pairs on either side of the blowhole. They communicate together to produce ultrasounds. The air passes with the nose canal from one bag to another and alters the diameter of the canal between the bags to vary the frequency emitted. It is a wind instrument. But to acquire the power of a sonorous sound, the sound emitted first echoes inside and at the crown of the dolphin's head, in a concave, adipose cavity that works like a sonorous converging lens. The sound is then beamed precisely to the desired location.

This system of echolocation is associated with another system that creates sounds that are audible to us. The frequency of these sounds is formed by a complex system that forms a proper language; 400 different sounds are known to us. It is probably the most effective communication language after Man's. A technical instrument is put to work here: the dolphin's larynx. Formed like a duck's beak, it is an extension of the trachea. It can emit frequencies in the range of 100 to 20,000 Hz. These sonorous emissions, audible to the human ear, are the result of a vibration of laryngeal pseudolips located in the trachea, somewhat as in birds. This has nothing to do with the emission of ultrasound formed in the nasal cavities.

The Caruso of the seas

The most remarkable songs are those produced by the Caruso of the seas: the humpback whale. This name is reserved for male whales only. They produce sounds that can be heard within a ten-kilometer radius. Sometimes they sing for hours on end. Water is their preferred medium for their vocal transmissions. They dive head down; then they freeze. Their bent tailfins give them excellent stability. Once in position, this sea world choir gets underway and they sing. Groups of individual whales band together and harmonize to form a chorus. They tune their "treble clef" in a few minutes. If a gatecrasher happens by, he is welcome to join in, but must adapt his frequency to that of his new mates. The humpback whale is one of the only species able to modify what it has learned over the years. This Caruso of the seas marks its territory and seduces its mate with its harmonics and its impressive singing. It seems to take real pleasure in vocalizing. The titmouse, the humpbacked whale, the dolphin—all have in common a seductive language.

The perfect ear: restricted to musicians

The perfect ear is one that can recognize the exact pitch of a note. It is a gift. Having demonstrated the highly developed temporal and frontal lobes of musicians' left hemispheres, K. L. Ohnishi makes the point that the perfect ear is not hereditary. Apparently, the apprenticeship of music from a tender age is propitious to its development. For the perfect ear is dependent on the left brain. The locations of music and of words are intimately bound here.

Left brain, right brain: is there really a difference?

Perception of sounds and harmonics by the left and right brain is quite different. The left brain's sonorous information is geared to receiving wide bands carrying few frequencies that can change rapidly. The right brain is more specialized in the reception of harmonics, its filter is more finely geared. Information is slow to take expression. Thus, attention to speech and analysis of solfeggio are left-brain, while attention to harmonics and melodies are right-brain. You can test this on yourself. While singing, cover your right ear, then your left ear. Your listening-in mode is different. One is harmonic, the other analytic.

Mechanics and audition

Where vibration and chemistry meet

A sound vibration is the result of energy being transmitted to air molecules and pushing these molecules bumper-to-bumper as it were, creating a shock wave or ripple wave. This vibratory energy is conveyed first by the external ear or auricle, then by a hollow, air-filled canal—the external acoustic meatus—down to the eardrum. In Man, the external ear serves only to channel sounds. Dogs have mobile external ears; they can move them without turning their head. Their hearing is outstanding. We have lost this faculty, although remnants of the muscles that mobilized our ear still exist behind our external ear.

This vibration, this multimolecular energy, hits the eardrum every four hundred and fortieth of a second in the case of an *A* note. The eardrum, fine membrane that it is, transforms this airborne impact into a vibration of its membrane with the same rhythmic frequency. The external ear serves to concentrate sound: it's a sort of acoustic magnifying glass. Thus, the vibratory energy that reaches the eardrum, a mere 8 mm in diameter, is transferred to the middle ear via the vibrations of the tympanic membrane. In the middle ear, we are still dealing with a mechanical transmission system, formed in this case by the ossicles. Until this point, sounds are airborne and vocal vibrations are conveyed without any transformation. But they're about to enter the inner ear, which has a fluid environment.

The stapes communicates this mechanical energy via an oval surface to the fluid medium that then acts as a receptor for the cochlea. The fluid in the cochlea transforms this mechanical energy into chemical energy in the cells that line the cochlea. At the point where the stapes closes the cochlea at the base of the spiral, which is significantly wider at its base than at its top, high-pitched sounds are received. Low-pitched sounds are received at the top. The cells that line the cochlea absorb these shockwaves progressively, from the bottom of the cochlea to its top. Think of it as the cochlear keyboard. This wave will then transmit the pitch of the voice to the brain. Pure magic! Thanks to a few millimeters, Man can hear frequencies in a range of 20 to 20,000 Hz. If you listen to loud music, you may hear afterward a persistent high-pitched whistling sound that's irritating. Why is this? The shock of this trauma is first absorbed by the first cells of the cochlea, at its base. The cells that are responsible for recognizing high-pitched sounds. Thus, they are first in line to receive the sonorous blast so damaging to ciliated cochlear cells. This whistling in your ears tells you that the cells have suffered and that the vibratory mechanical trauma is still ongoing. Hunters and amateur players of loud music regularly injure their cochlea. Its cells will inevitably be destroyed in the long run, and, with them, the perception of some high-pitched frequencies. The frequency most vulnerable, and therefore most often affected, is at 4,000 Hz.

The sound wave, specific stimulus of our auditory organ, is first airborne. (its speed of propagation is 340 meters per second at a temperature of 16° C. This speed increases by about 60 cm with every 1° C increase in temperature.). We are able to distinguish a frequency of 256 Hz from one of 257.5 Hz. But below 64 Hz, our hearing is not as efficient: it will only pick up variations of 3 Hz. Above 4,096 Hz, we can pick out a difference of 23 Hz. Our best performance is linked to frequencies in the range of 128 to 1024 Hz. That is the register of human speech.

The length of the sound wave gives the pitch of the sound, for example, in the case of the *A* note, 440 Hz corresponds to 440 vibrations per second. The pitch of the note is perceived thanks to the cochlear cells. Cells at the base of the cochlear keyboard recognize high-pitched sounds, those at the top recognize low-pitched sounds. These same cells are equipped with surface hairs that are immersed in the cochlear fluid. The more these hairs, or cilia, move under the stimulation of the vibration, the greater the power of the sound. Thus, these cells capture both frequency and power and send this double information on to the brain.

Sound is, therefore, subjected to a series of amplifiers along its journey: first the external ear, then the external acoustic meatus. It hits the tympanum, this 50-mm² doorway to the middle ear. Now it is the ossicles' turn to amplify the signal and, last in line, a tiny surface at the base of the stapes, called the oval window, all of 3 mm², allows an excellent recovery of the airborne mechanical energy by the cochlear fluid, which then conveys the information to the ciliated cells of the auditory organ.

If you press your forehead to a vibrating metal bar, you can hear the vibration. Yet the sound has not come into the ear via the external ear. It is the bone of your skull that conducts the sound. The transmission is through bone. The cochlea receives the information directly from the bone surrounding it, and not through the classical auditory system (external ear–middle ear), which is an airborne system.

The ear protects itself

The ear is able to protect itself. When a very loud noise is emitted, it arrives as usual at the eardrum, conveyed by the ossicles. Here, if the sound is too loud, two little muscles are brought into action. They act as shock absorbers, avoiding auditory trauma. The first muscle is attached to the stapes, anterior to the spot where the sound wave is transmitted to the cochlea. When this muscle is inflamed, audition is painful. All sounds then seem too loud, unmuffled. The second muscle is the muscle attached to the malleus, near the eardrum. The two muscles are thus located at both ends of the ossicle chain. The human ear is most sensitive to sounds in the 1000 to 3000 Hz range, with a power of 30 to 40 dB.

The middle ear contains an essential element: the eustachian tube. This tube between the middle ear and the back of the nose allows ventilation of the tympanum (the cavity of the middle ear), thus ensuring equal pressure on either side of the eardrum. If you fill a drum with water, the pressure on either side of its membrane is no longer equal. It will vibrate badly, the sound is altered. After traveling by plane or swimming underwater, you might have experienced uneven pressure in your ear. You have the impression that your ear is full, you hear badly through it, even after pinching your nose and trying to "blow" against the pressure. Because of rapid differences in air pressure between ground level and high altitude, or between high and low pressures in water, your hearing is deformed. Why is this? As with a musical drum, the pressure on either side of our eardrum must be the same, otherwise you have hearing problems. When the pressure is unequal, the tympanic membrane is sucked toward the side where the pressure is weakest. Instead of being supple, it becomes taut and rigid. The tension inflicted on the eardrum causes pain. You hear less well, certain frequencies no longer pass through, notably the higher frequencies. The eustachian tube is sometimes affected when you catch cold: hearing diminishes, singing is affected because of poor retro-control. If the cold persists, a serous otitis (liquid in the tympanum) can form, penalizing the professional singer. At this stage, the pain will have vanished, but hearing is impaired.

At other times, conversely, the eustachian tube may stay too open. Too much air is then conveyed to the middle ear. Hearing becomes painful when you reach high notes singing. You can hear yourself echoing. You are subjected to two different vibratory phenomena, one being vibration received from outside the body, the other from inside the body. This phenomenon is caused by a defect of the orifice of the eustachian tube that is level with the back of the nose. It no longer closes when you speak. Normally, the orifice of the eustachian tube opens when you yawn, chew, or blow into a blocked nose, and closes naturally when you speak or sing.

Hearing your own voice: two different circuits

You can hear your own voice through two different circuits. When you pronounce a word, it goes from your lips to the external ear. That is the external circuit. The internal circuit directly connects the vibrations of your larynx to your ear via bone, sometimes via the eustachian tube.

The ear must first hear, learn, and then recognize frequencies before you can sing in tune. Understanding the words you hear is essential. Sometimes you pick up a conversation without understanding what's being said. Understanding the spoken word is known as vocal intelligibility. When it's lacking, the cause may be impaired stereophonic reception, causing a difference in auditory quality between the left and the right ear, or defective cerebral integration. Of course, there's always a third possible explanation: "he has no head."

B *for Bernard,* P *for Patrick*

Verbal expression depends on the country we live in, on the language we speak. The human voice, for all six billion of us humans on Earth, ranges between 100 and 3000 Hz. This range is, of course, shaped by sociocultural influences. The frequency range will be higher in Russia than in France. It will be more musical in Italy than in Germany. The frequency of the spoken word is an essential consideration for telephone operators. The receiving band of a telephone is between 300 and 3000 Hz. When you speak to a friend on the telephone, your voice will only be heard within this range: it's the classical conversational range. Yet your voice can create acoustic errors. Of course, the auditory "reflex" will correct most errors. A badly heard syllable will immediately be reintegrated into its global context. That's what happens with ventriloquists, as we shall see. Also, certain words can be confused, especially if they're not in your mother tongue. Thus, "bit" and "pit" may sound alike, obliging us to spell out *B* for Bernard, *P* for Patrick. Why? Vowels carry our voice. Consonants do not vibrate, they merely punctuate articulated language. *B* and *P* are consonants that cause a vibration inferior to 300 Hz, the lower limit of the telephone frequency band. Their vibration is only 150 and 200 Hz, respectively. That's why these confusions can arise. The same goes for *s* and *f*, which are whistling sounds with a vibratory frequency above 3000 Hz. This is why we also end up spelling out *S* for Simon, *F* for Francis.

Chaos and harmony fuse in the ear

The ear receives the frequencies, vibrations, and noises that are part and parcel of the human voice. These sound vibrations are in fact a mixture of noises and pure frequencies. A frequency is a pure, isolated pitch: a single vibration, uniform, normally defined as the fundamental sound. What we call a noise is an irregular sonorous vibratory movement. No fundamental can be attributed to it. It is a real melting pot of several vibrations with different, irregular, and unpredictable tonalities. The human voice is made up of a mixture of these two elements: frequencies and noises.

12 tonalities create more than 500,000 auditory variations, which conductors may detect

In this voyage through evolution, only birds and cetaceans have developed musical song and a sonorous form of communication governed by some very complex codes. Not all animals have ears. Some have ears, but are deaf, like the cobra. The cobra feels vibrations through its skin; its ear is its entire covering. Fish perceive very low frequencies through the same mechanism. According to the species, the register heard can be very different. The elephant detects infrasound, the dolphin ultrasound.

During our evolution, we may have lost a little of our auditory acuity in the ultrahigh and ultralow frequencies, we may have lost the ability to orient ourselves in the dark, like bats, or to detect a drop of blood in a pond, as can certain animals, but we have developed our phonatory communication like no other species. For all that a primitive code exists among animals, no other species has developed the verbal code that our remarkable phonatory machinery facilitates. But this machinery is not sufficient on its own. Our hearing is indispensable and its precision remarkable; 12 tonalities can create more than 500,000 auditory variations, which certain orchestra leaders are capable of detecting!

How can "the orchestra man" integrate such a mass of acoustic information? He reads solfeggio like a novel. For him, musical notes are phonemes, verses are chapters. It isn't music he hears, it's a story that he understands as it unfolds. We have seen that words are memorized mainly, if not exclusively, in our left brain, whereas our visual memory is in our right brain. Precocious musicians have highly developed verbal and visual skills. Learning music before the age of twelve fosters a balance between harmony and rationality. It enables better memorization both of the spoken word and of song. Having thoroughly learned his musical language, the artist is now able to be creative, using the tools of his left brain and the emotion of his right brain.

Professional musicians are unmasked by medical neuroimaging. As they listen to Beethoven or Bach, one can observe a preponderant use of the left brain, as if they were listening to the diction of the music rather than to its harmony. They are reading the notes of the melody, much as a nonmusician reads a text. The musician then transposes the colors of the notes on to canvas and creates an artistic work.

Surprisingly, if you are not a musician and you listen to music, neuroimaging will reveal activity not in the left brain, as in the violinist, the pianist, or the conductor, but in the right brain. Indeed, you aren't reading music, decrypting it; you are merely listening to its harmonics. When you're listening to the wind rustling in the leaves, you're not analyzing the speed of the wind. 52 white ones and 36 black ones, that's the keyboard that the pianist transforms into Chopin's nocturne. Therefore, you're not listening to the individual notes, but you are tuning into the melancholy.

The conductor: Admiral of the musical vessel that sails before the wind of emotion

I go to the Bastille Opera to attend a general rehearsal of *La Traviata*. I sit in the third row behind the master, James Conlon, who sports a black polo shirt. The musicians are not in tuxedos. The lyrical singers are in costume, in order to experience the conditions of a live representation. (Indeed, the costume can alter the vocal technique of the artist.) I feel privileged to be able to enjoy the special atmosphere of a general rehearsal before opening night. The master takes advantage of this opportunity to correct last details. A soprano violinist is off by half a tone; the master's eyes and left hand request him to harmonize at once. The soprano singer is not where she should be on stage; a brief nod of the head suffices for her to understand the orchestra leader's request. James Conlon is actor, producer, musician, and conductor all rolled into one. The maestro's ear corrects the alto violinist with a wave of his baton, rectifies the rhythm of the double bass players on his right, appreciates the correctness of the soprano, and seems to indicate to her to emphasize the *legato*. I observe him living his music, his left hand aimed toward the heavens, his right hand holding his baton. The partition is in his head.

One can't help but be impressed by the volume of acoustic messages he is bombarded with and by the passion he invests in trying to reach perfection in the interpretation of this work. Admiral of this musical ship, he sails before the wind of emotion.

Chapter 7

Voice and language

The voice is a language with an immaterial support.

The origins of Man's articulated language have left their fossilized mark on our planet. Although the scrawls of writing allowed us to materialize our oral traditions, writing only goes back a few thousand years. The study of the endocranial molds of hominids, of their tools, and of the DNA clock gives us reason to believe that articulated language made its appearance several million years ago. This would mean that the ape-man never existed. The monkey never evolved into Man, but Man and monkeys have a common ancestor from which two separate lines of descendants—human and monkey—are issued. Both have a language, but only Man talks.

As from birth, our voice is ready for use

The brain still evolves after birth

During an ape's first three months of life, its brain experiences major growth. In Man, this growth is spread over the first fifteen months of life. The neurons multiply. The number of interconnections increases vastly. Billions and billions of synapses are formed. The different parts of the brain get their respective cues. Thus, in the first two years of a child's life, its education, apprenticeship, sociocultural environment, and family relationships will cause certain areas of the brain to become more developed than others. This

117

phenomenon is particularly marked in musicians. But however impressive the brain's development during these first fifteen months, in the six-year-old child, the brain is still only 95% developed. It will continue to evolve, slowly but surely, in more subtle ways, until the age of puberty, when reproduction becomes possible. From then on, the brain's development continues almost imperceptibly until the age of 20 to 22 years. Language is common to many species on our planet, albeit in different forms: chemical substances exchanged between certain bacteria, the origin of our pheromones; the chatter of songbirds; or the voice, unique to *Homo vocalis*, privileged mammal.

How to explore the voice commander: Cerebropolis

Neuroimagery is revolutionizing our knowledge. At the start of the 1970s, radiography, invented in the late 19th century, underwent a metamorphosis. Allan Cormac and Godfrey Hounsfield, Nobel prize-winners in 1979, perfected computer-assisted tomography X-ray imaging, better known today as CT-scanning. Later, in the 1980s, Paul Loterbur developed magnetic resonance imaging, or MRI. Here, the image is produced not by rays going through the body and passing information on to the computer, but by its own magnetic resonance. The machine induces a variable orientation of our body's electrons that sends out different signals that are captured, digitalized, and displayed by the computer. In the context of the study of the voice, functional MRI, or fMRI, enables us to see, track, and decode the mysteries of our brain while it's vocally active. The image becomes dynamic. It registers the activity of cerebral areas. It enables us to pinpoint and analyze the exact functional location for vision, reading, speech, and song. This analysis can be undertaken from a tender age. The danger of irradiation is nil.

Positron-emission tomography, also known as PET-scanning, provides even better screening of the cerebral indices involved in the projection and creation of the voice. The technique used here is most ingenious. It makes use of our body's energy requirements. First a solution of glucose—our brain's source of energy—is injected, along with harmless, relatively mild radioactive particles. (Another approach makes use of radioactive gas inhaled by the subject.) The subject places his or her head in a ring that detects radioactive gamma rays. Active areas of the brain consume energy and therefore use up more glucose than less active areas. The radioactive molecules all cluster in the active areas, enabling us to read, in real time, on X-ray film sensitive to gamma rays, the activity of the areas called into action: the speech center, or the song center, for example. The computer captures this information, makes sense of it and prints out a brain-scan image. This database provides an analysis that is not only three-dimensional, but also takes the time dimension into account. These four-dimensional techniques have revolutionized the scientific domain and allowed us to track functional aspects of the voice very precisely in vivo.

Observing the brain talking in the three-month-old infant

At the dawn of this third millennium, in 2002, G. Dehaene-Lambertz and S. Dehaene, of the Necker Hospital in Paris, researched the language function in human infants from the age of three months. The research looked to establish the pre-existence of a language function in a sample of 20 infants—14 baby girls and 6 baby boys. Equipped with a helmet, the infants were made to listen to a woman's voice for 20 seconds. This was followed by a 20-second-long silence. The voice spoke as would a mother to its infant. The same recording was repeated for 20 seconds, and then passed in reverse after another 20-second pause. What happens?

The fMRI confirms right and left activity of the brain in the temporal lobes. The activity of the left brain is much more intense. Reference marks that are well-developed in the adult brain are already visible. But there's more. The recording of the woman's voice activates another area of the brain when played normally, but not when played in reverse. This part of the brain is the seat of the memorization of language, the frontal right area, well-known in adults. Previously, this area was believed to develop only after puberty, adding to our panoply of cognitive functions. This is the area of complex memorization, of control, attentiveness, reflection. Thus, the infant's brain is ready to gear up to facilitate the ontogeny of language, the ontogenesis of the voice and its cerebral interconnections. In a few months time, if these areas of the infant's brain, ready for use, are stimulated, language and thought will blossom.

Voice and the influence of language

Man is born an artist

Each culture has its own language. Yet one can't help but be struck by the extent to which nations are influenced by their language. Russian or Germanic languages are often as rigorous as their climate. In Brazil, people like to show off their bodies rather than their clothes, the voice inhabits their music and gestures, they have dancing in their veins. But artistic expression, be it German or Italian opera, the frescoes of Lascaux or Chinese engravings, indicates that Man is born an artist.

The voice is passed down the generations

Verbal communication is imposed on us from our first day on Earth. Like the newborn dolphin ejected into the sea and able to swim immediately, Man's offspring is thrown into the world of the voice and gets to know its vibrations, the medium of communication of the voice. The stimulation of its genes sets off the irreversible evolution of the left brain's intelligence, of the right brain, of the limbic system. Since the 1950s, the cognitive sciences have provided a multifactorial approach to the human voice that associates linguistics, psychology, philosophy, biology, and, more pertinently, neurobiology. The voice influences how we approach others, how we relate to our inner self. It changes over time. For all that its apprenticeship is necessary, the voice is nevertheless spontaneous and natural, both innate and acquired. Learned. Stimulation by others is essential to its germination in the very young. Steven Pinker is partial to the theory that language and voice are instinctive and require very little apprenticeship, a polemical theory given the fate of the wild children we know of. Certainly the voice, unique to the human race, has provided us with a communication tool. But this vocal instinct is surely light-years apart from the instinct that guides migrating birds over thousands of kilometers, acting as an internal compass that has a specific cerebral location with a single, dedicated function. Our voice calls upon a host of interdependent, multiple factors.

Questions arise: Did language evolve out of the evolution of mammals? Is the voice innate or acquired? Does our voice create our thoughts, or does it just convey them? Is its structure scientific, Cartesian, and reproducible, or is its structure artistic and unique? Does it rely on a voice born from chaos for every phoneme, every sentence, every silence?

The innate voice: not just innate!

Noam Chomsky was a fervent supporter of the "instinctive" approach to language. The approach is certainly intriguing, but it merits careful reflection, because although neurotransmitters and the secretion of endorphins are undoubtedly involved in the creation of a poem or an operatic aria, it also involves another ingredient we call emotion. The "instinctive" approach is too reductionist; to deny the artist his Muses is to deprive him of his dreams, or worse still, to deny his existence.

Sentences are formed from familiar words, but the combination of words is constantly renewed, never the same. Each sentence is a new creation. A bit like Molière's "Bourgeois gentilhomme," who spoke prose without knowing that he did. Sentence construction is regulated by grammatical rules that are specific to each language. Noam Chomsky observed that young children develop a grammar that mimics that of people close to them, long before they learn any grammar at school. This complex regulation seems to be innate or hereditary. Grammatical logic is part of a universal grammar. It ensures that we understand each other and, as Wilhelm von Humboldt said in 1936: "Language makes infinite use of a finite language." If no anthropologist has yet come upon a people on our planet that do not speak, are we to conclude that the voice is innate? The existence of a hereditary predisposition to the development of the voice appears possible, but does the "voice" phenomenon kick in the same way as the "walking' or 'running" phenomena kick in, namely, instinctively? Such a conclusion seems a little facile.

The mouth-to-mouth of the voice's evolution

Genes in our DNA characterize a set of factors. However, these factors may never materialize if they're not stimulated. The human voice and its language also produce a transmissible element that can undergo mutations, be destroyed, or created afresh: the word. This unit of cultural transmission evolves freely. It enables language to evolve continuously with no anatomic or hereditary support. In this context, the evolution of the voice progresses "mouth-to-mouth." Culture is peculiar to Man. It is not handed down through our DNA, although it can be compared to DNA, notwithstanding the fact that after ten generations, our culture and our language have evolved, whereas our DNA is practically unchanged after millions of years. In the human species, language evolves much faster than our genetics. This has accelerated our faculty of understanding and our intellectual grasp. Hereditary transmission is of a different order. Its scale is that of planet Earth's. DNA has been its vehicle for hundreds of millions of years, and only the clock of time, associated with natural selection, makes its evolution possible. André Laganey makes the rather obvious point that the theories put forward by Lamarck and Darwin five decades apart, in 1809 and 1856, respectively, don't provide all the answers we seek: "All is transformed in nature, words more so than the rest." This cultural world structured by the verb, the word carried by the human voice, is indispensable to Man's education. For almost seven million years, *Homo sapiens* has owed his survival to his environmental world of communication with his peers.

Words are Atoms of the voice and of the space-time dimension

The language of DNA

If the life story of *Homo vocalis* is tied in with DNA, he owes his survival to his voice. Genes have their origins in DNA. Some scientists claim that DNA has something that closely resembles a unique language and grammar. DNA, or deoxyribonucleic acid, is made up of four molecules, called the molecules of life. These four nucleotides—adenine, thymine, guanine and cytosine—can recombine ad infinitum in 64 different combinations called codons. Is the temptation to compare these codons, these multiple associations that confide the secret of our existence to a double helix, to a unique language, not wonderfully troubling and mysterious? For the DNA chain is punctuated by genes that mean "stop," by others that mean "start again," by silences, by groups of genes that are synonyms, by others than are homonyms, by a gene that forms a sentence, by yet another that forms a chapter, or by the gene of *apoptosis*, harbinger of death. The chapters in this particular book are called the kidney cells, the heart cells, or the eye cells.

The voice is entropy

The arrow of time exists also in the language of words. It is Man's survival. The notion of irreversibility in the context of time's onward march is easy to grasp: a plate falls, it breaks. It will never reconstruct itself, even if time were to accelerate to the speed of light. A spring turns into a river, the river flows to the sea. It can never flow back up to its source. The same is true of the word: once pronounced, it cannot return to the neocortex. The voice occupies both space and time dimensions. The voice is entropy. Our brain is both subject and object, so is our voice. It becomes the tool of our inner world of fancy, after having been its master. Animal communication exists, but it always has a precise, concrete goal. Its language is systematically addressed to some living being out of a need to feed, to defend, to attack, to dominate and, sometimes, to seduce. Never out of a desire to indulge in a little introspection. Only Man has existential doubts.

We each have a lexicon sitting in our brain that enables us to speak to others or to ourselves. The lexicon contains both the words we know and a rule for combining these words: grammar. The word can be considered as a linguistic unit. In the sense that an atom is something that can't be divided, the word is the atom of the voice. The atom of language, the smallest indivisible unit, is the phoneme. The morpheme is the smallest meaningful unit of language.

What power does a word have? In 1972, Moulin used a well-known example involving the word *re-embarquons* ("let us re-embark" in French). Let us emulate it with the English word "re-embarks." Four phonemes make it up: *re* (again), *em* (inside), *bark* (floating object), and *s* (third person singular). Thus, several meanings are encased in these four phonemes. To say the word "re-embarks" out loud requires hardly any breathing effort; yet "re-embarks" is pregnant with meaning. In relative terms, the power of the word, tool of our thinking, as a "signifier" is five times greater than the power required to voice it. Words accelerate our ability to communicate and spare our energy. Yet a word can also be used just as a symbol, to suggest something: just saying the word "rose" is enough to conjure up its scent.

The rhythm of words and phonemes

Rhythm

The vibratory wave transmitting the word "rose" enables us to decode the message. The message can sometimes trick us, because one wave may hide another. Our ear, receiver of the voice, absorbs the acoustic energy, its harmonics, its noises, its vibrations. The difference between two spoken messages will depend on the pitch, intensity, and musicality of the spoken phonemes. This can sometimes cause us to hear something that wasn't, in fact, said. Instead of "rose," we may hear "prose." Steven Pinker carried out a remarkable experiment on this intriguing aspect of vocal transmission in 1981, an experiment well worth sharing here.

The sentence "Where were you last year?" was subjected to acoustic distortion, producing archaic sounds and overemphasizing its musicality and harmonics in odd places. Subjects were asked to listen to the distorted recording without being forewarned that it had been distorted. It came across to them as sounds from another world, probably beeps. No further interpretation of the recording was attempted by them. A second group of subjects listened to the same recording after having been informed that the recording had a meaning. Surprisingly, these subjects realize that a human voice had been distorted and modified. A quarter of the subjects are able to identify the entire sentence. Three-quarters recognize at least three words.

The brain, thanks to the ear, decrypted the distorted sounds and extracted something intelligible out of it, something that could be interpreted thanks to the brain's internal lexicon. The left brain (Wernicke's area) and the right brain (the frontal area), together with the limbic brain (seat of our intuition) enabled certain subjects to reconstitute the entire original message, despite the information having been masked.

Infants will only acquire a voice if they are exposed to a specific language, or to several languages. It's through hearing a language spoken that they are able to create their own voice. The construction of words and sentences requires the acquisition of a grammar that is specific to each language. The grammatical dimension of language is indispensable to the construction of sentences and to their comprehension. The acoustic signal given by the musicality and prosody of the spoken sentence is also a necessary element if the listener is to understand the speaker. What we have here is in effect a linguistic stimulation of the brain that triggers the apprenticeship of the language of the voice's own ontogeny. The voice transmits a string of phonemes. Singly, they mean nothing; it is their combination that allows the words to be understood, that gives away the sense of the sentence. In this forging of the human voice, linking one word to another, and to another, and to yet another creates the ability to think. The musicality and rhythm of the phonemes can change the sense of a word, even if the syllables are still the same. Take the following two sentences, they don't have at all the same meaning:

"This move is loved by you."
"This movie is loved by you."

Hearing 15 phonemes per second

Multiple stimuli enable us to hear someone's voice, as we've seen. All these stimuli charge down the external acoustic meatus of the ear and invade our neurons, which then transmit this information to the depths of the brain. The mechanical vibrations turn into chemical and electrical molecules. This vibratory alchemy is what links us to our true Self and to others: to our inner self, because our inner voice is one of the sources of our creativity; to our listeners, because they keep our voice alive. Our brain capacity is amazing. We can make out up to 15 phonemes per second or up to 40 phonemes per second with training. The conductor is a most remarkable example of this. He can detect an "off" note of the alto violin on his right, of the clarinet on his left, of the piano close by. He does so in one-fifteenth of a second, because he distinguishes the three instruments individually. No computer, even today, is capable of such an exceptional feat. No machine is able to recognize the voices of several people talking at the same time.

Phonemes and words

300,000 words maybe, but how many phonemes?

Thus, Man's resonance chamber, of which the vibratory source is the larynx, can mechanically produce words by combining different phonemes with specific musicalities and rhythms. Phonemes are the acoustic units of the word, whereas syllables are actually linguistic units, known also as "mores." A more is a unit that has a root meaning. It can actually be smaller than a syllable (the Japanese language has many of these), as long as it still has a root meaning.

We may have invented 300,000 words, but we don't have 300,000 ways of moving our mouth. Only 40 buccopharyngeal movements enable us, by combining them, to pronounce a word. Our 40 phonemes correspond to 40 vocal mimics, each of which produces a specific vibration of the vocal cords.

Our voice is characterized by its power, its pitch, its prosody, and its sonority, as well as by the humming formed by the echoes of our vocal cords in our voice box. Because multiple factors are brought into play, we never produce exactly the same frequencies when we give voice to an *A* note for ten seconds.

When we listen to synthesized music, we know it has been synthesized, because the perfection of the harmonics causes it to be identical for twenty seconds. The artificial voice is less pleasant to our ear. Somehow, it's "too perfect." This is why a new generation of musicians using synthesizers are introducing imperfect sounds, in fact an eighth of a tone every half-second, to come closer to the human voice.

Producing a phoneme

Seven elements make up our vocal mechanics:

The first is the larynx, of course, and the next three are part of the tongue. The fifth, tied directly to the tongue, is the velum palatinum or soft palate, which alternately opens or closes the nasal cavity. The nasal fossa is the sixth element: indeed, if you have a cold, you sound nasal. The seventh, but not least, element being the lips, exit door of our voice.

The most important element: the tongue.

It has three parts to it: the tip of the tongue, its body, and its base. The body of the tongue, its central part, arches to form an "i" sound (pronounced "e"), or stays flat to form an "a" sound (pronounced the "*a*" of master). According to the consonant, the tip of the tongue nestles against the top or the bottom teeth. In Man, the base of the tongue at the back of the mouth is very developed. It can move toward or away from the larynx. It opens and closes the nasal cavity and, together with the soft palate, allows nasal sounds like "n." A strong, jerky movement of the base of the tongue also enables consonants like "b," "p," or "k," that are almost like a percussion. Contraction of the tongue shortens the voice-box lengthwise. If the larynx moves upward, the voice becomes very high-pitched; this is what happens when a tenor sings. These high-pitched sounds are much easier to produce in the case of an "I," because the tongue is then dome-shaped and placed high. The larynx is pulled upward, the frequencies are higher. But in the case of an "*a*," the opposite is true. The tongue drops down in the mouth cavity and pushes the larynx down, the pitch is lower. A high-pitched "*a*" is more difficult to produce.

Thus, we see that harmonics can be modified according to the vowel produced. In order to sing *a, e, i, o, u* at the same pitch, we have to adapt the height of the larynx in relation to the height of the tongue and of the soft palate. To explain this data mechanically, let's give an equivalence: because of its shape, suppleness, and moisture, because of its plasticity, which allows it to lengthen and shorten, our vocal tube amplifies certain frequencies, but erases others. The greater the distance between the lips and the vocal cords (meaning the larynx has moved downward), the lower the pitch. The shorter the distance (the larynx having moved upward), the higher the pitch. Here is a simple example: pour some water into an empty bottle. At first, it will make a very low-pitched noise. As the bottle becomes fuller, the noise becomes more high-pitched, because there is less and less air in the bottle. The sound also varies according to the shape of the bottle, as each shape amplifies certain harmonics at the expense of others. For example: hold an "*a*" for five seconds and move straight on to an "*i*" for five seconds. Involuntarily, you will have raised the frequency of the "I," because you won't have corrected the height of the larynx modified by the position of the tongue, as previously described. You have just performed one of the first basic exercises in singing. Repeat the exercise, this time keeping the "a" and the "i" on the same frequency. To get better results, begin by doing the exercise with your mouth closed. That way, only the vocal cords come into play.

The lips bring the final touch to our voice box. Associated with the teeth, they make the voice sound young or old. They put the makeup on your vocal sound. On the telephone, they can betray your emotion. If you smile while you speak, your friend on the line is sure to tell you that "you sound in fine form." He can't see you smiling, but he can guess that you are, because a smile is more than a facial expression, it also gives expression to the phoneme. You have just put an interpretation on a spoken word.

Does the voice have a common denominator according to the language?

There is an "Earth" language: all languages are its dialects

The use of words and their symbolism imposes rules in the ways that phonemes, phonology, grammar, and syntax are brought together. This is the common denominator of the voice. Something has always struck me in my travels abroad. You listen to a foreign language that you don't understand, yet its intonations and prosody give you some basic sense of what's being said. You almost have the impression that the human voice is itself a vocal language: Earth language, or Earthen, and that all the languages on Earth are its dialects. This is what prompts S. Pinker to state that were an extraterrestrial to land on our Blue Planet, it would ask what the rules of "this language" are, not what the rules of English, Italian, or French are.

The same applies to artificial languages: Certain contemporary works of fiction have created their own vocabulary, their own language. In Tolkien's *Lord of the Rings*, the elf language he invented is very seductive, with its own structure and what seems like the sketch of an invented grammar. In the film *Star Wars*, we are able to understand the androids and other characters of the outer Empire invented by George Lucas, because of the intonation, musicality, and rhythm of their dialogues.

Your vocal resonance must harmonize with your living quarters

Does climate play a significant role in the different dialects of our planet? Suppose you live in a cavern in a cold country. You're well-covered, huddled with others close to the fire. Your voice adopts a relational resonance suited to this close proximity, as you're almost touching each other. Your vocal resonance must harmonize with your living quarters. Speaking in a grotto isn't the same as speaking in a cavern or an igloo, the echo is different. Your dialogues won't display the same harmonics. People obliged to take refuge from the cold in sheltered spaces speak differently from people who live by the sea on an island beach in New Caledonia or out in the open in the African savanna. Equally, the language spoken by people living by the sea is different from that spoken by people inhabiting dense tropical forests. Our voice colonizes space, it forms a bridge between men. It chooses its phonemes according to the lay of the land. For example, low-pitched, rhythmic sounds go down well in equatorial zones. The colonizing of space is probably one of the reasons why different languages developed on Earth. Our planet's geographic differences have influenced the anatomic structures of our features, of our voice box, of our vocal cords even, and therefore, of our voice. Did you know that most women in South America have nodules on their vocal cords, whereas this is relatively rare among Japanese women?

What is the lifetime of a language: extinct languages and living languages

The same vocal colonizing structure influenced the social life of the group and allowed the development and enrichment of the individual to benefit the group.

Without doubt, this stimulated Man's intellectual evolution. The subtleties of certain words in certain languages are not repeated elsewhere. The meeting of these terrestrial dialects allows an emotional evolution that is unique in the living world. Linguists agree that the lifetime of a language is around 5,000 years. Yet ancient Hebrew, Aramaic, Chinese, or Sanskrit don't seem to be on the verge of extinction. These languages have survived in spite of numerous threats. No doubt the scarred derivatives that survived these attacks enabled the creation of new dialects. Thus, extinct languages can be defined as languages that have become closed systems; they no longer grow, they don't evolve and thus they no longer allow the creation of new words.

Living languages contain the dynamics of their own future. They are a part of our space and time dimensions. Not only do we learn them, we also transform them, modify them, "modernize" them.

Bilingual children, ambidextrous in their use of language: highly gifted?

Alice and Shigeru

Alice and Shigeru come to consult me. Young Alice is nine years old, young Shigeru is eleven. They are accompanied by their Japanese father, who speaks French with practically no accent, and by their French mother. They lived in Japan for five years. In France since two years, the children have been steeped in a "bicephalic" world. They both have a mild case of rhinopharyngitis. Within minutes, we're far off the subject of their sore throats: they bombard me in perfect French with questions about my computers, my endoscopic cameras, the unusual mechanics of my Pentax endovideo-camera (they're familiar with the brand). My curiosity is aroused by these children, by their linguistic gifts, and their patently alert and brilliant minds. Having answered their questions, it's my turn to question them. I ask them which language they prefer to speak in. They answer unhesitatingly: "Whatever, French or Japanese." "What language do the two of you most frequently speak together?" Alice answers: "Almost always French. But if we don't want others to understand us, we speak in Japanese." Shigeru adds: "I agree, but when we fight, I speak in Japanese."

I resort to a simple test to try to detect whether they have a mother tongue and a secondary tongue, or whether they have two mother tongues. "Add $3 + 4 + 5$. What's the total?" The answer immediately comes back in French: "12." I then ask their father to ask them, in Japanese this time, to add $2 + 7 + 8$. The answer is just as quick. They inform me that they also learned English at the age of four with an English nanny. I ask them in English to add $2 + 5 + 6$. There is a slight hesitation for a few seconds while they translate the numbers mentally back into either French or Japanese, do the sum, get the answer, and translate it back into English to give it to me. So they have two maternal tongues, French and Japanese, and a second language, English.

Let's try and fathom what goes on in the heads of Alice and Shigeru. From a tender age, they will have developed both languages concurrently in their Broca's and Wernicke's areas. The mother tongues are inscribed in practically the same zone of their brain, as their response-time in either language is the same. However the cerebral projection of English, which they learned later, is farther back. Indeed, learning two mother tongues before the age of four causes the projection of the two languages to be identical, they get superimposed. The fact of having learned English at a later stage means that its integration is less efficient. Alice and Shigeru integrated French and Japanese before the age of four. They can do mental sums in both mother tongues with the same speed. If this integration creates cerebral circuits, are these identical? In the case of children who are bilingual since birth, Broca's areas are indeed superimposed. This was demonstrated by Kim, Relkin, and Hirsch in 1997 through PET-scans and fMRI. Mastering and speaking different languages is a faculty only Man has.

If the second language is spoken after the age of five or six, its cerebral projection does not map perfectly onto the mother tongue, it is slightly farther back in Broca's area. The later a foreign language is learned, the longer a person will take to make mental sums in that language, proof that its cerebral projection is even more posterior. A bilingual child must continue to practice both languages. If one language is dropped, its neuronal circuits will die out and will have to be re-established if the child takes up the language again at a later stage.

The mystery of Mario

This brings to mind a moving anecdote. Mario, a theater comedian with a very low-pitched voice used to understudy numerous actors, consults me for a very hoarse voice. For his seventy-five years of age, he is quite a character and is keen to recover his stage voice. I detect a polyp. He agrees to be operated on under general anesthetic. The operation, using laser technology, lasts under thirty minutes. Everything is satisfactory, there's no malignant lesion. The anesthetic wears off and the patient recovers consciousness. Imagine my surprise when he addresses me in Greek! He seems to be asking me a question and then makes a long comment. A good ten minutes go by before Mario, who is Greek by birth, but speaks perfect French, finally talks to me in French: "Is it cancerous?" I reassure him. The temporary disappearance of his French intrigues me. After consulting a neurologist friend of mine who is fascinated by language, the answer seems almost obvious. The anesthesia probably brought about a slightly decreased oxygen input to the speech center of the brain. The "Greek" area received more oxygen than the "French" area. Each language area had kept its integrity, its memory, its linguistic lexicon intact for over sixty years. A few days later, I saw Mario again and asked him how long it had been since he'd spoken his native language: "Doctor, I left Greece nearly sixty years ago. I was brought up here in an artistic environment in which we spoke only French. I practiced my mother tongue during this time only when singing." Little by little, the French language, its musicality, its intonations had stimulated his neurons. His "Greek voice" went into hibernation. Its cerebral projection received less stimulation, therefore it atrophied slightly. To a degree, his second tongue overdeveloped its cerebral projection. But the mother tongue is still present.

By analogy, a cerebral microinfarctus can bring about the loss of a second language learned after the age of five to seven years because the projections of these second languages are only about 8 mm apart, based in areas of the brain that are distinct but very close to each other.

To each language its own phonemes

As a one-year-old, Man's bilingual offspring can distinguish between the different prosodies and musicalities of the two languages, and inscribes them definitively in his brain. He will lose fewer phantom phonemes than a monolingual child. The "phantom phoneme" is a phoneme that hasn't been stimulated. It disappears around the age of two or three. Up until this age, we can pronounce any language. Past this age, pronouncing the phantom phonemes may be difficult, if at all possible. For example, I'm incapable of pronouncing correctly some of the words that Shigeru spoke in Japanese. The ability to pronounce any phoneme under the sun disappears around the age of three. This is also when the toddler learns to differentiate properly between the two mother tongues. So the apprenticeship is smooth and painless for the infant and very young child. He isn't more gifted than other children, it's not a case of the left or right brain having a genetic predisposition for languages; quite simply, it's because our brain has extraordinary assimilation capacities when stimulated from a tender age, be it for music or for the spoken language. That's why bilingual children are often thought to be highly gifted.

As a suckling infant, the bilingual baby is perfectly conscious that two languages are being spoken to him, but he presents a slight handicap as against the monolingual baby: his latency of response when spoken to is slightly longer. By the time he's three or four years old, he has caught up with the monolingual baby in this respect. He may be considered slightly "backward" in his language development between the ages of two and three. Yet this isn't the case. On the contrary, this apparent backwardness is only superficial; he has already acquired many phonemes that are lacking in the monolingual baby's vocabulary. He has activated additional neuronal circuits.

PET-scanning has demonstrated the superimposition that characterizes the truly bilingual child. But it has also demonstrated that when a second language is learned, the degree to which it overlaps the projection of the mother tongue will be all the greater the earlier it is learned and the greater the degree of competency achieved. So must we conclude that the brain varies the overlap as a function of how this second language is used? We can draw an analogy here with the reflex action of a tennis player's forehand or backhand, which deteriorates if the player gives up tennis for a few years. The answer is probably yes.

Thus it is that the bilingual or trilingual child will have no accent later. He will know instinctively how to manipulate silences, rhythms, and harmonics when he speaks in his mother tongues.

His vocal attitude and physical expression won't be the same in each language. His apprenticeship from an early age, his multiple vocal ontogeny, stimulated his brain and initialized the territories specific to each language and to the musicality of each language. Because of this unusual linguistic development, the bilingual child is often much quicker to observe and anticipate things. Stimulating the areas of the voice increases the voice's individual characteristics.

The order of words: treble clef of our voice

From the age of two onward, the toddler learns five words a day. This learning process is essential. He integrates with surprising ease not only syntax, but also grammar. How important are grammar and syntax for language? Put simply, it is equivalent to having the notes of a solfeggio without knowing what clef to play it in. The treble clef and the bass clef (*G* and *F*) are the grammar, the chords provide the syntax. Note that when a multilingual person listens to a foreign language, he is often able to identify, despite not understanding a word that's said, whether the language is Anglo-Saxon or Chinese. Our brain has a decoding strategy for analyzing the human voice in all its peculiarities.

The cerebral structures of the human voice are relatively slow to mature. Until we're four years old, Wernicke's area evolves significantly; thereafter, the rate of growth slows down. Only audition, in place even before we are born, enables us to start integrating already the audiophonatory loop. Our auditory maturity reaches its puberty by the time we're seven years old. The world of music is integrated at the age of four. There is no point in trying to get a child to learn music before this age. The worlds of speech and writing are integrated around the ages of four and five. This vocal puberty materializes itself through the cerebral development and maturation already described in the chapter on the brain. The corpus callosum, the bridge between our two hemispheres, loses nearly 70% of its neurons in the infant's first four months after birth. This allows the left brain to establish its ascendance. By the time this four-month-old infant reaches adolescence, new connections have been stimulated and the corpus callosum has grown in size again.

The voice fosters new circuits with specific cortical projections. Each person's cognitive, sociocultural, and intellectual development is dependent on these stimulations.

The musicality of words is a language

Music is also a mother tongue

Thus, the musicality of words ferries more meaning than the words themselves. The rhythm of a language enables us to build frontiers between its words. When we speak in our mother tongue, we are able to inscribe its natural rhythm, we know the indices that segment a sentence. When we learn a foreign language after the age of five, we often unconsciously impose the rhythm of our mother tongue on it. For example, a Frenchman will "chop up" his English into syllables. And an Englishman will speak French without giving it its proper syllabic segmentation.

It seems that infants are able from birth to create, understand, and learn one mother tongue, but probably also several mother tongues, something that hasn't yet percolated through into our education customs. Some phonemes exist in certain languages, but not in others. For example, certain "mores" of the Japanese language, with their very singular musicality, don't exist in French. They're learned from birth. For the first nine months after birth, babies are able to distinguish these phonetic subtleties in any language. This ability then begins to decline between the ninth and twelfth month. Vocal perception becomes less finely tuned. No longer will the baby be able to make out naturally the peculiarities of phonemes that are new to him. He will be unable to form consonants spontaneously if they don't belong to his mother tongue. He loses all phonological contrasts not already in his linguistic universe. If he hasn't heard them, he won't be able to reproduce them. It's as if he becomes deaf to them, phonologically deaf. These lost phonemes, these phantom phonemes are present during his first years. It's as if the newborn infant has in his brain the entire range of phonemes that exist or could exist, a palette complete with all the colors of all the languages and dialects in the world. But if they are not used and are not stimulated, they're nearly always lost after the age of seven. Yet there are exceptions.

The phantom phoneme

Phantom phonemes are fossil phonemes. For the first months after birth, the infant is able to integrate all phonemes in existence. Little by little, his neuronal circuits lose this dexterity. The phonemes that the baby hasn't heard will be printed in the memory center for the voice, in other words the part of the brain that houses the language and motor areas that allow this spoken language. But they won't switch on when the spoken language will begin to emerge.

For example, it's practically impossible for a Frenchman to acquire the correct pronunciation of certain Dutch or Russian words, unless he happens to have an excellent musical ear. The richness in auditory contrasts of these two languages is much greater than in French. Of course, this is not to say that we are insensitive to the expression of these unknown phonemes, but our analysis of them is delicate, difficult, and often deformed by our mastery of our mother tongue. We are incapable of reproducing unfamiliar phonemes. Our mother tongue imposes its own phonemes on our voice, creates them, and masks phantom phonemes.

The wrong word, substitute for the real word

I was witness to this phenomenon at a congress in Bangkok. The story isn't without humor. I'm about to make a presentation on vocal surgery. This is in mid-July of the year 1992. I'm sorting out my slides and I ask one of my Thai colleagues, in English: "Where is the slide room?" He doesn't seem to understand. I try with a better accent. He still doesn't understand. I point to my slides and gesture, at which point he exclaims: "Ah! where is the *glide* room?" For him, glide sounded like slide. He didn't know this phantom phoneme "slide." From hereon, I always ask for the glide room.

Your turn now: try the following experiment. Tell one of your friends: "I had quite a "fwight." Ask him to repeat the sentence. He's sure to have understood "I had quite a fright." It won't occur to him to repeat after you "I had quite a fwight." Why? Because your apprenticeship of phonemes doesn't include the combination "fw," it doesn't exist in the English language. Your internal dictionary in Wernicke's area, and your language structure in Broca's area have never recorded the word "fwight." This phantom phoneme is immediately replaced with a real phoneme that makes sense of the word in its context. We'll encounter these verbal hallucinations again in the section on ventriloquists.

The voice: echoing landscape of our language

The acquisition of language is determined by the strength of our lexical memory, our memory for words; this enables us to build our own cerebral dictionary. Two fundamental elements make this task easier: semantics and phonology. Semantics link words together, allow the construction of sentences, give them meaning. Phonology gives color to what we hear, provides sonorous landmarks, gives harmonics their rhythm. The production of a sentence capitalizes on the contributions from both of these clever characteristics of language.

When we speak, when we create a sentence, the attempt that launches the sentence continues incrementally, accompanying the effort to its conclusion. In other words, our language is construed in real time and in situ. It is fueled by its own creation. One word calls for another and stimulates the improvisation and creation of new thoughts. Our own voice influences our language, enriches it; hearing it facilitates the creation of the next sentence. The echo of our voice sometimes becomes the mistress of our imagination. When I speak to you, I can hear my own voice. While I talk, a retroactive analysis process is going on, with a response time of one-fifteenth of a second. The speaker that I am must decide for himself the importance of this retro-control, absent in cases of voodoo, as we shall see later. Our voice and language summon up the audiophonatory loop. No doubt it would be more exact to call this process, which enables the autocontrol of our verbal expression, the phonophonatory loop.

Did you know that in your everyday language, 80% of what you say uses no more than 500 syllables? Which they are depends on your maternal tongue. But whatever the maternal tongue, 80% of what we say is built with 500 syllables.

The word you produce depends on the area of the brain called the temporal planum. The person listening to you is stimulating the exact same area of his cerebral cortex. This has been verified by PET-scans. McGuire in 1996 and Skipper in 2005 also demonstrated that if the person listening to you then repeats exactly what you said, it will activate the exact same region of his brain: the left and right temporal planum. We call this "mirror neurons." This would tend to prove that voice, audition, and language are intimately bound; this we already knew, but neuroimaging confirmed it for us. The left and right temporal planum also enable us to read lips.

From genetics to voice and language

The child is predisposed

From the age of six months, the infant recognizes the vowels of its mother tongue, but more so the musicality of its vowels. By twelve months, he begins to form words, for example: "mu–mmy." He associates the two phonemes to enable the phonotactical coercion required to produce the word. This approach to musicality is surprising. We find it also in whale songs. Man's infant, at the age of sixteen months, begins to speak. At twenty months, he organizes words, at twenty-four months he builds sentences, at thirty-six months he is perfecting his grammar.

Everything is in place, but it was not clear sailing. Vocal ontogeny is running its course. Indeed, babies don't speak from birth. Three days after their birth, they still don't speak, yet foals run and dolphins swim. This child of ours progressively establishes his phonatory mechanics through the external stimulation of the left brain; his harmonics, and his sensibility to these, through the stimulation of his right brain; and his intuition through the stimulation of his limbic brain. The harmony of all these elements depends on the audiophonatory loop and the pneumophonic balance. So much of the matrix of the human voice is still a mystery to us waiting to be unveiled!

Does a gene of the voice exist?

Our thumb, acting in opposition to our other fingers, gives us exceptional dexterity, far greater than that of the chimpanzee with his hand. This primate also presents a pale imitation of Broca's and Wernicke's areas, but these only play a minor role in the chimpanzee's vocal expression.

Broca identified the language center of the brain in 1861. It was perfectly visible under the microscope. In the third millennium, will we be dissecting the depths of the molecule? Will scientific discoveries enable us to get to grips with our genetic heritage, 25% of which we owe to our cerebral activity? Are chromosomal, genetic, and molecular microanalysis about to deliver the secrets of the human voice?

Presently, the exact origins of the voice remain an enigma due to the complexity of the creation of articulated language and its neuronal circuits. Nevertheless, a gene called *FOXP2*, located on chromosome 7, has been isolated. In August 2001, in *Nature*, Cecilia Lai of Oxford compared this genome in a British family hit by a severe speech dysfunction, and in another patient from a different family that also presented speech dysfunctions. The same gene was responsible. Thus, it seems that the gene *FOXP2* on chromosome 7 is the one that ensures the coherence and intelligibility of the spoken language.

In August 2002, Wolfgang Enard and Svante Paabo go further: they establish that the same gene is also involved in facial expression, lip movement, and manner of speech. Going by the DNA clock, this gene seems to have appeared 200,000 years ago, around the time of our African Eve. And yet cranial molds show traces of Broca's areas that go back much further in time. Could this be only one of the genes of the voice, and not *the* gene of the voice? Richard Klein, of Stanford, makes the point that another mutation 50,000 years ago probably enabled the rampant evolution of our language. This gives me goose bumps. Does this imply that a genetic manipulation involving a graft of this gene *FOXP2* could make a mouse talk?

Are language dysfunctions innate or acquired?

Dyslexia has genetic origins involving mini-cerebral malformations that bring about cognitive deficiencies. The genetic hypothesis concerning dyslexia may seem reductionist, but it has the merit of illustrating that dysfunctions of the voice can have a biological cause. When the infant develops his language, the biological structure of his brain doesn't go down the normal evolutionary path. The phonological processing is faulty. This causes his behavior to modify. The cerebral asymmetry is less pronounced than is the norm for right-handers. The left temporal planum is also less developed. The corpus callosum is comparable in size. Neuroimagery reveals weaker activity in the area dealing with spelling. There is a genetic component, but the brain's amazing capacity to rebuild neural connections enables this anomaly to be rapidly mitigated through apprenticeship, application, and re-education, until it becomes negligible.

Already in 1960, Noam Chomsky put forward the hypothesis of a genetic component of the voice that would encompass language, syntax, and grammar. His pertinent analysis has the merit of raising the question of a gene of the voice. All languages have a grammar syntax, with often similar rules. Is this natural assimilation a phenomenon of a particular transcription of DNA, or is it just the product of a learning process handed down through the generations for several million years?

Twins

Natural clones, twins provide us with a partial answer to the question of whether the voice is innate or acquired. Philip Dale carried out research in Washington on 3,000 twins, with surprising results. 540 of them, that is, 18%, were backward in their language skills. The explanation derives more from environmental factors than genetic factors. These twins live as recluses. They speak to each other, but not to others. Their relational world shrinks, reducing their learning opportunities. Often they create their own language. The vocal areas of the brain are stimulated from infancy by relating to others, by hearing different voices. Though the numbers could suggest a genetic cause (18% is indeed a significant proportion in this context), this is by no means a foregone conclusion, given the importance of vocal ontogeny. Remember what happened in the experiment ordered by Frederic II, the King of Prussia!

His voice is the same as mine: François and Michel, monozygotic twins, are thirty years old. They consult me for a hoarse voice. They are both dark, mustachioed, dressed almost identically. "Doctor, Michel and I both have broken voices. Even when we're hoarse, we sound alike." To which Michel adds: "It's a fact that our voices changed about three years ago." When I examine their vocal cords, I detect small cysts on both cords at exactly the same place in both François and Michel. Could the origin of the cysts be genetic? Probably! Research by Steven Gray has identified pathologies of the vocal cord that are tied to a specific genome, pathologies such as nodules, cysts, and certain granulomas. To get back to our twins, one works in a bank, the other is a sales representative. Despite six months of speech therapy, there's no improvement. I operate on the cysts, their voices recover within a few weeks, and as you no doubt guessed, they recover their vocal identity. They still sound exactly the same on the telephone. They wanted to sound the same.

Monozygotic twins have the same voice, the same expression, often, according to some, the same emotions. Of course, all their genetic molecules are identical. We're talking here of over one hundred million identical molecular resonances. Small wonder then, that their voices should be almost identical, even though the stimulation given to their genes from infancy need not be strictly the same, as they don't always have the same life experiences. Records show that even after twins have been separated for several years, they still have the same vocal intonation, the same gestures, the same tastes, and the same desires.

Asymmetrical lobes and right-handedness: advantage or disadvantage?

The dogma of the left brain's asymmetry resides in the X-sex chromosome. An experiment by Crow on 11,600 English children aged eleven years, provided the opportunity to study the symmetry of the left and right brain as a function of language. Right-handed children with a dominant left brain had acquired language rapidly and correctly. fMRI tests of ambidextrous children revealed a deficient laterality of the language function. In other words, the left and right hemispheres are almost symmetrical, doubling up the language functions left and right. There seems to be an activation of Broca's area in the left brain that corresponds to actual stimulation, whereas on the right side Broca's area is in fact a pseudo-area. The corpus callosum skips between the two hemispheres very quickly. This genetic predisposition is pregnant with consequences. Are we not confronted here with vocal schizophrenia? It's a fact that schizophrenia is twenty times more frequent in the ambidextrous population than in the rest of the population, who have one hypertrophied hemisphere. A gene controlling this beneficial asymmetry has been found on the X-sex chromosome. Once more, investigation of a pathology has enabled us to better understand the importance of cerebral asymmetry and its consequences. The incidence of schizophrenia is very high in Turner's syndrome, a genetic anomaly in which one of the two X chromosomes is lacking, bringing about an XO karyotype instead of the usual XX karyotype. Practically no cerebral asymmetry is observed. Perception of language is dysfunctional. Therefore, as Pierre Bustany has asserted, cerebral asymmetry seems to be a crucial element enabling speech. Right-handedness has dominated for millions of years, as illustrated by the traces of cerebral grooves found on the calvarias of craniums dug up in Tanzania.

Language and Broca's area: unique to Man?

It seems that, since its inception, our voice has been subjected repeatedly to DNA mutations and has also been stimulated by new genes and new neuronal circuits. According to Al Galaburda, the left brain of great apes presents an equivalent to our Broca's area and Wernicke's area. Moreover, neuronal junctions can be found all over their brain. This left-brain asymmetry apparently is used by the apes not only for phonatory communication such as calling out to each other, giving orders, and so forth, but also, as in Man, it intervenes in facial expressiveness, movement of the lips, and their voice box structures. However, their audiophonatory loop is little developed. Is this the first evidence that Man and apes had a common ancestor that passed directly on to Man the ability to speak due to a series of genetic mutations? From then on, Man would have developed his own voice and his language skills to the hilt. During the Fire Age and its fire-related wars, phonatory communication was primitive. But over the next few million years, the accumulation of verbal information handed down from generation to generation created its own evolution: *Homo vocalis*, the vocal man, made his appearance.

The symbols transmitted from father to son, from speaker to listener, progressively evolved among the social groupings and tribes. The creation of new symbols from the primitive phonatory melting pot thus far created became possible only once a minimal threshold had been reached. Communication between these men evolved in parallel with the emergence of new desires, of their will to communicate, to name things, and to understand the abstract. Certain scientists have claimed that sign language was the first step along the road to the human voice. This probably wasn't the case, judging by the complexity and abstract richness of sign language, which shares the same language center in the brain as our language. Thus, the left brain, devolved to its language functions, grows in size and volume.

Languages become extinct

Our spoken language is an integral part of us, but also of our evolution. It evolves continuously. In order to exist, it must be used by enough individuals to guarantee its reproduction, enabling it to impose itself in the face of other social groups, other languages. Survival presupposes the existence of a predator. The languages specific to certain Amazonian tribes have become completely extinct, swallowed up by the giant Brazilian language. Certain dialects of North American Indians and Australian aborigines have known the same fate.

The chronology of language after birth

Thus, the apprenticeship of languages from infancy is given its impulse, even in our distant ancestors, by the dominance in right-handers, of the left brain over the right brain. Whatever the race, whatever the language, whatever the continent, the chronology of the learning of the mother tongue or of the bilingual child is fixed and constant for all humans.

Chapter 8

The script of the voice: language and thoughts

We write our thoughts with our voice.
Language is its writing instrument.

Our voice inscribes itself in the spatial and temporal dimensions of a familiar universe, but sometimes it enables us to better understand ourself, to talk to our Self. It inscribes itself in our dreams, in a mythical and utopian world that signifies "nowhere," a place that doesn't exist. Our voice is the interface between our language and our thoughts. The human voice is endowed with a special power: the power to mask or reveal, through words and silences, the very depths of the Self.

Thoughts are the ethereal receptacles of our language, the light source of our imagination. Their birth in our space-time world several million years ago accompanied the appearance of the human voice. Abstraction is king in this universe of thoughts. It enables us to converse with the unreal, with higher beings that we adulate, with a single God or with multiple divinities that incite us to pray and thus to formulate our thoughts.

Language and thoughts collide with an iron bar

Phineas Gage is a construction worker on a Vermont railway line in America. The year is 1848. He crams powder into rock in order to blast a space for a railway sleeper. He's taken by surprise and the accident happens: the dynamite explodes too soon. A 1.80 meter-long iron bar embeds itself in his face and skull. It enters through his left cheek and exits at the top of the forehead, above the eye. Despite this terrible trauma, he barely loses consciousness. Everyone is astounded. How can he possibly still be conscious, with a metal bar in his head! John Harlow, a doctor in Cavendish, removes the bar. Phineas seems to have escaped practically unscathed. He walks normally, talks normally, his memory and intelligence are unaffected. Two months go by. He's back on his feet, perfectly autonomous. The scars on his face have healed. These astonishing facts are penned in an article describing a successful case, published in 1848 by the Medical Society of Massachusetts. As it happens, the case study is a little premature, as the life of Phineas Gage is about to take an unexpected turn.

Indeed, a few months later, people close to him notice some changes. He isn't the man they used to know. His physical envelope is the same, but his language and thinking have changed. The old Phineas was staid, polite, courteous, and straightforward. He is now irresponsible, vulgar, asocial, a brawler with exhibitionist tendencies. Unable to hold down a job, he gets fired. For the next twelve years, he leads the life of a tramp and dies in 1860.

Nearly a century later, in 1990, Dr. Hanna Demasion carries out a superb investigation of his cranial trauma. His case had remained an enigma until this neuroanatomist from Iowa University successfully calculated the exact angle of entry of the iron bar. Her work shows that the areas concerned with motor function and language never suffered any damage. The areas affected were the control centers for emotion and behavior. The iron bar had destroyed the anterior frontal lobe. This part of the brain controls behavior, among other things. If the right frontal lobe is destroyed, attitudes change, reasoning is modified, self-analysis is perturbed. The person's character, language, and thinking are altered. These functions have an anatomic basis that is independent of the voice. Language and thinking are intimately bound. They're indispensable to the dynamics and construction of our vocal personality and they convey our emotional self.

Language and writing

Writing is a concrete expression of our language and thoughts: a palpable form of our impalpable voice. Egypt and China provide us with two very special writing traditions. Their writing isn't merely a transcript of the phonetic sounds forming a word, it is much, much more. Seven hundred years before Jesus Christ, Egypt was already losing its influence. Hieroglyphs were falling into oblivion. By contrast, China succeeded in keeping its writing tradition alive for millennia. China is our Ariana's thread that links our graphical expression to our vocal expression. Chinese script is writing, because each character signifies a phonetic element; it's music, because it suggests a melody that gives different meanings to one and the same phoneme; it's also an ideograph, because it represents an idea or an object

The oldest Chinese writings known to us are from 1500 BC. They represent the object they depict, as do Egyptian hieroglyphs, Aztec glyphs, Hindu, Sanskrit, or figures assembled in groups. The symbolism of the drawing and the symbolism of the phoneme are intimately connected. Then come the purely phonetic languages— Aramaic, Hebrew, Arabic, Latin. In these languages, the phoneme is king. The graphic aspect akin to drawing is sacrificed to a purely phonetic rendering. For example, five phonemes constitute the words "electric torch": e-lec-tric-tor-ch. In Chinese, the corresponding image is: *tin - k'l- teng*, meaning "lightning-steam-lamp." Such symbolism has its limits. The verb and indeed all words in Chinese are invariable; the Chinese language can't support the development of over 250,000 words, of a feminine and masculine gender, of conjugations such as we have in the West.

For the first "signs" of writing, the first objective trace of words, we must go back about six millennia. The human voice is Man's only Ariana's thread over the past several million years. Man first made tools for his survival, then he made tools with which he created artistic frescoes, for example, the bulls and horses at Lascaux, then came Chinese writing with its phonetic, symbolic, and sonorous representations, and finally the phoneme, the basis of all phonetic languages, was invented.

Phonetic writing progressively succeeded other types of writing. But concomitantly, over the last century another form of writing, another form of expression, invaded our culture: audiovisual writing. The human voice—first recorded on wax at the turn of the last century, then on magnetic film, and finally in digital form, has migrated from the physical body. It has become an intrinsic object for people, something we observe and listen to on its own. Is the best example of this transformation not our use of the telephone?

When we read, we register the sense of a word in a quarter of a second. This visual capture of words activates the visual areas of the brain in the occipital and frontal lobes; these cerebral areas interpret what we read and this creates an "internal voice" inside of us. The occipital lobe connects with the frontal lobe in 200 milliseconds. The human eye can only individualize an image if the image persists for more than one-fifteenth of a second. Cinematic technology is based on these facts. An impression of fluidity is created, whereas, in fact, only 26 images per second are projected.

The voice: a very private instrument put to the collective use

The Tower of Babel shows its limits, for uniformity breeds desolation. The charismatic power of the voice, this private tool of ours put to public use, is impressive. Whoever has heard General de Gaulle or Martin Luther King will agree. Here, language imposes itself on our thinking through its symbols and musicality. The voice's charm impregnates our left and right cerebral cortex and evokes the symbols fed by our emotions. There is absolutely no evidence to suggest that languages are evolving toward a single language, and, indeed, diversity is the very source of our abundant creativity.

To talk is to possess a language supported by a form of logic and reasoning that are closely entwined. Until 1997, no objective research had enabled us to pinpoint exactly where or how this intimacy is enabled by the brain. However, neuroimaging, the modern equivalent of Sherlock Holmes' magnifying glass in the study of the brain and of the human voice, has revealed to us the precise cerebral projection of our logical and reasoning center. This direct observation, in real time, of reason and of the human voice in action is neuroscience's greatest victory. This enabled us to observe verbal interaction and the logic of language acquired precociously. When a subject is asked to repeat: "All men are mortal, Socrates is a man, Socrates is mortal," it induces specific cerebral activity observed in precise areas of the left brain. For all that the statement is a syllogism, it demands a significant effort both of integration of the spoken word and of reasoning. Neuroimaging shows that the logic faculty of the left brain is activated at the same time as an emotional reaction is triggered in the right brain. The right brain is where emotions and our sense of Self are "created." This research, carried out by O. Houde, shows the interaction between our two brains. Each has a specific role to play, each is indispensable to the other. This is also the case for actors, artists, comedians, or singers.

The human voice is not just a language exercise. It is self-creating, it feeds off its environment and off its own drive to evolve. Of course, its anatomic and mechanical structures are indispensable, but to assume that this is all that there is to the human voice would be far too diminishing! The mystery of our vocal emotion, the reach of our thinking as expressed by our voice, give such wings to our creativity that we're transported to the very limits of order and chaos.

Did you know that we spend nearly a quarter of our time talking? Our mental voice allows communication between our language and our thinking. Our internal chatter stimulates our creativity and anticipation exponentially. Indeed, this is what has enabled Man to survive for millions of years, braving predators and the climatic vicissitudes of our planet.

Our conscience, alchemy between the voice and the brain, between the emotional and the rational, between the scientific and the artistic, is not far off. When you speak, when you listen, you're judging yourself, yet this one-on-one involves only you. Your own voice can amplify your analytical acuity, but it can also intoxicate you and trap you into being egotistical. When we're victim of a stroke or a cranial traumatism, our verbal world shatters. Yet our voice, which seems such a natural, essential part of us, indestructible because impalpable, can forsake our body during an illness or if a part of our brain deteriorates. In a deep coma, our language and thinking are affected, but how much are we aware of? And don't some patients tell us, when they emerge from a coma, that their thinking faculties were unaffected? Anatomy and biology play only a supporting role in the creation of our spoken language, they are only a means to an end.

Our voice exists only through its contacts with other voices

Voice and conscience

Our voice hatches with our birth. It seems to go hand in hand with our conscious and subconscious minds. It provides us with the means for introspection. Where would psychoanalysis, as defined by Freud, be without it? It is both the portal of creation and the guardian of our memory. It feeds our individual memories as the collective memory.

Boris Cyrulnik specifies that in order to become aware of something, we must first come into contact with that something. This reflection gives us insight into the important influence of the environment on our spoken language and on the human voice. In light of this, the vertiginous acceleration observed in our spoken and musical universes for nearly three centuries now is hardly surprising. The human voice enabled the creation of new words, of new theories. One word bounces off another. It constructs our thinking and the edifice of our knowledge. What seems evident to us today hasn't always been so. The word "conscience," so simple and yet so complex, does not exist in Chinese or in Ancient Greek. It was invented four centuries ago. Our understanding of the human body, of anatomy and physiology, of phylogenesis, of the brain—we're only just beginning to make inroads here—enables us to speculate on the conscious and the subconscious, on the connection between language and thought. Yet since time immemorial, the infant has been endowed with this conscience, with this language, with this thinking faculty, without any knowledge of them.

The first words switch on our thinking, so that further down the road, the word can become the tool, and our thinking its master

Whether we are dealing with our perceptual conscience (sensing others), our reflexive conscience (introspection), our higher conscience, or the conscience that is continuously molded by our emotional and affective environment, this conscience of ours is always in perpetual conflict with our ego. Our voice is the link between them, whether it's controlled, ranting, or silent, whether it's our inner voice or our public voice. I may talk often to others, but I'm always talking to myself!

Within our core Self, our fossil brain—the brain that's evolved from the fish, the amphibian and the primitive mammal—has a contribution to make. It's as indispensable to us as our other cerebral functions. The brain and its language, like the heart, are always active, there is no respite for them from the moment of birth to the day we die.

What motive has been driving Man in this adventure between vocal harmony and emotional chaos? The outcome and the motive blend together, are entwined, fuse. The trails cross over, forming a labyrinth with a single exit: the imagination; and only one hub—the voice, the common denominator of our language and thinking.

Chapter 9

From the descriptive to the affective

As breath flows from Man's breast to his lips,
what alchemy transforms a sound wave into a word,
a melody, a vocal imprint?

A sound, its frequency, its vibration are the preliminary sketches of our acoustic universe

Sound and light have been associated since millennia in the harmony of our perception. Aristotle explains the echo as the reflection of a sound, and likens it to a sun ray bouncing off a mirror. But sun rays are photonic reflections, whereas vibrations are mechanical reflections; yet for the scientist, they are intimately connected. As light passes through the prism of a piece of crystal or through the water particles of a waterfall catching the morning sun, it decomposes into seven basic colors, and this phenomenon gave rise to our musical scale with its seven notes.

In the Middle Ages, people listen to bards. These move from castle to castle and their music, never written down, goes with them to their grave. In the 7th century, Paul Diacre, a monk from Mount Cassin, loses his voice. He can no longer preach. He feels he has nothing to live for anymore. After much praying, he invokes Pope Zacharia, who cures him. He is immensely grateful. He composes a hymn for the feast of St. John the Baptist, celebrated on the 24th of June, considered then as the day of the summer solstice. (A few centuries later, give or take a day or two, in 1982, June the 21st is designated 'Music Day' in France.) His hymn will provide the phonemes of the first musical scale: **Ut** *queant laxis* / **Re**sonare *fibris* / **Mira** *gestuorum* / **Famulituorum** / **Sol**ve *polluti* / **La**biti *reatum* / **Sancte** *Johannes* . . . , which means: "Remove the sin of your impure servant, oh Saint John that the marvels of your actions may resonate on the relaxed cords of our lips."

Two centuries go by. Around the year 1000, Guido d'Arezzo puts the definitive stamp on the writing of our melodies by establishing the solfeggio, with the scale *ut, re, mi, fa, sol, la*. This Benedictine monk of the Cathedral of Arezzo, between Siena and Florence, is a music professor and an outstanding teacher. He perfects the scale written by monk Paul Diacre and gives to us a musical alphabet that enables the music of Bach, Mozart, and Glenn Miller to reach us unscathed. The musical stave is extended from four to five lines.

This musical annotation is revolutionary. Notes and melodies can now be learned objectively. Reading and learning music in the absence of a master rehearser becomes simple. Previously, artists could only learn music alongside a mentor, and this apprenticeship could take years. In 1673, Bononcini transforms *Ut* into *do* and at the end of the 16th century, Anselme de Flandres nominates *si* as the last note of the scale. The scale is now: *do, re, mi, fa, sol, la, si*. The English and the Germans prefer letters of the alphabet; they replace *do, re, mi, fa, sol, la, si* with *C, D, E, F, G, A, B*. But the scale is given additional subtlety. Gregorian chanting is unique in that it accepts two types of tonality for the *B* note: a "flat *B*," half a tone above *A*, (or half a tone under *B*) and a "hard *B*," half a tone above *B*. In time, the "flat *B*" became "*B* flat" and the "hard *B*" became "*B* sharp" (*B* is one tone above *A*. Thus, the sharp raises the note by one-half chromatic tone and the flat lowers it by one-half chromatic tone.)

The acoustics of the voice

The light and the voice

In 1737, Jean-Jacques Dortons de Mairan, of the Academy of Sciences, renews the analogy between vibratory waves and light waves. The subject spawns a number of contradictory mathematical theories. Light, like music, is broken down into a scale with seven intervals: the seven fundamental colors. However, we have to wait for the 20th century before the photonic wave, or luminous wave, is acknowledged to travel in outer space as well as through air at a speed of 300,000 km/h. It literally cleaves the air. It continues to perplex and fascinate researchers, whose theoretical basis remains Einstein's relativity theory and its formula, according to which $E = mc^2$. Photonic rays travel through space and through our atmosphere. They are very different from sound waves, which need a support to transmit their vibration. Void doesn't transmit sound. If you place a loudspeaker under a bell and suck the air out from under the bell, even with your ear a few centimeters away from the bell, you won't hear it ringing. Reintroduce some air under the bell and you'll hear it ringing perfectly. The air on our planet enabled Man to speak and gave him his voice.

How does sound propagate?

Acoustic sound waves are none other than a series of jolts to microparticles of air; the jolts have a bumper effect on the microparticles, as when lined up dominos fall over in a chain reaction. When a sound wave is set up, air molecules move in successive wave forms that vary as a function of the original frequency. This wavecan propagate itself in air, water, glass, metal, or wood but never in void. Its speed through the air is 340 m/s at a temperature of 16°. Through water, it is 1,450 m/s, due to the greater density of water molecules; close together rather than scattered, they allow much faster transmission. For the same reason, steel has a fast transmission speed of 6,000 m/s. Through the bone of our skull, our voice propagates at 3,500 m/s. This doesn't play a significant role when we speak, because although our own voice is transmitted to our ear at a speed of 340 m/s both internally (by the bones in our head) and externally (by our outer ear), the distance to the eardrum is so small that the brain perceives and integrates these two inputs of information concurrently, only a few thousandths of a second apart.

Sound must reach a minimal threshold for it to be registered by the eardrum. This auditory threshold corresponds to an amplitude of 20 dB. At 100 dB, sound is close to our auditory pain threshold, while at 160 dB, it's highly aggressive for our ears and can cause hearing traumatisms such as buzzing, tinnitus, and temporary or permanent deafness. If you have two loudspeakers in your lounge, both emitting 100 dB, the total volume of sound is 104 dB, not 200 dB. This is because decibels are calculated as a function of the logarithm of atmospheric pressure (aP), they aren't cumulative. A pneumatic drill raises 140 dB, a crying baby 110 dB, the ticking of a clock 30 dB, ordinary conversation 40 to 50 dB.

Frequency is the number of vibrations per second translated into hertz (Hz). For example, on a piano, 440 Hz, or 440 vibrations per second, is the pitch of A3, the musical note *A* on the piano's third octave. Human conversation can range from 100 to 4000 Hz. An octave is divided into 12 half-tones. The interval between 100 and 200 Hz corresponds to one octave, as does the interval 200 to 400 Hz, 400 to 800 Hz, and so on.

The secret behind the power and vibrations of our Voice

The larynx: a wind and string instrument

Man is unique in having his very own musical instrument: his exceptional larynx and its exceptional resonators. They are the only one of its kind on two counts: they constitute the only instrument we know of that is both wind and string, and this instrument is also unique in that it produces both words and melodies. Our vocal cords are symmetrical. We have two: one on the left and one on the right. They open when we breathe and close when we speak. Placed horizontally at the top of the trachea, they are the source of vocal vibrations. They are made up of striated muscle, covered by a white mother-of-pearl mucous membrane. It's the rhythmic movement of the membrane that produces the vibration. The mucous membranes of the vocal cords vibrate in contact with each other: the left and right membrane undulate, separate, and move in again with great frequential accuracy. They set up a string of emissions, consisting, in the case of the A3 note, of 440 "air puffs" per second or 440 vibrations. This sound is then propagated upward above the vocal cords. Thus is the "original" sound of our laryngeal instrument born.

The vibration of the vocal cord mucous membrane

During voicing, our normally passive exhalation becomes active, enabling us to control our voicing. The outward air stream moves upward, propelling air puffs that are released from the vocal tract with every vibratory pulsation, every nth second, as a function of the desired frequency and power. The V formed by the vocal cords closes and vibrates during phonation (see Plate 12). The wave travels through the glottic cavity (the space between the vocal cords) of the trachea toward the resonators described later. But not all the vocal cord structures vibrate, only the surfaces that are in contact with each other—called the "free edges" of the vocal cord, on which the respective mucous membranes are located—and this sets up a controlled pulsation. The free edges periodically join up, close, and open again. If they don't make contact, they can't vibrate. The vibration is a strictly mechanical consequence of exhalation, it is not under the direct command of the central nervous system. The outward air stream bumps up against the vocal membranes that are blocking its path and mobilizes them in its attempt to clear them. We control our vocal muscles, we don't have direct control over the mucous membranes of our vocal cords.

The power of our voice derives from our breathing

The force of our exhalation gives power to our voice and to the vibration of the vocal cords. The amplitude at which the mucous membrane vibrates determines the amount of power created. The greater the amplitude of the cordal membrane is, the stronger the voice; conversely, the smaller the amplitude, the weaker the voice. Controlling the exhalation will be the key here. The tone and length of the vocal cords are also under our direct voluntary control, as we're able to contract our vocal muscles at will.

Thus, the vibration of a single vocal mucous membrane is not sufficient to create a sound wave. It's the coming together of both mucous membranes that creates a string of air puffs, or micro-puffs, which then move up into the glottic space. These puffs set up a regular succession of "transglottic air waves" that propagate themselves up to the lips. This is also quite different from the way string instruments are played—consider the pinching of a harp string or the plucking of a guitar string—and, indeed, from the way wind instruments are played, like the clarinet, which requires contact between the lips and the reed. The larynx thus creates sound waves by virtue of the two vocal cords coming into contact and vibrating under pressure from the outward air stream. This makes it both a wind and a string instrument.

The minimum threshold for speaking

Launching the vibratory process requires a minimal initial degree of pressure and the dynamics to make it last. Daniel Bernoulli, a scientist in the 18th century, belonged to the second generation of an illustrious family that included nine scientists. His treatise on hemodynamics published in 1738 established him as the founder of this branch of science, and gave us a better understanding of the physiology of our laryngeal instrument and how certain traumas of the voice can be avoided. The "open and close" cycle of the surface of the vocal cords depends on the pressure of the air being expelled and the elasticity of the mucous membrane: this is known as the Bernoulli effect. "The pressure of a fluid diminishes as fluid gathers speed." In other words, the higher the speed of the flow is, the lower its pressure will be. The undulating movement of the vocal cords occurs in three dimensions.

Thus, when your voice fails you—and this happens frequently among singers, politicians, or judges—take a good breath to unleash the power of your voice and the first vocal vibrations. Your audience must be with you from your first utterances, as you need to captivate your audience from the start. The exhalation must set up a minimal amount of pressure to set off the undulation mechanism of the cordal mucous membranes. The two cords open while you breathe in, close and move into contact during phonation. The glottis (the space between the vocal cords) closes up, ready to assist in emitting sound within a few hundredths of a second. The lungs expel their contents through the tracheobronchial tree (see Plate 13). The pressure exerted by the airflow as it is expelled gradually opens up the glottis, or more precisely, separates the cordal mucous membranes as it pushes upward. The airflow meets with slight resistance from the elastic membranes. When the pressure reaches a certain minimal threshold, the glottis opens, the air stream is allowed through, the membranes separate and the pressure drops. At this point, the elasticity of the cords is stronger than the pressure of the air flowing through, so the cords move back inward to their initial position, in contact with each other; and the cycle starts again, hundred of times per second.

Every time you sing a specific note, you produce the same length, the same thickness, the same tension, the same elasticity of the vocal cords.

Every time you want to sing a note at exactly 90 dB, the same expiratory pressure will be produced. The bow glides on the violin string. Its light pressure produces a soft sound. If the pressure is stronger, the sound produced will be louder. The vibration is felt by the hand guiding the bow. In the same way, if you close your vocal cords too tightly, constricting them, you prevent them from vibrating. If you don't close them sufficiently, they won't be in contact and again, no vibration will be set up.

Producing a *fortissimo* or a *pianissimo*, an *A* note or a *C* note, requires constant precision-work and permanent fine-tuning. It takes a lot of hard work to make it sound easy and natural. Intimate knowledge of the mechanics of the larynx enables better control of this complex instrument.

Minimal contact in order to vibrate

For a bow to produce a sound on a violin, it must be in contact with the string. If the two don't make contact, there will be silence, whether the two are one millimeter or two meters apart. A vibration can only be produced when the two are in contact. Equally, our two vocal cords must be in contact to produce a sound. If they are apart, whether they're half a millimeter or two millimeters apart, no sound will be produced. If a growth alters their vibration, the vocal alteration will be practically identical whether the growth is the size of a grain of rice, like a nodule, or the size of a small pea, like a polyp. The correlation between voice dysfunctions and the severity or importance of the lesion is low. If you have a large polyp that's still able to vibrate, you'll be audible; if you have a hard nodule no bigger than a grain of sand, your voice will be very affected.

Volume, shape, mobility, suppleness, degree of lubrication, vascularization—these are all essential factors contributing to the emission of vocal sounds. Sex influences the speed of vibration during speech. The average speed of vibration in men is 180 cycles per second or 180 Hz, as compared to 220 Hz in women and 250 Hz in children.

A single nerve controls speaking

The pneumogastric nerve is the only nerve controlling the opening, closing, and sensitivity of the vocal cords. It is the only nerve in our body that conveys contradictory information (both agonist and antagonist); if this nerve malfunctions or is severed, the vocal cords are paralyzed and the voice is altered.

The pneumogastric nerve enables our vocal cords to contract or relax. It determines their tension and length. They're short and thick with respect to low notes, long and fine with respect to high notes. This nerve also opens the vocal cords when we breathe and closes them when we scream, cough, laugh, cry, vomit, swallow, and talk.

The vibration of the vocal cords creates harmonics

Harmonics dress up the pure sound

Tuning forks emit a pure sound created by a single oscillation with no resonance. No harmonic is emitted. This is why the tuning fork serves as a reference for tuning music instruments and our voice. It has a unique vibration. This can't be said of our vocal cords: when the cordal mucous membranes vibrate, the resonances of all the elements that form them, elements that are far more complex than any musical instrument, are harmonized.

Each element of the vocal cord has its own resonance and reacts differently. All the resonances harmonize together around a common denominator: the fundamental tone, or F_0. Helmholtz defined F_0 as the singer's fundamental tone, and more generally, as Man's, this being the lowest natural frequency we can emit. F_0 causes the vocal cords and resonators to produce harmonics.

Harmonics are formed by the acoustic signal bouncing off the resonators. The first harmonic is double the fundamental harmonic

($F_1 = 2 \times F_0$). If F_0 is equal to C2, or 128 Hz, then F_1 is equal to 256 Hz, or C3; F_2 is equal to $3 \times F_0$, or 384 Hz, which corresponds to G3; and so on. Thus, when a singer listens to the tuning fork and reproduces the same note, what you'll hear is the note, for example, *A*, as well as an acoustic effect formed by the fundamental frequency, F_0 (the frequency of the tuning fork reproduced by the singer's vocal cords), plus the harmonics F_1, F_2, F_3, produced by the various elements that make up the vocal cords and the resonators.

The beauty of the voice: harmonics and noise

How does one explain the seductive powers and vibratory expression of singers like La Callas, Mario Del Monaco, Caruso, or Roberto Alagna? When singers of their caliber produce the fundamental tone in their vocal cords, it immediately sets up the production of secondary fundamentals, also called harmonic fundamentals. These strong harmonics, more powerful than others because of the reverberation qualities of these singers' resonators, are called the singer's formants.

A bel canto voice has twelve harmonics, whereas you and I (if you don't sing) only have four to six. But there is more to an exceptional voice than its number of harmonics. The quality of these harmonics is also important, and that is what most of us lack. In the bel canto, these harmonic fundamentals (the singer's formants) are the second, third, fourth, tenth, eleventh, and twelfth harmonics. Thus, six of the twelve harmonics of a bel canto singer are reinforced harmonics.

The singing formants are found around the harmonics of 2800 Hz in women and 2300 Hz in men. They lend brilliance to the voice and enable singers to project their voices several hundred meters. They require complete mastery of vocal techniques, as exemplified by Roberto Alagna, Luciano Pavarotti, or Renée Fleming.

But let's not despair. You and I also have formants when we speak and sing. We just have fewer of them. If you acquire a good vocal technique with a teacher, you too will find or create your singer's formants. Singer's formants are what make beautiful voices so special and powerful.

The sound and its harmonics produced by our vocal cords are accompanied by noise that has no vibration and is aperiodic. This noise is natural noise. Acoustic spectral analysis provides an objective profile of its parameters. The human voice is not all harmony, regularity, and control, it also includes a certain level of noise. You hear it in the background, subconsciously. It's the singer's breath, that "something" else that accompanies the voice. These irregular parameters contribute a singular stamp to each person's voice.

Let's not forget that only the cordal mucous membranes can produce a sound wave. The resonators can never spontaneously produce one. They modulate sound waves, they don't create them.

If an *A* note played on a violin or a piano seems familiar to you, bear in mind that it's actually not the note that enables you to recognize the instrument playing it, but the harmonics created by the instrument's resonance chamber. The chamber modulates the original vibration and personalizes it. Thus, the shape of music instruments, their texture, their structural elements, their design, and their elasticity all contribute to the originality of their signature. The acoustic print that enables us to recognize a sound—whether made by a piano, a harp, or a trumpet, a man's voice or a woman's voice—is always characterized by its harmonics (see Plate 14).

Theater, conference hall: the artist must adapt himself

When your larynx emits a melody, a sentence, or a poem, your voice invades the space around you. But the color of your voice will be different according to reigning conditions, such as heat or humidity. Your surroundings can change, modify, alter, or improve the sound and projection of your voice. Most affected are the speed of sound and the quality of certain harmonics. Opera singers and variety singers are well aware of this. An empty, cold opera house doesn't have the same acoustics as a full, heated opera house with a background noise level of 15 dB and an atmosphere moistened by the breath of 3,000 spectators. The resonance of the hall modifies our hearing experience.

Sound travels through air at 330 m/s at 0° C. This speed increases as the temperature rises. This is only logical: a thermal increase augments molecular agitation, which increases the speed at which sound travels. Its speed is also modified by the composition of the air. For example, in pure oxygen, its speed is 317 m/s, while in helium, it's 1,300 m/s. That's why you sound like Donald Duck if you breathe in helium; your voice becomes sharper, practically all the low-pitched harmonics disappear. The fundamental tone shifts upward, because the gas that's now stimulating the vocal cords is less dense than air and the air puffs therefore travel faster.

Thus, the lower the density of the air and the higher the temperature, the faster sound will travel. Also, the more humid the air, the more the harmonics will change. The acoustics of the room or hall are also an important factor. This is why before a concert, rehearsals are useful to bring into account the resonance of the hall, its atmosphere, its degree of echo, all of which affect each instrument differently. Normally, each instrument has an invariable location in the orchestra. The angle of reflection of the vibration behaves like a luminous ray: it invades the theatre or hall and creates its own vibratory environment. If you move a musician, you alter the orchestral harmony of the concert. The positioning of the singer is equally important. The singer must have optimal control over his voice, which can be affected by the concert hall, the reigning heat or humidity, his place on stage, and the quality and number of spectators. His audiophonatory loop is constantly on the alert. The orchestra is familiar with all these parameters. This is why musicians tune their instruments once the public is seated, and again after each interval. During a concert, the hygrometry increases, the air becomes heavier, the tonalities drop. The success of a concert depends at least in part on the adaptability of the professional singer, the musicians, and the orchestra leader. The singer only requires a few tenths of a second to adapt to his surroundings. It is himself he has to evaluate; he is the instrument he must tune!

From a technical point of view, for our ear to distinguish two distinct phonemes, these must succeed each other with a minimum interval of six seconds. If the phonation rhythm is too fast, it affects intelligibility. Equally, our ear cannot distinguish two frequencies if they're not at least one-fifteenth of a second apart.

Thus, when an actor voices a word at the theater, the sound travels at 340 m/s. It meets an obstacle not less than 34 meters away, which means the sound he has to evaluate has to travel 68 meters to come back to him. If the reverberation is shorter, the sound will be less intelligible. This may all seem very mathematical or theoretical to you, but these parameters explain why you can often be disappointed by your seat at a show. The quality of reception is very different depending on where you sit. Opera fans know exactly which seats to book in order not to miss a single harmonic of their favorite diva! We have all experienced certain theaters that have such bad acoustics that the dialogues or songs become unintelligible. Happily, this isn't frequent. Indeed, the best-known theaters like the Comédie Française, and operas houses such as la Fenice in Venice, la Scala in Milan, or l'Opéra Garnier in Paris are built like a vibratory amplifier, with an elliptical vault that amplifies all vocal harmonics. Thus it is that in the final act of *La Traviata*, one can hear Cyrano de Bergerac whispering on his sweetheart's balcony and one can make out Violeta's *pianissimo* as she lies on her bed.

The stage-set of our voice and how to explore it

The violin, shaped by Man since Antiquity, has been around now for some 3,000 years. Like most musical instruments known to us, it has three key elements: a vibratory body (the string), an engine or source of energy (the bow gliding on the string, which produces the note), and the amplifier or resonator (the body of the violin).

In our vocal instrument, the vibratory elements are the two vocal cords, one on the left and one on the right. They are an integral part of the larynx. The engine is the exhalation emitted by our air duct, namely our lungs, bronchi, and trachea. The amplifier or resonance chamber begins just above the vocal cords and ends at the lips (see Plate 15).

The laryngologist endeavors to devolve to its owner his or her original vocal print, as it was before an aggressor altered it: an infection, an inflammation, a tumor, or in the case of voice professionals, the more subtle manifestations of stress or vocal strain.

To do so, how will the laryngologist investigate this wonderful voice instrument?

Can we look at the voice?

The Ancients were already fascinated by the voice. We owe our first anatomical sketches of it to Leonardo da Vinci. In 1834, Dr. Elvey received a Gold Medal prize from the Royal Society of London for his invention of an instrument that could be pushed down the throat to inspect the vocal cords. This instrument associated a number of mirrors with candle light, which wasn't very practical. Twenty years later, a scientific revolution saw the light of day.

For years, Manuel García had been obsessed with the idea of being able to observe the larynx during speech or singing. Born in 1805, this well-known singing teacher is nearing his fifties. The mystery of the human voice intrigues him: his sister, la Malibran, is a diva—to what does she owe her great voice? How does the vibration of the vocal cords come about? Son of a Spanish singer of international renown, Manuel enjoys a brief career as a baritone before losing his voice. This dramatic episode puts an end to his stage-life at the age of thirty. He then decides to further his understanding of our laryngeal instrument. In 1854, during a stroll in the gardens of the Palais Royal in Paris, a ray of sunlight bounces off the pommel of his cane and dazzles him. It strikes him that the vocal cords might possibly be observed using a system of mirrors to bounce light into the depths of the throat and larynx. He hurries to Les Établissements Charrière, a manufacturer of mirrors for dentistry near the Odéon. He buys a mirror costing six francs. He hardly has eyes for the palace that has been the residence of Richelieu, of the Empire, and presently, of the Duke of Orléans. Neither does he notice the cafés crowded with nobility. He rushes home to his private hotel on the Place de l'Odéon, and discovers his own vocal cords: laryngology is born. Within a few years, his reputation as a singing teacher spreads throughout Europe.

A few years later, in 1861, Charles Bataille writes the first account of phonation. Edison invents the phonograph. The voice is now recorded, it is 1877. Then, at the dawn of the 20th century, cinematographic techniques see the light of day. They enable scientists to develop the stroboscope, which simulates slow motion. This is used to illuminate the vocal cords, adapting the frequency of the flashes to that of the vibration emitted. Thanks to the artificially slow motion, the phenomenon becomes observable. The secret of the vibration of the vocal cords is out at last. In 1939, Jean Tarneaud writes one of the first treatises on phoniatrics, then in 1958, Paul Moore and Hans von Leden present in America the first cinematographic images of the vibration of the vocal cords, images that revolutionize the scientific world. Later, the invention of fiber optics enables the larynx to be viewed through the nose instead of through the mouth. The introduction of instruments into the mouth is thus avoided. By the same token, the buccolingual articulation is unaltered, lip mobility is normal, phonation is natural. A fibroscope is introduced into a nostril. It goes down the left or right nasal fossa, past the back of the uvula, down the throat between the tonsils on either side, and so straight down to the roof of the larynx.

In 1981, I perfected a dynamic vocal exploration technique that allows multiple aspects of the larynx to be observed. It becomes possible to look at the action of the voice during phonation and singing, associating five perfectly synchronized techniques, and to record it on magnetic or numeric supports. This exploration integrates recordings from pharyngolaryngeal fibroscopy, stroboscopy, the position of the head in relation to the thorax, the electrolaryngogram, and the spectrogram.

1. Nasopharyngolaryngeal videofibroscopy enables us to observe the mobility of the vocal structures without introducing any instruments into the mouth that could perturb its mobility.

2. Stroboscopy enables us to observe lesions that can only be diagnosed in slow motion, notably minute cancerous lesions or mini-cysts.

3. Positioning the head correctly in relation to the thorax avoids drawing erroneous conclusions from a posture-induced asymmetry of the vocal cords. Indeed, the voice is altered if the head is turned slightly right or left during the examination, or if it's in either hyperflexion or hyperextension. In these instances, the alteration is caused by the larynx-neck-thorax alignment, not by a laryngeal pathology.

4. The electrolaryngogram evaluates the resistance and quality of vibration of the epithelium of the vocal cord mucous membranes.

5. Finally, the spectrogram provides us with the individual's acoustic identity card. It analyzes the fundamental tone, the harmonics, and formants, more developed in singers.

This vocal exploration provides us with the voice's identity card: the vocal print. Thanks to this approach, pathologies caused by voice strain can now be identified. After a few minutes of vocal practice, small veins begin to swell, nodules and thick mucous fluid form. In the same way as cardiac pathologies can be screened by testing cardiac effort, thereby avoiding heart attacks, an inauspicious vocal strain can be detected before it results in a lesion of the vocal cords.

The larynx: more than just vocal cords

The neck encases the larynx. In men, the Adam's apple makes the larynx easy to spot. A number of muscles suspend the Adam's apple between the head and the thorax. The muscles draped around it are indispensable to our vocal expression. Just under the jaw and above the Adam's apple is a small, isolated bone in the shape of a horseshoe: the hyoid bone. It serves to make fast the insertion of the tongue muscles and ensures their impressive mobility. A vertical posture is a technical element of importance to voice professionals. Their neck muscles are particularly tonic. This vertical posture is made possible mainly by the cervical vertebrae, with their familiar forward curvature. A singer's voice can be affected by tightness of the neck muscles, or by cervical arthritis.

Creating three octaves

Is one of the four strings of the violin vibrating? The finger that's pinching it is putting it under tension, changing its length, thus producing the desired frequency. Surprisingly, whereas a short violin string produces a high pitch, our vocal cords produce a low pitch when they shorten and a high pitch when they lengthen. Man and his instrument, two directly opposed modes of functioning. Why?

Our vocal cord becomes finer when it lengthens and thicker when it shortens. When the finger pinches the violin string, the string diminishes or increases in length, but its diameter remains unchanged. Therefore, the frequency of a cord is determined both by its length and by its diameter. Logically, if you can't change its diameter, you have to change its length (as happens with the violin). But when the cord lengthens and its diameter decreases, it necessarily produces a higher pitch (this is the case with the vocal cord or when an elastic band is stretched). We owe this insight to Manuel García.

The vocal cord is a striated muscle. This enables it to become thinner and longer for high frequencies and fatter and shorter for low frequencies. Its elasticity guarantees the speed with which it adjusts to a new frequency. Its length, thickness, tension, and elasticity are intimately connected with the specificity of each frequency. Mastering this is one of the professional singer's hidden skills.

When the vocal cord emits a frequency, it creates a single vibratory wave, known as a sine wave. This sine wave is in harmony with the opposite vocal cord. When you stretch several meters of sailing rope between two fixed points and set it off undulating, the initial undulation sets up several waves, or sine waves. Pathology can upset the harmonious working of our vocal cords; like the sailing rope, the vocal cord ends up with two or three waves along its length, instead of a single one. A nodule or a polyp can be the cause. The voice then sounds hoarse. In other cases, the vibratory synchronicity between the left and the right vocal cord may be affected. This can happen for a variety of reasons: an allergy, an infection, an inflammation due to gastric reflux. In rarer cases, a neurological problem entailing the superior laryngeal nerve can be involved. With age, the vocal muscles can also atrophy asymmetrically and this also affects the vibratory symmetry of the vocal cords

The human brain is a true marvel, as precise as a clock maker!

A beautiful voice depends on three interconnected imperatives linked to the vocal cords

All three, namely *vibration*, *closure*, and *lubrication*, are indispensable (see Plate 16). They are the three key words to have a nice voice.

Vibration: if the vocal cords don't vibrate or vibrate only partially, voice quality will be poor.

Closure: if the vocal cords don't touch, no sound will be produced. No sound, no voice.

Lubrication: vibrating at 200 to 300 vibrations per second, the vocal cords must be lubricated, otherwise they break within a few minutes. As they begin to overheat, they dry out. At that point you feel the need to clear your throat.

Rub your hands together just ten times per second, and you'll notice how warm they get. The same happens to our vocal cords.

Our vocal cords are protected by a shield

The larynx is a very mobile organ. This mobility is necessary for swallowing and for phonation. The larynx is shaped like an upside-down cone with a truncated base. The neck muscles surround it and the cervical spine at the back structures it. It is made up of muscles, epithelium, fibers, bone, and cartilage. It's a precision instrument. The two vocal cords, horizontal, symmetrical, and perfectly mobile, are its noblest elements. They are protected by the thyroid cartilage (from the Greek word *thyros*, meaning "shield"). This shield is closed at the front along a ridge in the neck that one can palpate, and opens out posteriorly onto the neck cavity. It is formed by two cartilage wings that join up at the front. The Adam's apple on the thyroid's upper edge is none other than the result of the calcification of this cartilage, which is unique to Man. The calcification is brought on by male hormones. This makes it easy to tell a man's throat from a woman's throat.

The thyroid cartilage rests on the only complete ring in our body: the cricoid, from the Greek word *krikos*, meaning "ring." Fixed firmly in place and immutable, it sits at the top of the trachea. Such is the architecture that surrounds and protects the vocal cords.

The shape of the larynx and vocal tessitura

The anatomy of the larynx, its structure, its dimensions often correlate with a person's stature. For example, we have noted a frequent correspondence between the shape of the larynx and vocal tessitura.

Tenors are usually stout, with a thick-set neck and well-developed neck muscles. The larynx juts out a little, its angles are rounded and the thyroid cartilage is more open at the back. The Adam's apple is less prominent. The larynx is in the shape of a squat cone, with a broad base. The thyroid cartilage is less developed than in baritone or low bass singers, and the membrane of the cricothyroid (a muscle between the thyroid and cricoid cartilages) is short and very strong, symptomatic of a powerful head voice.

Contrast this with bass singers, with their tall, slim silhouette and long larynx. Although well in proportion, the thyroid cartilage in this instance is smaller in diameter and forms a tighter angle. The laryngeal cone is deep, literally plunging down into the vocal cords. The cords are very characteristic: long, powerful, darker than those of a tenor. The epiglottis is particularly fine. One could sketch practically the entire anatomy of the larynx simply by observing it through the fiberscope. The larynx is housed in a long, muscular, well-defined neck with clear outlines. The Adam's apple is prominent and of a good size. The large space between the cricoid ring and the thyroid cartilage enables the singer to pass with ease from a head voice to a chest voice.

Baritones are between these two types: tenor and bass. In women, the anatomical differences between the neck of a soprano and the neck of an alto are more difficult to spot from a simple visual examination. Of course, the above are skeleton descriptions, simplified for the sake of clarity.

Arthritis of the voice

The arytenoids move at the back and articulate with the cricoid cartilage. This small ossicle, already encountered in earlier chapters, is oddly shaped. It looks like a jug or a funnel and is broader at its base. *Arutainoeidês* is the Greek word for "shaped like a ewer" (a wide-mouthed pitcher). The vocal muscle is attached to it. The left and right arytenoids are joined by very powerful muscles. They allow opening and closure of the vocal cords. When these cricoarytenoid joints are affected or become dysfunctional, our verbal and musical world breaks down. The arytenoid is the only mobile part of the vocal cord. As we get older, small calcified elements caused by arthritis can form on it. Like the knee or the shoulder joint, the arytenoid is involved in a synovial joint. Thanks to its pyramidal shape, it slides, pivots, rolls, and rocks physiologically over the cricoid to allow glottal movement. It can be weakened or altered by an affliction, an inflammation, an ankylosis or a postoperative trauma following an endotracheal tube under general anesthesia. These afflictions diminish the mobility of the joint. The voice's timbre is affected, voice strain settles in and swallowing becomes difficult.

The larynx becomes stronger with age

From birth until adulthood

From birth until adulthood, our laryngeal instrument transforms itself and evolves. Puberty causes profound changes in men. By the age of 20, calcification of the thyroid cartilage has created a fully formed Adam's apple. There are also signs of calcification in the cricoid in both boys and girls. Its calcification is complete between the ages of 24 and 38. In men, the angle of the thyroid cartilage is more closed. It becomes hard, ossified. Its outlines are sharper, more prominent, straighter. It enables the development of greater vocal energy as the years go by. This is vital for singers, comedians, or lawyers. The laryngeal muscles insert onto a calcified surface, be it the thyroid or the cricoid. This provides them with excellent grip, greater stability, and more precise control of the vocal cord movements.

In women, the key cartilages of the larynx evolve differently. Around age 30, the thyroid cartilage shows signs of ossification. The protective shield has adopted a more open angle. The larynx is rounder, its lines more curbed, the angle formed by the vocal cords is more open. By the menopause, around the ages of 50 to 55, the thyroid and cricoid cartilages are 50% calcified.

The larynx and vocal training

The agility of the laryngeal joint and the development of the laryngeal muscles come with training. This applies as much to the variety singer as to the opera singer, the comedian, the lawyer, the politician, or the salesman. Although these voice professionals all make intensive use of their voice, their requirements in the vocal field aren't the same. By analogy, after five to eight years of competitive training, the crawl swimmer and the breaststroke swimmer have a different morphology; their athletic respiratory resistance is similar, but the two styles have honed different muscles. For any voice professional, the importance of systematic vocal training, at any age, cannot be overemphasized.

The thyroid and cricoid cartilages are joined by an articulation that is highly developed in singers. It allows the larynx to rock and facilitates the passage from high to low frequencies. Put your hand on your larynx or Adam's apple and sing an *i*, first in a high pitch, then in a low pitch: you should feel your thyroid cartilage going up, then down. This is made possible by the joint between the two cartilages (the cricoid and the thyroid). This maneuver enabled the cricothyroid cartilage to tighten (for the high frequency) then to slacken (for the low frequency).

We have just described the solid structures of our laryngeal instrument, which you can think of as the hull of our vibratory vessel. Let's not forget the epiglottis, the fibrocartilaginous lamina that caps the larynx. It us made fast by two ligaments that stretch out from the arytenoids, looking like the stays holding up the mast of a ship.

Honor to whom honor is due: the vocal cords; their private life—acquired or innate?

Two strings and a nail

The left and right vocal cords insert at the front into the angle formed by the thyroid cartilage, where its two immobile wings join up. They are solidly attached to this meeting point. At the back, they insert into the arytenoids, which are mobile. To get a better idea of their shape, imagine a nail to which two strings are attached. The attachment point at the front fixes the strings. They can only spread open at the back. This creates a horizontal V that opens and closes at the back. The V of our vocal cords closes to enable us to cough, swallow, sneeze, cry, sing, or talk. It opens to enable us to breathe.

A specific stage of development

What is the intimate secret of our vocal cord? The synchronicity of the two cords is perfect, just like that of our eye globes. When one moves, the other moves in exactly the same way. Before acquiring their adult dimension, they grow and change up until puberty. In the two-year-old, the vocal cord is 6- to 8-mm long. By the age of nine, the cord is 12-mm long, by puberty, it's 14-mm long. But don't expect equality between the sexes here. Women's vocal cords are on average 17-mm long and 3-mm wide; men's are on average 24-mm long and 4-mm wide (see Plate 17). Yet in our clinic, we have seen male bass singers with vocal cords that are 26 or 27-mm long, and female alto singers with vocal cords that are 20-mm long.

The extraordinary structure of the cover of the vocal cords: the mystery of the vibrations

The muscle of the vocal cord is striated, just like the biceps. It gives height and power to the voice. The cordal muscle is covered by an epithelium layer that enables it to vibrate. This mucous membrane, or epithelium, consists of two layers of cells, as it does in other mammals, until we reach our ninth or tenth birthday. Then, after puberty, a third layer of cells forms.

Man's cordal epithelium, with its free edge formed by a complex cellular structure with three distinct layers, is therefore unique in the mammal world. Dogs, for example, have an epithelium with only two layers. Maybe that's why they rarely lose their voice. It's a fact that polyps of the vocal cord are very rare among dogs and children.

Certain cordal lesions change between childhood and adolescence. This happens with nodules. Because the vocal cord continues to grow until puberty, and sometimes even later, a nodule is very rarely operated on in a child. Its frequency in little boys and little girls is the same. But after adolescence, over 99% of boys no longer have nodules, compared to 60% of girls. Mother nature has been at work. A posteriori, this is as it should be. The vocal cords have grown, the third layer of the epithelium has restructured them.

But the vocal cord is not just a striated muscle and a mucous membrane. It's a little more complex than that. In the 1990s, Steven Gray discovered the secret of our extraordinary vocal suppleness and of the agility of both the cordal muscle and the cordal mucous membrane. This noble part of the mucous membrane and its submucosal layers contains elastic fibers (in addition to muscle fibers) that underpin the quality of the vibration, collagen fibers that guarantee tissue nutrition, and also some things called proteoglycans, veritable molecular springs between these fibers. These molecules absorb vibratory shocks in order to give them better thrust, amplifying them like a trampoline or a spring mattress.

The cordal mucous membrane slides on the thyroarytenoid muscle (the vocal cord muscle) thanks to a space known as "Reinke's space." This natural exploit is conditioned by the laminar structure of this submucosal area. The expelled air mobilizes it, makes it slide, vibrate, undulate on the underlying tissue. For comparison's sake, pinch the skin on top of a finger joint. Hold the skin tightly between your fingers as you move it about; notice how supple it is as it slides over the muscle. If the joint were inflamed, the skin would lose this suppleness, and you could only partially bend or extend a finger. The agility would be altered. Worse still is when a wound causes retractile scarring; then the skin can't even be pinched, it remains stuck to the muscle, flexing the fingers becomes difficult, if at all possible. This agility is also altered after a burn trauma. It's the same with your vocal cords: you lose your voice when the mucous membrane stays stuck to the muscle, it's then lost its agility. Unable to slide, it can no longer vibrate correctly in relation to the underlying structures. Thus, a beautiful voice is only possible if the mucous membrane of the vocal cords is well hydrated, tonic, and supple. It must be able to vibrate along the whole length of the vocal cord, without any adherence. So the vocal cord possesses a mucous membrane, a space that enables it to slide, a ligament with a lamellar structure and a striated vocal muscle.

What role does genetics play?

The vocal cord is submitted to the influence of genetic factors. Nodules and "furrows" called *sulci vocalis* on the vocal cords (anomalies of the mucous membrane that alter the vibration) can be hereditary, just as they can be a cultural phenomenon. Intensive stimulation of the mucous membrane in a population at risk can bring about an alteration of the vocal cords. In these families, the synthesis of the collagen and elastin fibers has a low threshold of resistance to vocal effort. Language structure and musicality are also important.

Anna: "My voice splits in two."

Young Anna is 21. Her voice has been husky since childhood. It is weak and sometimes produces two vibrations simultaneously. "My voice splits in two," as she puts it. Her work brings her into contact with people. Her voice is now a handicap to her. Both her vocal cords display a furrow (sulcus vocalis), a malformation of the mucosal and submucosal membranes, which have not developed properly during her childhood. I detect a deficiency in the vibration, in the sliding undulation over the vocal muscle; also, the epithelium has only two layers, instead of the usual three. Has nature not completed its work? Anna informs me that her two young brothers, Pierre, 21, and Bertrand, 12, as well as her father, also have unusual voices. Having examined the family, I find that they all display, to varying degrees, the same malformation of the cordal mucosal and submucosal membranes. There's a genetic anomaly at work here, with a variable penetrance of the gene; the mother's voice is normal. Despite numerous speech therapy sessions, there is no improvement in Anna's and Pierre's voices. The mucous membrane is too affected. I operate on them in order to inject a substance that will recreate a sliding space between the muscle and the only existing mucous layer. The injection works well. Reinke's space, the sliding zone between the muscle and the submucosal layer, is reinstituted. Pierre's and Anna's voices are greatly improved. Thus microsurgery of the vocal cords can at least partially correct Mother Nature's omissions. This surgical option is very important given the worldwide rise of the media and verbal communication in this day and age.

Sanchi, a Brahman priest, and the Ganges delta

This anecdote brings to mind a trip I made to India, during which I ended up operating on several families that presented this very same pathology, all from the region of Bengal. In February 2003, I arrived in Pune, a town about 150 km from Bombay, to attend a congress during which I was to demonstrate operating techniques at the University Hospital. The people brought to me to be examined all showed the same anomaly of the vocal cords as Anna, namely a furrow or *sulcus vocalis*. Their voices were hoarse, chopped up by frequent vibratory cuts. Why this sudden desire for a cure, for a different voice? The congress may have stimulated the demand, but I felt there was more to it. These patients had known each other for years, their ties went back over several generations. They lived in one of the sacred regions of India, a humid region bathed by the Ganges delta. What had happened? Were their voices abnormal? But with respect to what, or to whom?

Bombarded by the media, invaded by the Western world, and by films and ads portraying actors with clear voices, certain groups of this Bengalese population had experienced a shift in values. Of the people I had examined, I only operated on one-third, namely people whose voices were inaudible and a real handicap to them. The other two-thirds weren't really handicapped by their voices in their day-to-day activities, their motivations were more worldly, driven by fashion. Their voice was normal in relation to the family members accompanying them. There was, therefore, no reason for me to change their verbal personality.

All seemed simple enough.

Then one Wednesday morning, around 10 AM, enters one Sir Sanchi, 81 years old, dressed in a *dotii* (a beige and white robe), and sporting a *tika* (a red mark on the forehead). "Good morning," he greets me. His voice is hoarse, his English very pure. His head is wagging gently, his hands are joined palm against palm. A beige-white rope running from hip to shoulder indicates him to be a Brahman priest and emphasizes his noble, slim figure. I'm impressed by his stature—1.90 m—and his piercing gaze. He follows my every gesture, my every word. "My voice bothers me in my prayers, in my daily activities," he tells me. His four children are at his side. They share his opinion and confirm his predicament. "How long have you been like this?" "Nearly eleven years, after straining my voice singing," he answers. He sits in the examination chair on the sixth floor of the hospital. I have there all the instruments I need to make a precise diagnostic. In case of need, the ceiling fan in the light blue room, worthy of a Humphrey Bogart film with its peculiar atmosphere, is my link with Asia in this scientific and medical environment. I detect a furrow on Sanchi's left vocal cord. His age and a scar due to an earlier trauma have probably altered his voice. There's undoubtedly a family predisposition at work, as his son also has a husky voice. What am I to do? A detail reveals the answer to me. He explains: "I would like to have a clear voice, I've never really had one, also less dryness. *Atcha*? (which means okay)" An operation would change his voice, upset his emotional world, and interfere with his internal vibration. I explain my reticence to operate him and ask him to consult with his family. I'm wary of operating on his voice, so perfectly suited to the spirituality emanating from this Brahman priest. A voice unusually charged with emotion. His veiled, feeble voice fits his persona, dominated by affect. The next morning, he agrees with my decision. I'm not to operate on him. He and his family thank me. Sanchi specifies: "It's true, my voice carries the scars of this life." By this, he meant no doubt, given the spiritual context of his life, that his reincarnation in a future life would keep the vibratory print of his present life.

The alteration to the mucous membrane of Sanchi's vocal cord probably ensued after a hematoma that had caused retractile scarring of the cord and destroyed the vibratory sliding space. There remained the question of the dryness of his throat. Loss of lubrication might have caused this. With advancing age, it can bring about vocal fatigue. It is the same with our eyes; if there are no tears to wet them, they become dry. This causes microulceration of the cornea, as well as keratitis (an inflammation of the cornea) and conjunctivitis. The same phenomenon can occur with respect to the vocal cords. Calluses form on the cordal mucous membrane, which can become ulcerated and may form a polyp. Where nature has provided us with tears for our eyes, for our vocal cords it has provided us with glandular cells above and below the cords. These cells keep the mucous membrane moist without inundating it. At times, these glandular cells are on the vocal cords themselves, causing cysts to develop. In Sanchi's case, with advancing years, the glandular cells had diminished in number, causing his throat to be often dry.

In Anna's case, an operation was justified because her social life was affected; operating on Sanchi would have altered his personality, and, therefore, was not justified.

The breath, energy source of the voice

A cathedral-like apparatus

Looking at the voice, you have the impression you are looking at a vocal cathedral. We've just described the vibratory heart of this cathedral, but its energy comes from our breath and breathing apparatus. Our lungs provide its energetic power.

We breathe in and breathe out in an incessant coming and going. This breathing begins in the lungs. It is activated by the elasticity of the lungs, by the diaphragm, the muscles of the thoracic cage, of the chest, of the abdomen, of the back, and pelvic basin. These complex elements enable air to be conveyed outward from the alveoli toward the bronchi and the trachea. The trachea ends at the point where the larynx meets the cricoid cartilage above it. An adult breathes in and out 17 times per minute. Each breathing cycle enables the man in the street to inhale 500 ml of air, whereas at rest, a singer inhales 1.5 liters (L).

The full capacity of the lungs, in other words the maximum amount of air you can force yourself to inhale and exhale, is 4 to 4.5 L for men and 3 to 3.5 L for women. In singers, the figure is 5.5 L for men and 4 L for women. However, some air always remains in the lungs. This residual lung capacity is around 1 liter. When you breathe normally, the inhalation and exhalation phases take up, respectively, 40% and 60% of the breathing cycle. But when you talk or sing, the breathing-in phase is much faster, much shorter. Then, it is only 10% of the breathing cycle. When you're talking, the exhalation phase takes up 90% of the cycle.

The air machinery: a masterpiece in voice professionals

You speak only while you exhale. The vocal cords have to change shape in order to emit different sounds and this interferes with the resistance to the air being expelled through the glottis, between the vocal cords. The bellows have to adapt themselves immediately if the voice is to remain stable and free of breaks between two different pitches. This fantastic "air machine" of ours, called a support by some, a prop by others, brings into play a variety of factors, the mechanism of which we're only just beginning to understand. The respiratory mechanism has to be working normally in order to expel air from the lungs. The command center for this is our spine, not our cranial nerves. (The spinal nerves radiate from the nervous system of this vertebral axis. These same nerves, arising between the third cervical vertebra and the second lumbar vertebra, command the complex respiratory structure of our organism.) Well known to opera singers, the abdominal girth muscles and the perineal muscles that are under the control of these spinal nerves contribute to the power of the sung voice. Singers have to learn how to work these specific muscles in order to develop them for singing.

The power of singers' voices and the length of their career is determined in part by their vibratory body, the larynx, but also, and more importantly, by their mastery of their breathing. The bellows are located in the thorax, a vast cavity with little room for fat or muscles. All is ready to welcome the voice's energy: air. Tiny little intercostal muscles surround the left and right lungs, which are large and elastic. This muscular network is an architectural structure of high precision. This retinue of striated muscles, which are under our voluntary control (all striated muscles, except the heart, are under our voluntary control), is completed at the front by the pectorals, level with the breasts; at the back, by the trapezium, located high up, above the thorax.

As for the part above the diaphragm, the thorax, is a marvel of nature. The usual name for it is the thoracic cage. It's composed of 12 pairs of ribs centered on the sternum at the front and on the spine at the back. The insertion point between the ribs and the sternum is elastic and supple; it only calcifies around the age of 60. At the top, the thoracic cage is overhung by the clavicles. At the bottom are two floating ribs (the two lowest ribs of the thorax). Voice professionals, and especially lyrical singers, have a thoracic cage that's shaped like an upside-down cone. It usually presents a very slight narrowing above the two floating ribs. The thoracic cage is a two-time mechanism: an exhalation phase accompanied by tightening, compression and constriction and an inhalation phase accompanied by dilation and expansion. Everything is synchronized to minimize energy consumption while maximizing efficacy.

The left lung is smaller than the right lung, because it accommodates the heart. The functional unit of the lung is the alveolus, the last bulwark between air and the inside of our body. It is an energy factory that extracts oxygen. The alveoli are tied to small bronchioles that are, in turn, tied to their source bronchi. The source bronchi are below the trachea. The trachea, 10-cm long and 2-cm wide, is formed at the front by a cartilaginous half-ring. This cartilage acts as a shield. This half-ring joins up with its posterior half, which is supple and elastic, not rigid, to form a complete circle. But the posterior half can dilate when we cough, shout, or sing. An inflammation of the trachea or the esophagus can constrict this part of the trachea. Tracheitis or mucus can make our breathing loud and wheezy, and affect the voice. When we speak, as we only speak during the exhalation phase, this mucus can make its way up to the vocal cords and cause a coughing fit.

Harmony in our breathing rhythm

The inhalation and exhalation phases are accompanied by a sliding motion of our lungs in the thoracic cage. This all happens harmoniously thanks to the pleura, a thin serous lamina that allows this incessant coming and going to carry on unhampered, averaging 17 inhalations and 17 exhalations per minute, or 34 thoracic lung movements in total. A simple infection of the pleura brings on pleurisy, which makes breathing difficult and singing impossible. Practicing a sport that harmonizes breathing and muscular effort is really important. Our bellows enable our wind and string instrument to work. All of its muscles, be they the intercostal, abdominal, or perineal muscles, participate in expanding the thorax. Inhalation is an active phenomenon, the diaphragm then sinks down and the thoracic cage expands. Exhalation is a passive phenomenon, a natural consequence of the elasticity of our respiratory structures. Is the last breath we take not an exhalation, and the very first, an inhalation?

We inhale through the nose or through the mouth. When we sing, the inhalation is shorter. The quality of the inhalation is reflected in the timbre of the voice. However, when we sing the exhalation is longer, it can last 20 to 45 seconds. Voice qualities such as intensity, timber, and regularity depend on perfect control of the exhalation. Singers are people with a perfect mastery of their wind-machine, their oxygen factory, their rhythm, and their vocal cadence. The normally passive exhalation phase becomes active, mastered, and controlled during voicing. Asthma can upset the voice; it's a pulmonary disease that takes our breath hostage and thus kidnaps our vocal power.

The diaphragm: frontier of the thoracic and the abdominal world

The diaphragm is a muscular-membranous lamina fine in the center and thick on the periphery. It inserts itself all along the bottom of the thoracic cage. Thus, it separates the thorax from the abdominal cavity, providing perfect insulation. A few holes in it allow vessels and the esophagus through, without this affecting its efficiency in any way. The heart and the two lungs rest on the diaphragm. The digestive organs and the liver lie beneath it. Thus, a weakness of the diaphragmatic orifice, where the stomach meets with the esophagus, allows the infamous hiatal hernia through. This happens frequently in people over the age of 55 (due to a weakening of the diaphragmatic muscle) and provokes gastroesophageal reflux. Acid flows up from the stomach toward the esophagus and up to the larynx. Its acidity can burn the vocal cords and provoke laryngitis. This acidic reflux is a cause of voice strain and frequent clearing of the throat, which is painful for the person doing it, but also for people in the immediate vicinity. This reflux can bring on chronic coughing, called sometimes "nervous" coughing. When you are stressed, the stomach contracts and produces more acidity than necessary. The reflux becomes chronic and causes the vocal cords to dry out.

Indigestion can upset the voice

It's often said that we breathe with our stomach. The strap that surrounds the abdomen is made up of many muscles, called the abdominal muscles. The abdominal wall deserves its name. It controls our breathing. But we have to learn to use it, to build it up. The abdomen contains our digestive organs. An upset stomach, a bad meal, or indigestion prevent us from being fully functional, we're beset by flatulence and colic. The diaphragm sits atop these organs. Therefore it is perturbed by these intestinal happenings. Abdominal breathing is hindered and can be painful. The pelvis just below the navel also plays an indispensable role in vocal control. A woman's voice can be perturbed by painful menses, a sensitive ovarian cyst, or a uterine fibroma, which, if large, can interfere with the muscles of the pelvic floor. There again, menstrual pains radiating into the lumbar region, the groin, and the navel can make singing difficult. Does the pelvis not provide support for singing a counter *ut*?

The power of the breath of the voice

On stage, facing their public, singers are perfectly aware of the importance of breathing and of a braced posture. Suppleness of the lungs and elasticity of the diaphragm are crucial. Singing teachers often tell their pupils to brace their pelvis to be firmly rooted to the ground. The pelvis is the receptacle for the energy behind vocal power. The ring of muscles formed by it supports the female uterus. It enables the impressive surge of vocal energy of the tenor. The perineum is no larger than the palm of a hand, but it's the seat of strong elastic muscular resistance. Did some singers not say to Dr. Wickart, Clemenceau's renowned laryngologist, in the 1920s: "Wait till you hear the pair of B flats I'm going to pump out in the second act!" The inspiration—both lyrical and erotic—for this promise, derives from the sensation of resistance that tenors experience when producing a *B* flat. They draw their vocal power from their perineum. The *B* flat is without a doubt one of the most difficult notes to sing; it can even give singers a fleeting impression of vertigo. The whole body vibrates.

A vertical posture is a *sine qua non* for a beautiful singing voice. The major contributor to this verticality is the bony framework provided by the cervical, thoracic, and lumbar spine. It provides a solid edifice to which the body's muscle trains are attached, much like the mast of a ship with its sails and roping gear, and this allows the pneumophonic tube to develop maximal efficacy. But once she has acquired the technique, Violeta sings magnificently and with a lot of emotion, even though she is lying down.

How sound becomes voice: the resonators

The story of a string, a hole, an empty room and a piano

In 1840, in Munich, Professor Pellisson takes a string from his piano and fixes it to his bedroom wall. He pinches it and gets little response. He goes next door. He makes a small hole in the wall, level with the string, and places the piano's resonance box against the hole. He returns to his room. He pinches the string. This time he hears a superb sound that's recognizable as coming from a piano. Proof, indeed, that the piano string alone is not sufficient and that the resonance box is an indispensable item.

One of his colleagues has a similar idea, though easier to carry out. In his acoustic laboratory, he takes a single violin string and fixes it between two nails. He slides the bow over it, to no avail. Precious little can be heard. He surreptitiously brings close the resonance box of a violin made by him. The sound produced is mediocre. He does the same with a Stradivarius: the sound produced is sublime. Proof, this time, that though the resonance box is important, the quality of the resonance box is primordial. The Stradivarius admirably reinforces the vibration of the four strings. Nothing can beat its resonance.

As extraordinary as it may seem, man's vocal cord presents analogies with the Stradivarius. This violin has a unique design. Its belly is in spruce, its inner lining is of maple wood. The distance between these two boards is remarkably precise. They are joined together by an odd piece of wood called the sound-post. Together, the 83 pieces that make up this violin, perfected by the violin makers of Cremona in the 17th century, create harmony and form a majestic sound amplifier. The resonance is heightened by the fibrous and linear composition of spruce, which enhances the propagation of the vibration.

The human vocal cord presents an analogous structure. Here too we find fibers. They are numerous and lie parallel to the vocal cord. These collagen and elastin fibers, linked together by proteoglycan molecules, play an essential role in the quality of the laryngeal sound. Nature has ensured that the mucous membrane that produces the vibration of the vocal cord is endowed with a submucosal layer that reinforces its resonance. This is the first resonance chamber of the human voice.

Hi-fi, resonance, and harmonics

Resonance chambers behave exactly like your hi-fi when it receives the fundamental tone of the singer you are listening to on the radio. The radio doesn't alter the fundamental tones of the melody, but its equalizer acts on certain of the low, medium, or high harmonics by stressing them or diminishing them with acoustic filters. The song sounds more pleasing to the ear because the musical timbre has been modified, but the musicality is unchanged. This is the role of resonators, they stress certain harmonics and change the vocal timbre. The harmonics are influenced by the mold of the resonators. These natural acoustic filters can change shape—the pharynx can contract or dilate, the velum can lift up or lengthen, the tongue can lengthen or pull back—and are modified by the moisture of the mucous membrane that lines the resonator and plays a determining role, both in the reverberation of sound and in its relievo, before it takes its final shape at the lips. The resonators have two roles: on the one hand they form the harmonics, as we have seen; on the other, they form our articulated language, our vowels and our consonants.

Vowels are proper to Man

Vowels are the indispensable link between consonants that enables the production of a word. They are the fundamental building blocks of the voice. We must differentiate two types of vowels: the first is a direct result of a change in length of our resonance chamber, as when *a* and *o* become *ou* (see Plate 18). The second is more the consequence of different movements of the tongue, as in *e* and *i*. The vocal spectrograph or sonograph, first described by Edison in 1896, allows vowels to be analyzed precisely with reference to their different harmonics and intensity.

A vowel creates several harmonics. All harmonics do not have equal strength. Some come across as louder, more audible, more distinct thanks to the resonators. Each vowel produces an amplification of certain harmonics and formants that is specific to that vowel and defines it.

Formants are the fingerprints of the vowel. They are different for an *a*, an *e*, an *i*, an *o*, or an *ou*. All vowels have two formants that are more marked.

The vowel *a* has four formants, of which the third and fourth are intense. It requires complete closure of the pharynx by the velum. The air is expelled only through the mouth as the nasal fossa are closed. The tongue lies flat on the mandible, allowing the formants to blossom forth maximally.

The vowels of professional singers all have four formants. The third and fourth formants are less intense, more fragile, more tenuous, sharper, and this gives charm and warmth to the sound and enriches its timbre. Formants enable singers to project their voices beyond the front rows and to be heard over 20 meters away. When the recordings of tenors are analyzed, the remarkable strength of all four formants, and not just the first two, is obvious. Formants evolve with the passing of years; they become richer between the ages of 20 and 50 and decline after the age of 60. There's a loss of suppleness, the buccopharyngeal agility decreases, the muscles and mucous membrane lose mass. The loss is more obvious if vocal training is abandoned.

Consonants

Like vowels, consonants are formed in the resonators during exhalation. But they are not, strictly speaking, vibrations. They create sounds, more specifically, irregular sounds with few harmonics. During speech, their duration is variable, in the sung voice they're brief or very brief.

Two different mechanisms produce consonants: an explosion of air between two elements of our resonance chamber or an incomplete closure between two elements of the resonance chamber.

In French, acoustically speaking, there are three main types of consonants: fricatives, sibilants, and nasals. When they precede a vowel, they're long, as in "ma*mmmm*an." The consonant sound is regular and variable. It can superimpose itself to the fundamental tone in what is known as voicing, because the vibration of the vocal cords contributes to the production of the consonant, as in *v*, *z*, or *m*. Here, the consonant sound is accompanied by the vibration of the vocal cords as they approach each other. The fundamental tone then helps to distinguish the consonant better. Consider "zoo" and "Sue," "veil" and "fail."

Some consonants can seem tricky. Imitators make use of them, not to mention certain comedians, such as Louis Jouvet and Roger Blin, who stuttered and used their handicap to advantage to make it their personal stamp. Indeed, their vocal rhythm and pronunciation are very distinctive. A case in point is Louis Jouvet's "Hhello (microsilence) mmadam."

In English, consonants are plosive: *p*, *b*, *t*, *d*, *k*, *g*; fricative: *f*, *v*, *s*, *z*, *h*; or nasal: *n*, *m*, *ng*. Plosives produce a brief and intense sound, lasting around 15 milliseconds. They have no harmonics. In comparison, the vowel following a plosive lasts 1 to 2 seconds.

Some consonants are produced not only by the resonator, but also by to a quick opening and closing of the vocal cords. These are called "voiced" consonants, as opposed to "voiceless" consonants, which are produced with the vocal cords open. Some consonants are inaudible and voiceless, like *w* in *who*; others are inaudible and voiced, like *w* in *we*, also *r, w, l, m, n, ng*.

Plosives can smack the lips together, producing the bilabial consonants *p, b,* and *m*; however, *m* is softer, more sustained, not as explosive. *F* and *v*, produced between the teeth and the lips, are called labiodental.

Some consonants bring the tongue into play: *t, d, s, z, n,* and *l* are alveolar consonants, they bring the tip of the tongue in contact with the alveolar ridge; *th* or *the*, the dental consonants, are produced with the tongue between the teeth; *k, g,* and *ng,* the velar nasal consonants, solicit the velum.

The soft *r* as in *rear* is produced with the tip of the tongue curled somewhat back behind the alveolar ridge and approaching the roof of the mouth, which is hard and can't vibrate. This is a retroflex consonant, not to be confused with the rolled *r* found in Spanish, which is formed between the tongue and the posterior part of the velum and uvula, both of which are supple and able to vibrate. Thus it is that if the uvula is removed surgically to prevent snoring, a rolled *r* is no longer possible.

To be a musician or to snore: it's one or the other

Jean-Pierre, his hunting horn and his peaceful nights

Jean-Pierre is an international lawyer. He snores so loudly that his wife is considering adopting separate sleeping quarters. This voice pro decides to undergo an operation. He consults a colleague and is operated on to relieve the snoring and allow his wife to get a good night's sleep again. The operation removes the uvula and a part of the soft palate (see Plate 19). Weeks pass by. His wife is sleeping well again, he no longer snores, the intervention has been a success.

Nevertheless, a few months later he comes to consult me for the first time. "After half an hour of pleading, my voice tires, instead of concentrating on what I'm going to say, I find myself wondering how I'm going to get through to the end of the session." But the request of this very charming man gets more original: "My throat becomes dry, I often speak Spanish with my clients and I find that

I can't roll my *r* anymore. But Doctor, it gets worse, and this is ruining my life."

He pales, a light sweat pearls his forehead: "Please go on." He gets his breath back: "I love music and I play the hunting horn, but not since the operation. However hard I try, I can't get a sound out. All the power of my exhalation goes out through my nose. I get the impression that my mouth is no longer insulated, that somehow the surgery removed the separation between the back of my throat, my nose, and my mouth." He opens the case beside him and takes out a superb hunting horn. He shows it off as if it were a piece of art, then tries to play it. Indeed, no sound comes out. The description of his pathology is worthy of a clinical case study. Fibroscopic analysis of the area operated on reveals nothing untoward. Technically speaking, the surgery was performed correctly. Thus, the uvula has gone, the soft palate is retracted, it's dry and has lost its lubrication. But I want to understand the mechanics of the velum better and bring to light all the factors pertaining to his mute performance with the hunting horn.

I decide to observe him through the endovideoscope, which is introduced through the nose and slides through to the back of the nasal fossa, over the velum and its scar. I ask him to play and to try really hard to produce a sound with his hunting horn. Impossible! What has happened here?

His spoken voice is satisfactory. The dryness of his throat is to be expected, as the surgery has removed one of the most important lubricants of the resonance chamber, namely the uvula. Located in the center of vocal cathedral, it permanently moisturizes its surroundings with a fine spray. The rolled *r* is produced through the vibration of the uvula and its contact with the wall of the pharynx at the back, therefore his present inability to speak Spanish properly is perfectly logical, as his snoring was caused by the strong vibration of the uvula in contact with the pharynx. But there's more to come. After hearing my explanations on how and why his problem has arisen, he begs me: "Doctor, please make me a new uvula." The surgery had penalized the musician.

More precisely (the velum has two parts: a soft mobile part and an anterior, harder part that lines the bony roof of the palate), how do the uvula and the soft palate intervene when this wind instrument is played? I explain to Jean-Pierre that these two elements, the uvula and the soft palate, help to close the nasal fossa at the back. When the hunting horn or the oboe is played, the outward air stream arrives with full force into the mouthpiece during the exhalation. The pressure required to produce a sound on the hunting horn, the saxophone, the trumpet, or the clarinet is impressive (just check out Louis Armstrong's cheeks). It requires very precise control of the air pressure as the air is expelled. If the velum or the uvula can't completely close off the nasal fossa, as they should, as much as 5 to 50% of the air escapes through the nose. Beyond this percentage, the spoken voice becomes nasal, with the characteristic phonation presented by the hare-lipped child, who requires plastic surgery. This should not be confused with the quacky "Donald Duck" type of nasal voice that you typically develop when you catch a cold, or if subjected to sinusitis and have a deviated nasal septum.

Jean-Pierre's voice was perfectly satisfactory, but the nasal leakage, though mild, was sufficient to make it impossible for him to play his favorite instrument. He could no longer properly close off his oral cavity from his nasal cavity. Unfortunately, it is not possible to rebuild an uvula. As time goes by, the velum might recover some of its suppleness and enable this musician to indulge in his passion again.

To play the clarinet or to snore, it's one or the other

Jacques is an ardent lover of jazz music. He plays the clarinet remarkably well and has done so for many years. As chance would have it, he consults me on the same day as Jean-Pierre, and only an hour after him. His story could have been similar. This musician and lawyer snores loudly. His wife can't bear his snoring any longer. He has come to consult me about an operation of the velum. Which is it to be? It's one or the other: snore, or play the clarinet. He decided. I'll let you guess which he chose.

The voice echoes and blossoms in its inner cavern

Man's vocal cathedral is unique

It isn't immutable nor is it fixed; it can be modified and adapted. Man's voicing is created in the larynx, then moves upward in the aerial cavities of the resonators. The odyssey of the vibration begins level with the mucous membrane of the vocal cords, at the false vocal cords or ventricular bands. These are symmetric and meld with the vocal cords a few millimeters above them. The laryngeal ventricles are between them and the vocal cords. These ventricles are minute: 5 mm deep. They reinforce the vibration. They are too small to play an important part in the resonance chamber. However, they help to lubricate the vocal cords. The ventricular bands are vestiges from our evolution. We touched on their role and importance in chapter 2 on Evolution of the voice. Men can develop these ventricular bands. For example, if you do a lot of weightlifting, the ventricular bands are frequently solicited to create extra thoracic pressure on the air trapped in the lungs. This sport is absolutely not recommended for voice pros! These elements perturb the vibration on its ascension from the vocal cords, because the false vocal cords become too muscled and hypertrophic. The same applies if you play the oboe, the clarinet, or a similar instrument. To be both singer and oboe player or trumpet player is tough, unless you happen to be Louis Armstrong. He had an edema and a hypertrophy of the vocal cords, which explains his very unusual voice.

Let's pursue our path. We arrive in the resonance chamber unique to Man. Two materials compose it: rigid resonators made of bone and cartilage, namely, the sinuses, the nasal septum. The mastoids (a bone of the cranium located at the base of the ear). The malleable, supple, extensible, and compressible resonators are the nasal fossa, the tongue, the pharynx, the mouth, and the larynx. These supple cavities modulate, deform, and sculpt the sound that becomes voice. The movements of the inferior maxillary and the tongue are by far the elements that most modify our resonance chamber, together with our lips.

The palate includes the soft palate, which is a posterior extension of the hard palate, and which forms the percussion surface of the resonance chamber. It is this surface that reflects the vibrations created by the vocal cords. At the back and above the uvula is a small cavity, the cavum, seat of the adenoids, small lymphoid growths in the nasopharynx. The adenoids normally disappear around the age of seven. If they don't, the voice becomes nasal and they cause mucus to form, which drips into the throat. If you block your nose, the vibratory wave no longer reaches the upper resonator. This dampens the sound produced, because no harmonic is able to blossom in the upper half of the face. A deviation of the nasal septum can have the same consequences.

Claudine cures her sinusitis by singing

Claudine, a soprano coloratura, takes care of her sinuses in a most unexpected way. This professional singer in her forties consults me because her voice has been bothered by mucous fluid on her vocal cords. This problem arises every spring and autumn. "As you know, for years now I've been bothered for two to three weeks in April and in October. But this time I've had the problem since the beginning of April (we are now in June). Also my sinuses are hurting, just below the eyes. I didn't come to see you earlier because I normally manage to clear it in 48 hours with some specific singing exercises. This time it hasn't worked." I must admit I was a bit perplexed as to how singing exercises could clear sinusitis, if that's indeed what she'd had. I asked her for more details. "When practicing certain vocalizations in a low frequency, I could feel a vibration in the sinuses and a stream of mucous fluid would slide from the sinuses into the front and back of my nose." This soprano had literally created a specific resonance in the bony walls of the maxillary sinuses and these frequencies had encouraged the evacuation of intrasinusal fluid, in the same way that grains of sand move in the same direction and homogeneously across the surface of a table when subjected to vibrations that have a specific rhythm.

Lowering a spy-microphone into the sinuses and throat: do we hear something?

What sounds are produced in the sinuses when we sing or talk? In the 1990s, it occurred to me to place a miniature microphone on the end of the Pentax videofibroscope. I then explored the left and the right sinuses. This enabled me to register the spoken and sung voices of ten singers of both sexes. The interior of their sinusal cavities is clean, empty, filled with air at ambient pressure. In other words, their sinuses are normal. Let's not forget that the sinuses present numerous resonance chambers. These include the maxillary sinus we're about to explore, also the frontal ethmoidal and sphenoidal sinuses. The latter isn't bilateral.

I'm eager to listen to sound from within the body. I delicately introduce the videofibroscope and its companion spy-microphone into the nasal fossa, then into the sinus. The recording begins. Each singer is asked to sing the same sentence from a well-known song. "Frère Jacques, Frère Jacques / Dormez-vous, dormez-vous? / Sonnez les matines, sonnez les matines . . . " The sound waves are analyzed in real time by the sonograph in an attempt to elucidate the mysteries of the facial harmonics. We record the sentence, first spoken, then sung. The result is surprising. The sinus was silent in all ten singers. The bone wall vibrates, for sure, but the interior of the "sinusal home" is sound-insulated (see Plate 20). I'm so taken aback that I repeat all the tests.

As Claudine just demonstrated to us, the bony wall is indeed isolated and has its own vibration. This may seem paradoxical, considering the number of times you hear singing teachers exhort their pupils to "project your voice into the facial mask." Yet there's nothing paradoxical about this exhortation. Set a tuning fork vibrating, stand it on your desk: your desk will resonate, which goes to show that the metaphor of projecting one's voice into the head is perfectly justified.

This scientific experiment takes me further down the path of understanding vocal vibrations. I lower my spy-microphone down to 5 mm above the vocal cords, right in the den of the larynx, where the voice is born. I ask these artists, who are exploring the "inner voice" with me, to say *a - e - i - o - u*, then repeat both spoken and sung versions of the sentence previously tested. What clues do you suppose the spy-microphone finds this time around? The sound brought back from this voyage into the body is even more unexpected: there's only one sonorous rendering of all five vowels and of the spoken and sung prose: "mmm," as when you hum with your lips closed. I bring the microphone up to the back of the velum: the vowels are barely audible here. I then place it in front of the velum, close to the tongue: the resonator has metamorphosed the "mmm," the vowels *a, e, i, o, u* are now plainly audible. In other words, without the resonators, the original sound emitted by the vocal cords is unintelligible.

The oral resonance cavity not only structures sounds during their ascension to give them voice, it also amplifies them. The more the resonator is able to make the best of its natural ability to amplify sound, the greater the quality and the power of the voice, and this for a minimum effort, without vocal strain. The sonorous fountain with its glottic source flows toward the front, toward the resonators. Its direction and shape will be modified most first by the epiglottis, then at the base of the tongue. Once past these humps in the internal landscape and into the anterior estuary, the vibratory flow can proceed unimpeded. It then bounces off the palate, roof of the mouth, palatine vault of the cathedral of our vocal instrument.

The tongue speaks with consonants and vowels

The tongue, which makes up the central part of our oral resonating chamber, is indispensable to the voicing process; it also plays a fundamental role in swallowing and equally in phonation. Without the tongue, no vowels, no consonants. Its agility is quite unique. Perfectly mobile anteriorly, it can move, change shape, curve, and lengthen at will. Its total mass is fixed, but the ways in which its volume is distributed in the resonance chamber are eminently variable.

The lyrical singer is well-acquainted with this phenomenon for having made use of it in numerous vocalizations. When the tip of the tongue becomes narrow and short, the back of the tongue becomes fatter. When the tongue spreads itself at the back of the inferior incisors, it seems smaller at the back. Thus, the greater the space taken up by the base of the tongue, the rounder the base, the farther back it drives the empty space above the vocal cords, and the more it diminishes the diameter of the vocal tract. Conversely, when an *a* is emitted with the mouth wide open, the tongue hunkers down flat behind the inferior incisors and the vocal tract is wide open. The singer then has maximal vocal power. When the base of the tongue moves backward and covers the larynx, the voiced sound is then accentuated. Of the stretching exercises for this region of our body's musculature, the one that best stretches the resonance chamber is yawning.

Lips: a "look" unique to Man

The lips produce the definitive phoneme and are at the frontier between our internal sonorous world and the external world of vibrations. Their appearance in Man is unique in the animal kingdom. Monkeys have lips that turn inward; they look more like discrete piping, with no sexual appeal for other monkeys. And Man? Only humans have lips that are turned outward, well-defined, and curvaceous. There are many anecdotes concerning women's lips. Certain fashion fads have dictated women's recourse to plastic surgery, to give their lips a sensuous and pulpous look through silicon injections. However, if not properly carried out, this "relooking" can sometimes perturb, modify, and alter the sung voice, especially with respect to consonants that require the lips to close, like b, f, p, or m. The lips finalize the phoneme. They're an essential contributor to the voice. The fact that one can lip-read is proof of this.

Teeth betray our voice's age

The mouth, exit of the voice, is demarcated by our teeth and lips. The mouth of an elderly person, if toothless and deformed, is no longer capable of forming certain phonemes. The lips stick to the gums and the tongue is unable to pronounce certain consonants. Dental hygiene is indispensable to keep a youthful voice, even if it means resorting to prosthetic solutions such as dental implants. Imitators wedge their lips between their teeth in a superb mimic of the way elderly people speak.

The instrument of the human voice is extraordinarily precise

The face, the voice, and the command

The face is a key part of the voice. Several dozen muscles assist in articulation, the main ones being around the lips and jaw. This edifice is under the control of our brain and an impressive armada of nerves that activate the mechanical lever of the resonators.

The great hypoglossal nerve (cranial nerve XII) gives the tongue its mobility and allows the formation of nearly all the consonants and all the vowels.

The trigeminal nerve (cranial nerve V) controls the mobility of the jaw. It modifies the spatial volume of our vocal tract. It also controls the sensitivity of the face.

The glossopharyngeal nerve (cranial nerve IX) controls the movements of the pharynx, part of the range of movement of the tongue, the mobility of the velum or soft palate, which influences the nasal quality of sounds, and its sensitivity. It also controls the production of saliva.

The pneumogastric nerve, also called the vagus nerve (cranial nerve X), controls the movements of the velum as well as the vocal cords. It also acts on the heart, blood vessels, lungs, and digestive tract. It's the nerve that reacts to stress. Reactions include gastric acidity and bile, a dry throat before speaking in public, a faster pulse before an important interview.

Finally, the facial nerve (cranial nerve VII) gives expression to the face, and controls the mobility of the lips, the final frontier of our vocal tract.

Of course, all this is subject to the very important role played by our breathing and by our abdominal muscles (this is the role overseen by the cranial nerve, that controls the movements of the neck and shoulder muscles, and by the spinal nerves, that control breathing and as well as other muscles).

A complex instrument for a complex emotional world

Singing, acting, pleading, or speaking in public require a vocal technique that's specific to each of these activities. A painting needs to convey emotion, but it is the end result of a technique that has guided the painter's hand on the canvas and has provided expression for his inspiration. In the same way, an actor or a lyrical singer must master the spoken voice or the sung voice. This mastery requires perfect knowledge of one's vocal instrument—only then can such knowledge be put at the service of one's emotions.

Chapter 10

From the affective
to the virtual

The myth of the virtual clone able to speak still exists.
But can emotions survive vocal cloning?

The first artificial voices: three hundred
years ago already

In the 18th century, scientists are fascinated by the concept of an artificial voice. Automatons of this period are equipped with human faces and a fake voice. Clock-making is at the height of its glory. Biomechanics produce the android. Each piece requires months of work, sometimes several years. The result is peculiar. The android performs for only a couple of minutes. Spectators are enthralled. In the 19th century, the magician Jean Eugène Robert-Houdin is without a doubt the best of his generation as regards the automatons he produces. They begin to disappear at the start of the 20th century, having kindled passions in the 18th century. Baron von Kempelen showed his first talking machine to the tsarina Catherine the Second of Russia. His passion for automatons led him to write a book on the human voice and its functioning. In his opinion, the reed used by many musical instruments resembles the human glottis (the reed can be single or double: if single, the piece of reed is placed on the mouthpiece, as in the case of the clarinet or the saxophone; if double, the piece of reed is folded over, as in the case of the oboe, and the player applies his lips to the reed and blows on it to make it vibrate). The Baron's machine can pronounce a few words, like "daddy," "mummy," "pantomime." He prefers to make it say a few words of Latin, French, or Italian, German being too difficult to reproduce. He has created his speaking machine out of a box, a rubber funnel that serves as the mouth, a second rubber tube that forms the nose, and an internal mechanism simulating the lungs: bellows. The tubes convey the air to the pseudo-mouth, which the Baron has equipped with a vibrating reed. A sound can be produced. A third lever modifies the resonators in the android's head. Abracadabra. The android "speaks."

The Abbot Mical, a renowned ecclesiastic eager to win the competition run by the Imperial Academy of Sciences in Saint Petersburg, manufactures two talking heads capable of producing sentences such as "the King brings peace to Europe." In this late 18th century, in which knowledge is taking precedence over religion, Lavoisier and Laplace witness the Abbot's scientific demonstration and are impressed by the talking heads. Aside from our two French scientists, however, everyone else thinks that, although the lips of the two heads move, the words that come out are often unintelligible and the voice is still harsh. Around 1850, an engineer from Grenoble, Jacques de Vaucanson, can't make his dream come true: he wants to make a speaking android. He manufactures a number of automatons, but none are to his liking.

These first mumbles of the robot demonstrate Man's fascination for the voice! We encounter this same fascination in numerous science-fiction writers, in today's films, in computer games. Androids still fascinate at the beginning of the 20th century, but techniques have evolved. Robots are able to express emotion. Artificial speech is well under control, but the robotic voice is still in its infancy. In a world increasingly sold on realism, the robotic voice must now bring to account vocabulary, syntax, and the expression of emotion.

The Golem: myth or reality

The frontier between mythology and fiction is a tenuous one. Between man and his cloned android, between Adam and the Golem, the mystery zone is thinning. The robot known as Hephaistos, son of Zeus and Hera, married to Aphrodite, is an inert mass of metal or clay. The word "robot" was first coined by the Czech writer Karel Čapek. It means in Czech: slave laborer. Man has been looking to control his own clone for years now, hankering after a manual technological extension of himself, as if transferring his ego to his creation. In mythology, the immortal gods make men, mortals who are in their service. Now Man wants to make his own puppets and play at being God. According to the 18th Song of the *Iliad*, in the eighth century B.C., Hephaistos was the first mortal to make his own robots, of which the best known are the two servants in gold who could think and speak and, therefore, could be considered human. Indeed, when we expect a robot to speak, we humanize it and want it to be intelligent. We're creating a being that's "almost" a living being.

In Psalm 139-16 of the Bible, Cain inscribed the word "*Emet*" on his forehead and uses the word "*golem*" in its original sense, which was "formless matter." The Golem was a human statue that also had the word "*Emet*," meaning "Truth," inscribed on its forehead. Take away one *e*, and it means "death." The legend of this clay giant that could not speak was revisited in the 15th century by the Chief Rabbi Loew of Prague, also called the Maharal of Prague. He would put a piece of paper in the mouth of the Golem with the Tetragramme written on it to make him work. Then, on Friday evenings, he would take it out of its mouth for the Shabbat. It was like loading a program in a computer! Still, today, many people visit his home.

The Golem is the Master's servant. He is mute. As history would have it, he grew inexorably. No longer could he control his strength. His destruction was unavoidable. His legend stresses the power of the word, the power of the voice, in relation to power over Life itself. The Golem obeys orders; therefore, he's just a clay slave whose only strength resides in his massive physique. The abstract, the word, thinking, have no place in his life. He doesn't have a life, because he doesn't have a language or a voice. Is the Golem not the ancestor of the automaton that Man wants to rule over? Is he not the ancestor of Pinocchio, who comes to life the day he's able to speak?

The artificial voice: emotion speaks through the imperfections of our voice

To synthesize the human voice as best as possible on a computer, we have to be familiar with all its mathematical formulas and have extracted and scored its melodic diagram. We need to understand not only the frequencies of the vocal expression, but also its silences. Then, through acoustic analysis, we can project onto curves thick and thin strokes representing the density of each fundamental element in the sound recording. When an *a* is voiced, the spectrograph displays several frequencies in different shades of gray. The computer is programmed to correlate each shade of gray with a specific frequency, a specific intensity, a characteristic noise. This vocal synthesis is represented three-dimensionally.

The spoken or sung language is not a succession of identical sounds. Consider the letter *a* in *daddy* and *father*: it's pronounced differently, yet the computer reproduces it as if the two were identical. Therefore, to artificially reproduce the exact phonetic representations of *a*, a succession of different phonemes have to be programmed in.

Pavel, a Russian orchestra leader I met at the end of the 1990s, is beginning to work on synthesized music. He tells me a surprising experiment. Basing himself on mathematical acoustic analysis, he synthesizes violins, cellos, the accordion, guitars, and so on. He programs a melody, then records it. He listens with tremendous sadness and a sense of failure: although the spectrograph's curve for this music is superb, the music grates the ear. Yet all is perfect—probably too perfect! All the *A* notes are precisely 440 Hz. All the violins have the exact same timbre. Such perfection is never achieved by an orchestra, usually the *A*s are either two hertz lower or two hertz higher, depending on the violin and on the degree of humidity in the studio. The fault lies with the recording, which could be a replica of a mathematical formula or a geometric curve. This isn't art any more—it's a photocopy. When Pavel leads his orchestra, he never gets the exact note twice over, never gets the same timbre out of an instrument. The genius of this artist was that he sensed and understood that this synthesized world was empty of all affect. Its error lay in its very perfection! He doesn't give up, he gets back to work. This time he adds a "chaotic" element to his virtual recording. He programs the computer to introduce a variation of plus or minus 2 to 4 Hz in relation to the desired note. The recording becomes human; it has recovered its emotional expression. Imperfection has enabled Pavel to make the music sound almost natural.

Dubbing: from the artist to the virtual

The spoken voice animates a synthesized character or a cartoon character. Dubbing brings these characters to life.

Dubbing artists are remarkable. They can take on the voice of a baby, of Mickey, Tintin, Bambi, or Peter Pan. Their partner is the cartoon strip. Finding just the right tone, the right timbre, the right affective silence that brings that extra something to the personality of the Lion King requires immense vocal creativity. The human voice makes these characters vibrate, makes them human, engaging. Real artistry is involved in this work, as evident by Luc Hamet's French interpretation of the impish Roger Rabbit: the vibration of his voice lends color and emotion to the character.

But the synthesized character can be given a synthesized voice. The study of the prosody of the voice when angry, when it smiles, when it's sad or happy, is the foundation of the virtual voice. The virtual voice requires that the mimics and lips of the protagonist be taken into account. The synchronicity between the voicing and facial expression during the filming of a cartoon strip is critical. The lips and facial mimics in the animated strip must reflect the melody and the sensitivity of the voice, and vice versa.

From the affective to the virtual—an achievement that hardly seemed possible fifteen years ago has come to fruition. The conceiver becomes the creator of a living virtual world. The computer alone contributes the image and the characters' voices. In its own binary language, it builds in the harmonics, the melody, the rhythm of the spoken or sung voice, its imperfections, accents, and silences, the facial expressions and character of the hero. But the prosody will differ according to the language used, according to whether the accent is from Marseille or from Paris, according to the words chosen to bring the idea alive. The number of parameters that have to be taken into account is just mind-boggling. That is the job of the master of the scenario.

In the 20th century, synthesized voices are found in an increasing number of applications: in cartoons, in automated messages on the telephone, on the Internet. If the synthesized voice is to move us, it can't be neutral. The fundamental harmonic alone isn't a sufficient indication of an individual's vocal print. The person's melody, vocabulary, and charm are essential ingredients. In the future, vocal synthesis will have to take these intangible parameters into account.

Part 2

Voice and Emotion

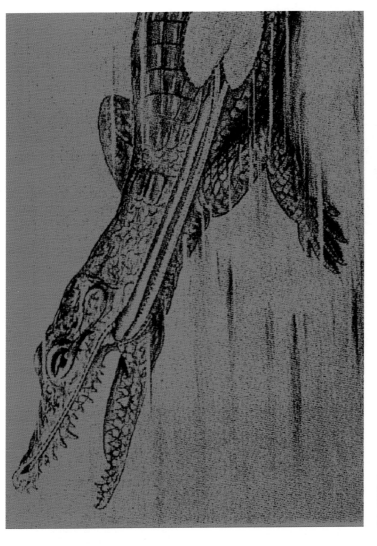

PLATE 1. The larynx protects the crocodile's lungs from the water. (Reproduced from the *Journal of Laryngology and Otology*, January 1931, with permission.)

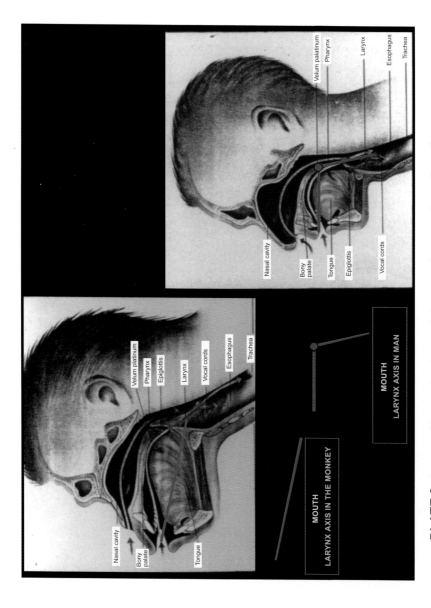

PLATE 2. Impact of increasing the angle between larynx and mouth on the resonators.

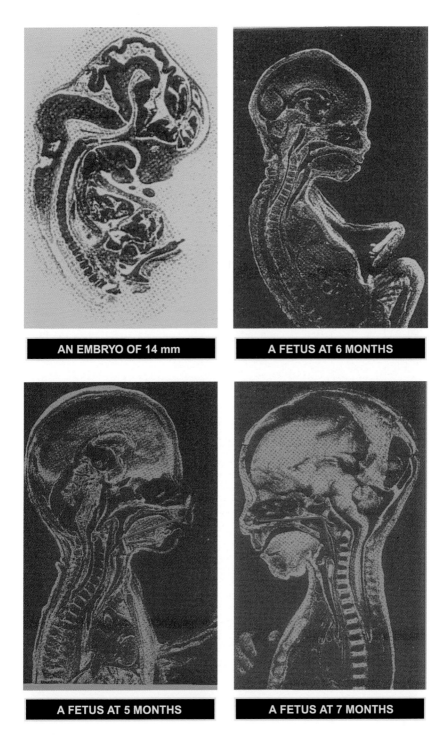

AN EMBRYO OF 14 mm

A FETUS AT 6 MONTHS

A FETUS AT 5 MONTHS

A FETUS AT 7 MONTHS

PLATE 3. A sagital view of the evolving angle between the mouth and the larynx in Man.

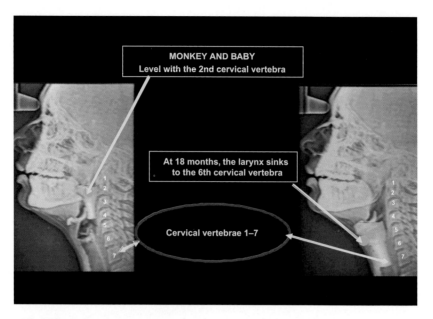

PLATE 4. The larynx descends from the 2nd cervical vertebra to the 5th.

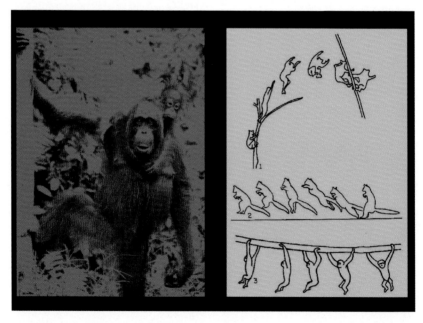

PLATE 5. Traction on the arms brings the upper part of the larynx into play.

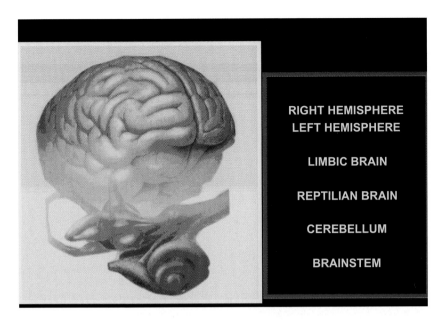

PLATE 6. Evolution of the brain.

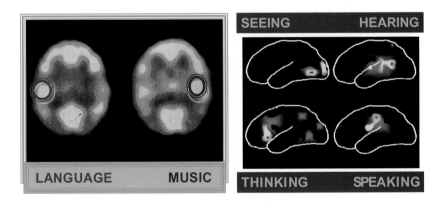

PLATE 7. Areas of the brain active in language, music, seeing, hearing, thinking, and speaking.

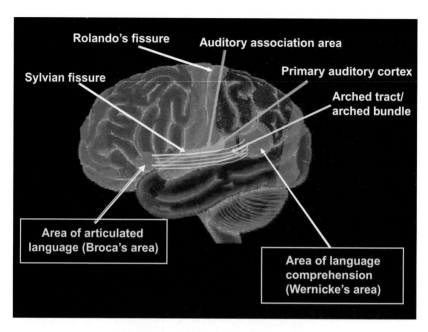

PLATE 8. The brain and its evolution.

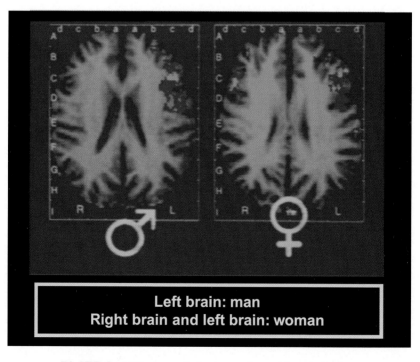

PLATE 9. Differences between male and female brains.

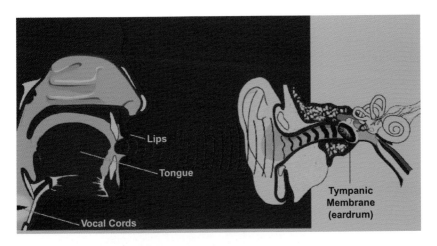

PLATE 10. The auditory-phonatory loop.

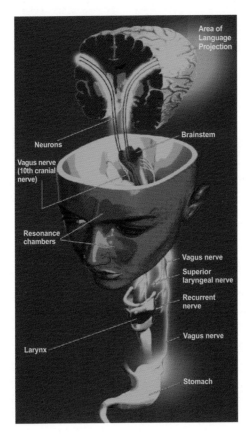

PLATE 11. The highways of the voice, showing the auditory tract and cerebral integration.

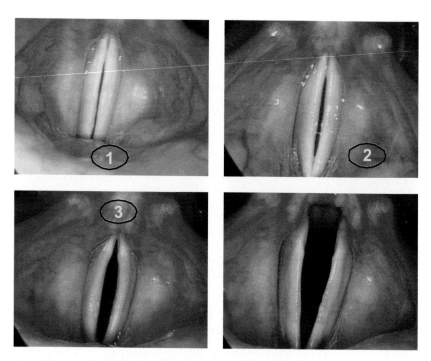

PLATE 12. Normal vocal folds shown during phonation (*1, 2, and 3*) and respiration (*bottom right*).

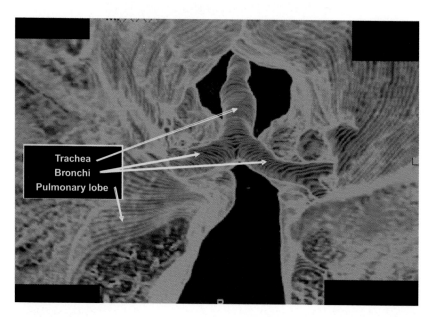

PLATE 13. The pathway of our breathing. (Photo courtesy of Drs. A. Castro and R. Gombergh.)

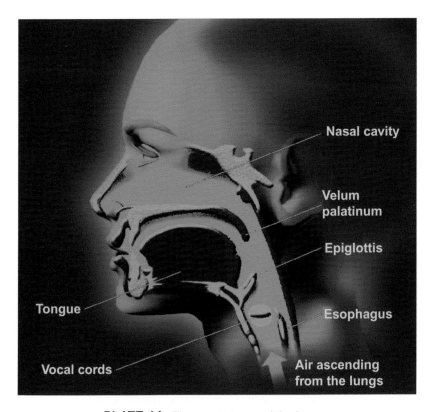

PLATE 14. The resonators and the larynx.

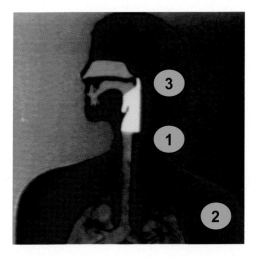

PLATE 15. The vocal apparatus, like a musical instrument, consists of three parts: 1. The vibratory body, 2. The vocal folds (energy: air → lungs. 3. Resonance chambers.

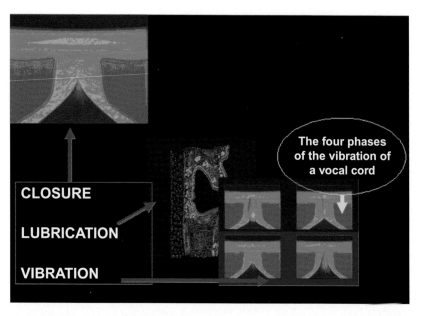

PLATE 16. The three key features of the voice: closure, lubrication, and vibration.

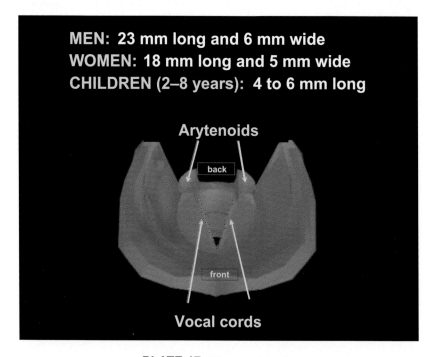

PLATE 17. The vocal cords.

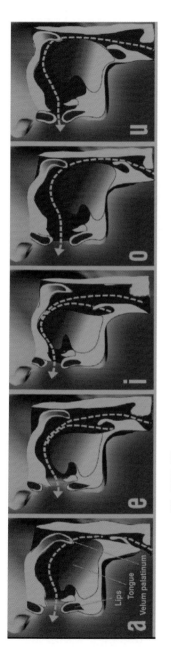

PLATE 18. The shape of the mouth while forming different vowels.

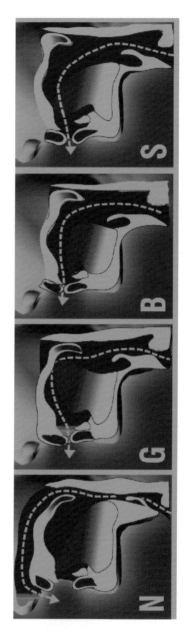

PLATE 19. The shape of the mouth while forming different consonants.

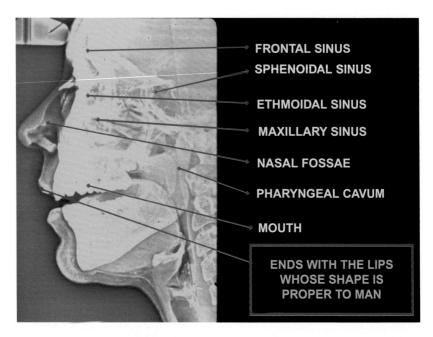

FRONTAL SINUS
SPHENOIDAL SINUS
ETHMOIDAL SINUS
MAXILLARY SINUS
NASAL FOSSAE
PHARYNGEAL CAVUM
MOUTH

ENDS WITH THE LIPS
WHOSE SHAPE IS
PROPER TO MAN

PLATE 20. Resonance chambers.

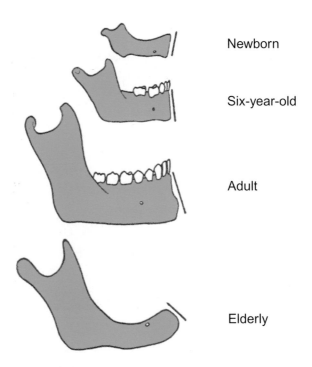

Newborn

Six-year-old

Adult

Elderly

PLATE 21. Evolution of the jaw as a function of age.

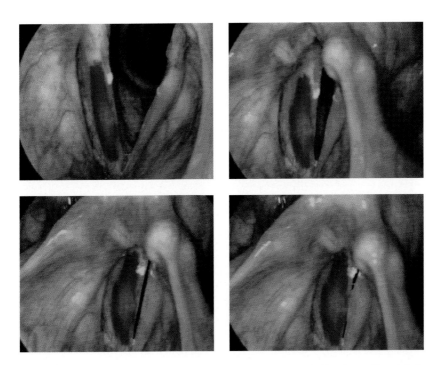

PLATE 22. Hematoma of a vocal cord results in loss of vibration, alters lubrication, and impedes closure.

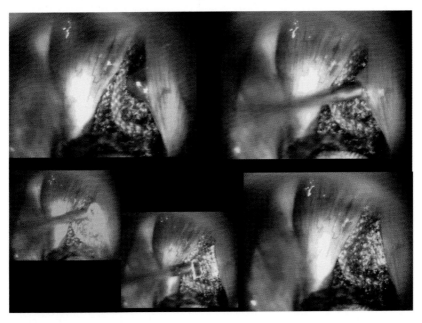

PLATE 23. Laser surgery showing removal of a polyp on a vocal cord.

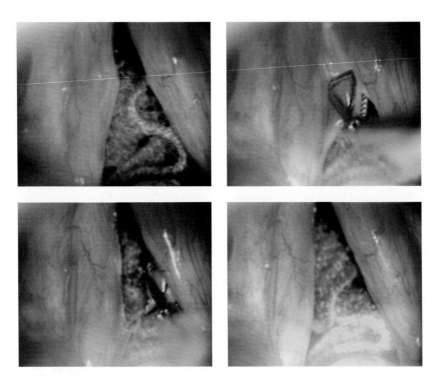

PLATE 24. Laser surgery showing removal of a cyst on a vocal cord.

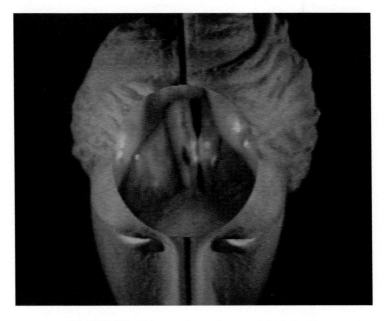

PLATE 25. Voice and emotion are intertwined.

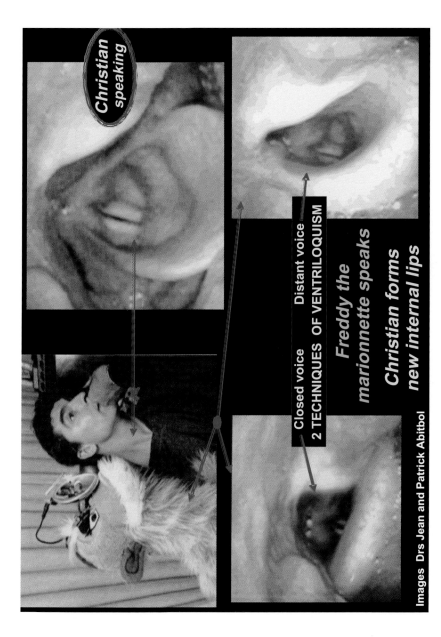

PLATE 26. The ventriloquist forms lips behind his lips, a mouth behind his mouth, to speak while giving the illusion of not speaking.

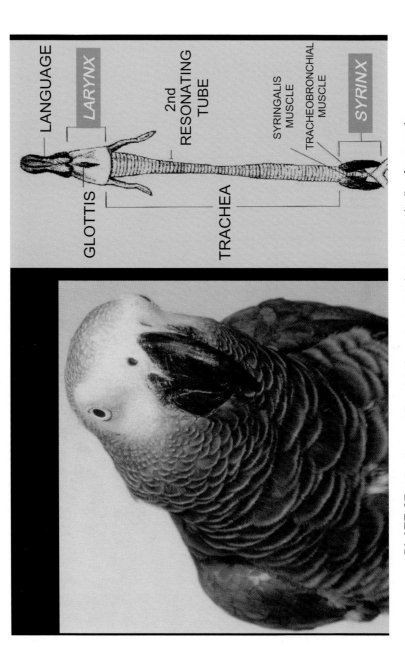

PLATE 27. Like the ventriloquist, the gray parrot does not use its lips for speech.

Chapter 11

Does the voice have a sex?

A man's voice, a woman's voice: genetics and hormones are the cross-links.

What separates the infant's screams from that sexy female voice or from that male voice that charms us so? How does the hormonal revolution of adolescence transform the voice? How does our genetic mapping stamp the verbal expression of our thinking and our emotional universe?

Voice and hormones: two words that clash, meet, and harmonize. The one is intangible, emotional, symphonic; a reflection of our being. The other is chemistry, a molecular formula, rational, purely scientific, perfectly understood, in which each atom has its predefined place with no room for improvisation, regulated by an impressive, well-oiled mechanism since millions of years. What is the link between them?

Hormones and chromosomes: not always in agreement

The voice is sexual. But is our voice's sex the same as our genetic sex? Is it determined by our XY, XX chromosomes, or by estrogen and progesterone hormones in women and androgens in men?

Our musical instrument, the larynx, is the target of hormones. It's hormone-dependent.

At puberty, the larynx undergoes a host of changes. These transformations are determined by our genetic heritage, but more so by our hormones. Indeed, the castrati, as we shall explain in a later chapter, retain a child's voice, said to be feminine. This ambiguous vocal "monster," who can make us feel ill at ease, is proof enough of the unquestionable impact of male hormones on our vocal cords, and of their determining influence on our male genetic print.

What are hormones? What is the influence of testosterone, the ruling hormone with respect to the quality of our voice? From the first appearance of *Homo habilis*, the differences between men and women point to a significant difference in physical mass. The male is twice the size of the female. His voice is different, deeper, stentorian. The female's voice is higher, weaker. This difference diminishes as soon as *Homo sapiens* enters the scene. Testosterone is the reigning hormone in Man's male infant. It triggers his puberty in his adolescent years.

The stag in the Chambord valley and the male hormones

Deep in the forests surrounding the castles of the Loire valley, near Chambord, a stag roars. This roar of his, in this month of October, the deer's rutting season, is unusual. He wants to sound aggressive. In fact, he wants to attract hinds in order to seduce them, but he also uses his roar as a weapon to intimidate his peers and establish himself as the dominant male. He is ready to form his harem. What is unusual about this acoustic message? It is accompanied by a bunch of related, precise signals that are the trademark of the stag. He rakes the ground with his antlers: this is a visual signal. He demarcates his territory with urine and sperm: these are olfactory signals. His roar is very low, very male: this is an acoustic signal. Its tone establishes him as the dominant male. You only hear this type of call during the rutting season. If you were to observe him through the branches, you'd notice his engorged neck and swollen testicles, symptomatic of a renewed important secretion of testosterone.

This male hormone builds his laryngeal muscles, lends power to his call, and seals his ranking. These attributes enable him to intimidate other males without having to fight them. The significant influence of androgens on his vocal print, on the power and frequencies of his call, without a doubt triggered the appearance of the secondary sexual attributes.

DNA undeniably and very precisely contributes these hormonal molecules. We are almost tempted to state that this built-in process is immutable. Does voice have a sex? If it does, is its character hormonal or chromosomal? Our voice changes over the years, it changes with our life story, with our appearance, and with our physique. It also changes as a function of our emotional environment. Where our fingerprint identifies a physical part of our anatomy specific to us, unique to us, that has no duplicate, our voiceprint reveals our personality, our innermost Self, our sensibility. It betrays our thoughts, reveals our sexuality. Let's try to follow the trail of the sexual voice. Let's retrace the steps of this miracle of Life, from the embryo through to the adult. How does our voice, impregnated with hormones and programmed by chromosomes, transform itself, construct itself, and create an identity for itself?

The infant's cries have no sex

There are male infants and female infants. They are easy enough to tell apart: the male has "it" all hanging out, the female has "it" all tucked away. But their cries are identical. In no way are some cries identifiable as feminine and others as masculine. Only at puberty will a sexual register impose itself on their voices.

The larynx is hormonal dependent and evolves with the sexual life of each individual. When you hear people speaking on the radio or on the telephone, you can identify their sex from their voices within a few tenths of a second. The voice is a secondary sexual characteristic. Of course, sex hormones influence it, but so do others. The thyroid hormones play a determining role in our vocal register. The thyroid gland at the base of our neck can become the seat of a goiter, basically a nodular increase in its volume, or conversely, it can become hyposecretive, in other words, its secretion of thyroid hormones becomes insufficient. The thyroid is indispensable to the evolution of the voice. It acts as do bellows on a fire, stimulating a majority of organs in our body and influencing our vocal timbre. In a serious case of hypothyroidism, the voice becomes harsh. The vocal cords present a slight edema and the vocal muscles become congested. This well-known pathology regresses as soon as thyroid extracts are administered. The voice recovers its normal register and its natural harmonics. However, the essential elements that modify the quality of our voice are our sex hormones: estrogens, progesterone, and androgens.

What are hormones?

The word hormone comes from the Greek *hormas*, which means "I excite" or "I stimulate."

From Aristotle to the present day: nothing much has changed

Hormones are secreted by discrete small masses of glandular cells. For almost two centuries, physiologists have been aware of the importance of these chemical mediators that ferry information via a molecule and facilitate the modification, transformation, and adaptation of their target organ—in this case the larynx, source of our voice. Four hundred years before Christ, Aristotle had already demonstrated that the castration of a male nightingale changes its singing to a much higher register. Nearly two centuries go by before Leonardo da Vinci, in 1543, takes an interest in the endocrine glands that synthesize hormones. Another three centuries go by. Claude Bernard, a renowned physiologist, takes an interest in 1865 in the role played by the liver. This huge gland not only enables the secretion of bile, but also synthesizes substances that are then secreted into the bloodstream to modify some of the functions of our organs. In 1889, Brown Sequart goes further. He asserts that "each cell of our organism secretes special ferments that are secreted into the bloodstream and via this medium, influence all other cells, which are thus made inter-dependent by a mechanism other than the nervous system." He injected himself subcutaneously with pulverized rabbit testicles to fight the rigors of age and recover a semblance of youth. According to his writings, he derived some benefit from this. It has since been accepted that certain glands feed a substance through their excretory canals into the bloodstream. This chemical message is a hormone. Endocrinology, the science of hormones, is born. The study of glands with internal secretions becomes a specialized medical field. The survival and normal functioning of our organism depends on it.

Hormones are molecular remote controls

The thyroid gland's role is to counter the aggressions of the outside world (the weather, cold, heat, stress). The role of our sex hormones is to enable our sexuality to adapt. Of all mammals, Man is the one with the greatest hormonal complexity—to such an extent that if our hormonal secretion is upset, it can cause irreversible damage. If no substitutes are provided for certain glands when these are suppressed, the outcome can be fatal. Finally, the precarious balance between our hormones is what ensures the stability of the living being. Their action is key for the evolution of our adolescence. Our endocrine glands, the main ones being the hypophysis or pituitary gland, the ovaries, the testicles, the thyroid, and the adrenals, produce a hormone inside the gland and secrete it through an excretory canal into our blood vessels. From that time onward, the hormone travels on these highways of our body to reach its target organ, which it stimulates.

The hormone stimulates a specific receptor organ, in other words the organ that can facilitate the desired outcome: adrenaline accelerates the heart, testosterone increases our libido. Only the ovaries secrete estrogen and progesterone, the female hormones, and then only if the ovaries have previously been stimulated by FSH and LH, the pituitary hormones. Finally, estrogens and progesterone will, in turn, stimulate one of their main target organs, the genital organs, and bring on the menses in a woman, if she still has a uterus. If a woman has had a hysterectomy, she has no uterus, and therefore no menses; the target organ at the end of the line has been removed. The consequences of the menses are definitively gone, but not the consequences of the sex hormones' effects on her organism. Thus, other target organs like the vagina, the breasts, or the larynx retain their tonicity and their hormonal rhythm.

In certain respects, the hormone is like a cordless remote control, but its operating method is molecular rather than infrared. An infinitesimal amount suffices for a significant impact. Where vitamins are an indispensable element in our nutrition because the body does not produce them, hormones are produced by our cells, but are just as indispensable to our survival. They accelerate, stabilize, or slow down their target organ. Knowledge of the chemical formula of these mediators enables us today to synthesize them and to analyze precisely their specific impact on our organism; more especially, it affords us a better understanding of the complex structure of our hormones' orchestra leaders, the hypothalamus and the pituitary gland, and enables us to treat hormonal dysfunction better.

The larynx: a target organ for multiple hormones

As a target organ, the larynx is warned by its specific receptors of the arrival of hormonal molecules. These receptors then synthesize the proteins for a precise action. Time has an important influence on hormonal activity. This fourth dimension plays a role not only in the evolution of Life, but also in our day-to-day life.

Certain hormones must be secreted at precise moments of our life: during our fetal development, at birth, or at puberty. Before, it's too soon, after, it's too late.

This remarkable internal clock of ours isn't yet fully understood. The thyroid hormones are a case in point. If they don't do their work in the first years of our life, this brings on irreversible physical and intellectual anomalies that can lead to cretinism. Should one later try to palliate this hormonal deficiency with artificial substitutes, it would be to no avail, the damage will have been done. Nowadays, very early diagnoses enable appropriate treatment to be prescribed in good time. But if the impact of our hormones dictates the need for a precise timetable, if they are to efficiently influence the evolution of our life, nowhere is this more evident than in a woman's menstrual cycle and our diurnal cycle. In our diurnal cycle, cortisone is naturally secreted by our body at the end of the day and in the early morning. These different secretions are controlled by an internal feedback system that avoids hormonal excess or insufficiencies through autoregulation.

Three chiefs rule over our hormones

Our mighty hormonal factory gets into gear at puberty. Three CEOs (Chief Executive Officers) manage it: the brain, the pituitary gland, and the hypothalamus. Their orders provoke hormonal secretions. The first CEO intervenes: our neurological center and emotional world pass information in the form of electrical impulses on to the hypothalamus at the base of the encephalon. This second CEO takes over to pass this information on to the pituitary gland. This third CEO now secretes substances and expedites them to the glands concerned. The informed gland then secretes its hormones and releases them into the bloodstream, where they will, on the one hand, migrate to the target organs and, on the other, inform the hypothalamus and the pituitary gland that all is well, that the secretion rate is satisfactory. This retro-control is remarkably precise and maintains our hormonal balance just as it should be, neither too high nor too low. When hormonal secretions are excessive, the hypothalamus and pituitary glands jointly diminish the stimulation of the gland concerned.

For example, if the pituitary gland detects an excessive level of thyroid hormones in the blood vessels that feed it, it will diminish its secretion of TSH, the substance that stimulates the thyroid gland. The stimulation of the thyroid gland then diminishes and the thyroid gland secretes fewer thyroid hormones. At this point, the pituitary gland receives fresh information: the level of thyroid hormones reaching it in the bloodstream has lessened. This information is taken into account and the thyroid gland receives more stimulation again. And so the cycle continues. This hormonal feedback acts like a thermostat: let's say you've set the thermostat in your bedroom at 20° C. When the temperature reaches 22° C, it activates the cooling system. When the temperature drops to 18° C, it activates the heating system. In either case, it stabilizes the temperature of the room around the desired temperature. It's an artificial feedback system that's self-regulating.

Hormones play an intermediary role between our brain and our various organs, notably the larynx. The pituitary gland, no bigger than a small pea, governs our survival! This subtle tuning between balance and imbalance ensures harmony at all times. In adolescence, a contusion of this gland in an accident can permanently affect a child's growth. A rapid diagnostic allows the ill-consequences of this lesion to be avoided through the administration of substitute hormones. In other cases, the pineal gland may not be properly balanced. Its secretion of one type of hormone may be anarchically excessive. Growth is perturbed. Here too, the imbalance must be quickly addressed to avoid the irreversible consequences of a pituitary dysfunction.

Puberty, vocal metamorphosis: male or female, the choice is made

Adolescence takes us down the path leading to sex-determined vocal frequencies. The adolescent, now virile, slim, and athletic, is ill-served by his shrill, unbearable falsetto voice. Meanwhile, the magic of evolution will have endowed others with the vocal vibration of a Caruso or a Callas, or simply the man-in-the-street, as much at home with his voice as he feels at home in his skin.

The hormonal revolution

At puberty, threshold between childhood and adulthood, our secondary sexual characteristics develop and, with them, the physical and psychological transformations specific to each sex. In the West, the average age of puberty is ten to thirteen years, in the East it's nine to twelve. The appearance of our sex hormones—estrogens and progesterone in girls and androgens in boys—triggers the development of the third layer of epithelium cells on the vocal cords. Thus, the harmonics of our voice become adult in part due to this third layer and in part due to the final development of the striated muscle of the vocal cords. As a girl becomes a woman, she develops higher harmonics, as well as some lower ones that she previously lacked. In boys, the action of testosterone on the muscular and mucosal structure of the vocal cords favors the appearance of new low harmonics and the loss of some of the child's high harmonics.

The hormonal revolution is more impressive in men. The shape and covering of the vocal cords changes, thickens, grows, acquires more volume, but the thoracic cage, lungs, stature, and brain are also evolving. In the West, men's left brain develops more than the right brain, whereas women maintain a certain equilibrium between the rational brain and the emotional brain. The consequences of puberty for the voice may be more obvious in boys than in girls, but they exist in both sexes. It triggers emotional changes that are usually appropriate to the person's physical appearance. In women, the voice drops by a third of an octave compared to girls' voices; in men, the voice drops by an octave.

Puberty can take a wrong turn

It can take an adolescent boy one to five years to acquire his adult voice. But puberty can take a wrong turn. A lack of harmony due to an imbalance between voicing and breathing caused by pneumophonic disturbances, in some cases, produces a voice that "goes off the rails," like a Tyrolean melody. Compared to women, men have greater lung capacity, a more developed cardiovascular system, a higher level of hemoglobin and red blood cells, more striated muscle mass. In the boy turned man, a falsetto voice that can't stabilize itself must be treated. It produces an anachronism between the apparent youth of the voice and the man's physical appearance. A difficult harmonization between voice and physical appearance is one of puberty's most delicate obstacles because the voice is seen to project its owner's personality! Therefore, one should definitely help adolescents to successfully complete this metamorphosis, should this be necessary. Speech therapy can help an adolescent with this problem to discover his adult voice, to control his exhalation during laryngeal voicing, and to adapt his behavior to his sociocultural environment.

The bend has been successfully negotiated: male or female, there's no ambiguity

In male singers, a well-defined head voice and chest voice make their appearance after puberty. These two vocal techniques bring into play the ligaments and muscles located between the thyroid and the cricoid cartilages, which are more developed in men. They allow the larynx to rock, and the previous calcification of the Adam's apple greatly facilitates this. The significant lengthening of the vocal cords in men also makes it easier for them to sing in these two head and chest registers.

In women, the process of puberty is less eventful. It flows more smoothly. The thyroid cartilage and the cricothyroid membrane hardly change. The vocal cord lengthens slightly and increases its muscle mass. Despite the formation of the third epithelium layer, the vocal cord remains very supple, with a fine mucous membrane. Small glandular cells keep the vocal cords lubricated and depend on feminine hormones (estrogens and progesterone). The ovaries enter their active period of reproduction. The first menstrual cycles appear. They become progressively more regular. After a few months, the voice discovers new high-pitched and low-pitched harmonics. The periodicity of the female hormones' secretions gives rhythm to the adolescent girl's life cycles.

The lunar cycle is orchestrated by the hypothalamopituitary axis due to the action of FSH and LH, two hormones that act directly on the ovaries to stimulate the secretion of estrogens and progesterone. Note that the menstrual cycle presents two distinct phases: a follicular phase between the first and the fourteenth day of the cycle, in which only estrogens are present—there's no progesterone— and a luteal phase between the fifteenth and the twenty-eighth day of the cycle, during which both estrogens and progesterone are secreted. In this context, ovulation occurs on the fourteenth day.

All is sweetness and light between the lunar cycle and the solar cycle

In both men and women, the sex glands have two functions:

1. The first is reproduction, through the formation of sperm in men and the preservation of the ovum in women.
2. The second is synthesis of the sex hormones: androgens in men, estrogens, progesterone, and a hint of androgens in women.

The female life span

In girls, the number of ova is predetermined from birth. This is the number of follicles, which exist only in the ovaries. The ovum has

23 chromosomes, but they are all X chromosomes. Therefore, the sex of the baby will be determined by the spermatozoon, which can be X or Y. In men, the testicles ensure the regular production of sperm almost until death. The male climacteric is delayed in some men until their eighties. Extraordinary but true: 1 cm^3 of sperm contains close to 200 million sperm, only one of which is required to successfully fertilize the ovum! What a scuffle to carry off the prize!

From the age of five months, the ovary of the female fetus is endowed with 7 million follicles. This number decreases to 2 million in the newborn female infant. By the age of puberty, the adolescent girl only has 300,000 follicles. Around forty, a woman is down to 25,000 follicles. By menopause, only around 3,000 remain. By the time a woman is fifty-five, she no longer has any.

The first menstrual cycle appears during adolescence. It's triggered by two hormones, FSH and LH, that launch the process of the life cycle. The lunar cycle harmonizes the next forty years. The active phase of the genitals has begun. After each menstrual ovulation, once the mature follicle has burst, a permanent scar forms on the ovary. Each cycle is punctuated by a physical, mechanical, and ovarian impact, but equally by a molecular, hormonal, and chemical impact, with repercussions on the entire organism. In mid-cycle, the ovum leaves its follicle, which remains in the ovary. As soon as the egg is released, the follicle undergoes significant reconstruction as a yellow substance that becomes an endocrine gland that secretes progesterone. The ovum floats between the ovary and the edges of the fallopian tube in search of a sperm. Thus, in this first chapter of the cycle, there's no progesterone, only estrogens are secreted. During the second period of the cycle, both estrogens and progesterone will be secreted. But, and this is critical, the progesterone can only act if the estrogens have previously prepared the ground and informed the receptors of the target organs. The yellow substance is eliminated on the eve of the menses, ensuring the production of progesterone is stopped. The sudden drop in estrogens and progesterone production brings on the menses. (Of course, if the ovum has been fertilized, the yellow substance persists and allows the uterus to play its role as foster mother while the placenta is formed and the fetus develops.) Here too, a feedback mechanism is in place. As hormones are no longer being secreted, the hypothalamopituitary axis is no longer being restrained; therefore, it relaunches the secretion of the two hormones FSH and LH, which in turn stimulate the ovary to begin again a fresh menstrual cycle.

Whereas men renew their sperm daily according to the solar cycle, women ovulate in tune with the lunar cycle.

A woman's voice

Three actors for our sex life: androgens, estrogens, and progesterone

Our three actors are similar in their molecular structure. Their skeleton is a steroid molecule composed of 18 carbon atoms, similar to cholesterol. Each hormone has a privileged role to play, a specific function. It can only fulfill its role in our body because of the existence of specific receptors fixed to the target organs of our body. Each molecule has a male or female influence. It triggers a modification of the mucous membranes, muscles, and bony tissues, therefore our laryngeal instrument, our voice, is also modified. It also influences the cerebral cortex, thereby influencing the brain. This influence is primordial at puberty and persists for the rest of one's life.

The feminine voice has exerted its charms since millennia. In the Greek civilization, Apollo and Orpheus discussed the merits of the athlete's worship of the body and of the powers of a siren's voice to soothe emotions.

Estrogens are flowing and the vocal timbre is sharper

The estrogens secreted by the ovaries have different implications for the larynx. They result in a slight thickening of the cordal mucous membrane, which creates greater vibratory amplitude. The voice acquires a good timbre. The desquamation of superficial cells is reduced, accompanied by a decrease in the need to clear one's throat and in the amount of laryngeal mucous fluid. The lipid cells under the cordal mucous membrane are stimulated. The voice becomes more supple (in the menstrual cycle, this is called the maturation phase with a proliferate action).

The cells of the genital and the cordal mucous membrane: are they different?

By 1982, receptors for estrogen hormones had been identified on the vocal cords and in the uterus. These separate objective findings were confirmed by J. Abitbol et al. in 1986 and 2004 by comparative studies of smears taken from the vocal cords and the cervix of the uterus, during the same day of the menstrual cycle.

The results were amazing; in both cases, the cellular aspect was identical. There was a perfect correspondence between the smears taken from the cervix of the uterus and those taken from the vocal cords. This correspondence had long been suspected. Given that both have the same type of mucous membrane, it is only logical that they should have the same cyclical impact. But now there was scientific, objective proof to support this. This is consistent with the observation that the voice can change with the menstrual cycle.

Estrogens: a broad spectrum of action

Estrogens also act on the mammary glands and its excretory canals to affect the growth of girls' breasts at puberty. Their action on the metabolism of calcium influences the bony and cartilaginous structures of our larynx. These structures increase or maintain global bone mass. Estrogens also improve the permeability of blood vessels and capillaries, which are very numerous in the vocal cords, thereby increasing oxygenation. They have no effect on striated muscle. They diminish the risk of Alzheimer's disease. They have an antagonist effect with androgens. Finally, for progesterone, the second, strictly female hormone, to be effective, the tissues must first have been impregnated with estrogens.

Progesterone appears exclusively in women: the voice is modified.

Progesterone provokes a thickening of the vocal cords. Unlike estrogens, progesterone only exists in women, not men. As its name indicates, progesterone is a hormone that enables gestation to persist (from the Latin *progestare* and *hormone*). It is secreted in the ovaries only during the active genital phase of a woman's life, from the age of fifteen to fifty-five. It prepares the mucous membrane of the uterus for the nidation of the ovum. That is its primary role.

With respect to the vocal cords, progesterone causes cells on the surface of the mucous membrane to slough off (a process called desquamation). It thickens the secretions of the gland located below and above the vocal cords, causing, during the four days preceding the menses, dryness of the larynx, the need to clear one's throat, less agility when singing, and a narrow register. If the voice is strained during this phase, nodules may form (these are small supple swellings of the cordal mucous membrane). Progesterone also brings on a slight decrease in the muscle tone of the vocal cords, and it diminishes, and may even inhibit, the permeability of capillaries. This causes the extravascular fluid, that is, fluid outside the blood vessels, to stagnate in the tissues of the vocal cords, bringing on an edema of the vocal cords, which remain swollen during the week prior to menses.

It is thanks to the estrogens that the intravascular fluid is transferred to the extravascular spaces in the surrounding tissues. Then, when progesterone is secreted, if the balance between the two hormones is satisfactory, the interstitial fluid will be well distributed. The edema of the vocal cords will be minimal. If, on the contrary, this is not the case, the progesterone will prevent the return of the interstitial fluid to the vessels, causing an edema to form. The progesterone in this instance closes the door of the capillaries and prevents them from draining the tissues.

This imbalance between estrogens and progesterone causes a cyclical edema in the last week of the menstrual cycle, caused by, the accumulation of interstitial fluid in the vocal cords. A similar process causes some women to have swollen legs before their menses.

Progesterone acts on the envelope of neurons

Everyone agrees that progesterone is secreted by the ovaries and was originally considered as a hormone involved only in reproductive functions. But N. Gago has demonstrated that it can be synthesized within the nervous system by neurons and glial cells. The progesterone has promyelinating and neuroprotective effects. Moreover, it can be synthesized locally in the nervous system by neurons and glial cells and can, thus, be considered a "neuro-steroid." It plays an astonishing role here. It activates the synthesis of the protective sheath of the neuron, the myelin sheath. The myelin sheath, a sort of protective sleeve that shields the nerve from all traumatic aggression and from differences in temperature, enables nervous impulses to be transmitted at a constant speed between the brain and its target organ. Nerves that have this myelin sheath conduct nervous impulses better and faster. As early as 1995, Ian Duncan of the University of Wisconsin lifted the veil on the action of progesterone on the brain, but not on its synthesis. The impact of this discovery led to a better understanding of ther-apeutic approaches to treating neurological diseases, or certain myopathies that alter the myelin sheath and, therefore, nerve con-duction, such as Lou Gehring's disease or multiple sclerosis. It seems that progesterone significantly slows the evolution of these afflictions.

At menopause, the brutal drop in progesterone results in a progressive slowing of nerve conduction that's barely noticeable. This slowdown is due to a relative lack of myelinization of periph-eral nerves, and as a result, singing is less well controlled.

The voice injured by hormones

A violent pain, then no more voice

One autumn Friday around 5 PM, I receive a phone call from the Bastille Opera House asking me to urgently examine the diva S. L., an international lyrical soprano with a remarkable track record and an outstanding vocal technique. The drama occurred during her third rehearsal of a Verdi opera, in the first act: she could no longer sing. Her voice was injured. I received her at 6:30 PM, accompanied by her impresario: "I'm dying, Doctor." This seasoned professional, used to a high level of stress and pressure in her working environ-ment, is convinced her voice has gone. It can't be due to stage-fright. Her impresario, Mr. R., tells me what happened. The diva prefers not to talk, she's too worried. "During the rehearsal, Mrs.

S.L. felt tired. She has been feeling tired for the past few days. But she insisted on attending rehearsals, to practice and to get to know the orchestra. All was going well. Today, I took her to the Opera House. She sang in a normal voice for a few minutes, without straining. But at one point she had to sustain a high-pitched note and she felt a violent pain on the right side, in her neck. I saw her grimace, but she carried on singing her lines. The tenor responded. During the forced rest of a few dozens of seconds imposed by the tenor's verse, she was able to catch her breath. When she sang again, her voice had dropped, the high register was gone, the *B* note and its *pianissimo* had evaporated: impossible to do the *vibrato*. Her voice had gone." I asked if she could talk. "Yes," he answers, but softly. But she couldn't sing any more. We interrupted the rehearsal, and here we are. Worried, she bursts into tears and asks me: "Is my voice injured?" I examine her.

But first, I'd like to share with you a lesson I have learned from experience. Artists know their voice inside out. They know perfectly well if one cord is vibrating badly. Their knowledge of their laryngeal instrument is remarkable.

When artists complain of a vocal problem, most of the time they are right. Which means that if I can't detect a pathology of the vocal cords, it doesn't mean that there isn't one, it simply means that I haven't found it.

Consequently, I have to keep searching, dig deeper, carry out more technical examinations, and remain on the lookout for a pathology.

Who is guilty?

S.L. points to her larynx with her finger to indicate the exact place where she felt pain during her vocal effort. Her finger is indicating the right vocal cord. Palpation of her neck is normal. It reveals no particular sensitivity. The videoendoscopic examination of her larynx gives me the key to the mystery. The vocal cords are moving normally, but where the left cord looks normal, the right cord is indeed injured precisely where she felt a violent tear. I can see a hematoma on the cord, a pocket of blood that has formed under the epithelium. The stroboscopic examination of her larynx reveals the history of this problem. The right vocal cord is bright red, engorged with blood, but it vibrates. It's not inert; it is supple. But it cannot lengthen and shorten. Its contour has changed. The precarious balance of this exceptional instrument has been damaged. What happened? How can a professional singer with perfect technical mastery and an irreproachable lifestyle be the victim of such a regrettable lesion?

To understand how this hematoma came about, we must delve into this diva's past, now being sketched for me by my stroboscope. We must hunt for clues. The diva, S. L., in her forties, is not on the pill. Her menses are normal. However, she informs me that four to five days before she gets her period, her breasts are sore, her legs feel a little heavy, her pelvis is sore, and her voice alters slightly. I ask her to be more precise regarding the changes to her voice. She answers with exemplary precision. "I lose 10 to 15% of my voice, in order to be heard above the orchestra I have to control my breathing better and brace my pelvis more than usual on stage to counter the weakness of my vocal cords. My register is also affected. I lose a half-tone to a tone in the high notes, but my low tones are still great. My vocal control is also affected at this time, I often clear my throat and feel tired. By the end of the performance, my larynx feels sore." I ask her to explain what she means exactly by control: "By control, I mean sensing the timbre of my voice. In that phase of my cycle, prior to the menses, the color of my voice is a bit more metallic, the vibrato is a little harder to hold. But especially, I find it hard to do a *pianissimo* on certain frequencies. I have practically no problem in the forte. It's changing from one harmonic to another that bothers me, that's a problem. I find it hard to control my full voice." I ask her: "Mrs. S. L., what phase of your menstrual cycle are you in now and in how many days do you think you'll get your period?" This was for me the crux of the matter. "In two or three days, doctor." I add: "Did you have time to warm your voice up properly before the rehearsal?" She thinks about this, then confirms my intuition: "No, I was already late, and on top of that the air was dry because of the air conditioning . . . " To all intents and purposes, the guilty party that had caused the hemorrhage of the vocal cord had now been flushed out.

This diva normally sings at 70% of her capabilities. In her premenstrual phase, just before her menses, she sings at 90% of her capabilities to produce a comparable timbre. But today, other elements perturbed her vocal musicality. The Opera House's air conditioning had dried the atmosphere. She was feeling tired. She informs me that she had also slept badly the night before. She had things on her mind.

The clue is not far

The reasons for the hematoma are getting clearer. The singer was suffering from a premenstrual vocal syndrome. My Sherlock Holmes magnifying glasses—none other than my endovideoscope and stroboscope—allow me to observe vocal cords. They tell me their secrets during vocalizations. In this instance, the examination reveals not the hematoma on the right vocal cord, easily diagnosed, but microvaricose veins on the left vocal cord, sign of venous fragility. The singer doesn't suffer from them. The cord vibrates normally. The danger they present stems from their fragility. Her vocal power damaged the right vocal cord. That brought on the hematoma. Indeed, four days before the menses, the vessels are more fragile due to hormonal influence. The lubrication of the vocal cords was perturbed by the dryness of the atmosphere. The microvaricose veins burst, but only under the submucosal layer. They burst under pressure during the very powerful vocalizations of this lyrical soprano in a high register, the result being the submucosal cordal hemorrhage.

Could she have avoided the misfortune, perchance?

There was no way of predicting this accident. It was the first of her career. The reasons for it are simple: for years now she's made it her practice to warm up her voice, to loosen up her vocal cords, to oxygenate her laryngeal muscles. But today, around 2 PM, she didn't have time to prepare her laryngeal instrument, due to some personal problem. It's just before her menses, and she's fragile. The reasons for the accident are now clear. To her fans' immense disappointment, her performances have to be cancelled. Her treatment begins. It's simple: strict vocal rest combined with sprays, phlebotonics, minerals, and anti-inflammatories.

Two weeks later, all was back to normal. I recommend to the diva a cyclical treatment of ten days each month, for a minimum of two years; also a regular checkup of her vocal cords, especially prior to her menses. The fragility of her blood vessels, the impact of the progesterone at the end of her menstrual cycle were partly responsible for her vocal predicament. This type of problem must have been known in earlier times, because since the 19th century, any female singer performing at the Scala Opera House in Milan could during the five days preceding her menses and during her menses cancel her performance and still receive her fee. Back then, the influence of the hormonal cycle on women's vocal cords was already known.

The vocal print sometimes gives away the start of the menses

The voice changes during the menstrual cycle

A premenstrual cycle is evident in all women. But only a third of these present a more noticeable edema of the vocal cords and swollen breasts, symptomatic of the precarious balance of the sex hormones. Women on the pill can sometimes present these same symptoms if the pill is biphasic (one containing both estrogens and progesterone).

What is going on? The case of Mrs. S. L., the diva, is a good illustration of the premenstrual vocal syndrome; however, she didn't present all the symptoms. The usual syndrome is an altered voice. This can be accompanied by a bout or recurrence of gastric reflux, brought on by a loss of tonicity of the esophagus. When the stomach contracts, if the cardia, or the part between the esophagus and the stomach, isn't perfectly tonic, it allows gastric fluids to escape upward. These acidic fluids reach the back of the vocal cords in the throat and cause dryness of the larynx. But you'll recall that progesterone is already having a drying effect on the vocal cords. This causes a posterior laryngitis, as well as an edema of the cordal joint. But no pain will accompany this because neither the pharynx nor the larynx has been hurt.

Your voice: it's psychological, Madam

The singer with a premenstrual vocal syndrome complains of tired-ness, of a loss of *pianissimo*, of an alteration in certain harmonics in the higher registers, of a deficit in the power of the voice, and of a veiled voice. Technology has confirmed the objectivity of these alterations of the larynx and has flouted the systematic response: "it's psychological, Madam" previously encountered when women consulted for this syndrome.

In some patients, I've also observed pharyngitis and cyclical sore throats that required vaporization of the tonsils with the help of the laser in order to avoid a monthly intake of antibiotics and anti-inflammatories.

During this premenstrual period, the formation of an edema can create or aggravate the formation of nodules on the vocal cords. This causes a hoarse voice for the six days prior to the menses and for the first two days of the menses. If this cyclical, episodic dys-phonia recurs too often or gets worse, the nodules also get worse. At first, they are soft and vibrate correctly. From one cycle to another, this simple nodule, the size of a small, supple button in the central third of the vocal cord, hardens. Now the hoarseness is per-manent. This problem always requires speech therapy to enable the singer to rebalance the axis between her breathing and the vibration of the vocal cord. Sometimes, these voice therapy sessions carried out by the "clock makers" of physiotherapy, namely, speech and language pathologists, are backed up by microsurgery of the vocal cords. This intervention becomes necessary if the voice remains impaired between menses, as this can seriously handicap a singer's career. However, it's then more judicious to operate on these pathological vocal cords well clear of the week preceding the menses, thus allowing the organism to spontaneously reabsorb the edema of the vocal cords just described, which normally disappears between the third and the twentieth day of the menstrual cycle.

The voice and pregnancy

A professional singer can sing remarkably well while two to seven months pregnant. The vocal cords are then nicely plump and perfectly lubricated. The quality of the vibration is improved. The hormones that accompany a pregnancy confer special warmth to the voice's harmonics. The voice is rounder, it carries well. It seems that pregnancy does beautify the voice. After the seventh month, the breathing support is impaired, which is only normal. The sole ailment that needs to be treated during a pregnancy is gastric reflux.

Menopause: with or without hormones?

Different times, different problems

During the menopause, this cycle is progressively disrupted. But this menopause that today is of interest to us all, has only relatively recently become topical.

In the Greek civilization, four hundred years BC, the menopausal woman didn't exist, or was an exception. The average life expectancy was twenty-three to twenty-seven years. Menopause still didn't exist in the Middle Ages. Life expectancy was then twenty-three to forty years. Only in the 20th century was menopause finally taken into consideration. Indeed, girls born in the 1980s can expect to live to the age of ninety-two! Menopause now corresponds to practically half a woman's life. By the end of the 20th century, France accounted for nearly eight and a half million menopausal and menopaused women. The importance of the voice, the development of verbal communication, interpersonal relationships, all point to the essential problem that the voice and the menopause are now beginning to pose.

Why these changes in a woman's voice around this period of her life?

During the perimenopause, ovarian activity diminishes strongly. The yellow body, or corpus luteum, forms only episodically. Her cycles are no longer regular. Progesterone levels collapse. The menopausal woman no longer has any progesterone, she no longer ovulates. Very few estrogens remain, since the ovaries are wasting away. Equally, the secretion of male hormones also drops off considerably. But their presence, now that they're no longer counterbalanced by feminine hormones, can sometimes cause the voice to become more masculine. Thus, the ovary becomes a simple endocrine gland with no reproductive function.

In the West, the menopausal phase normally lasts from the age of forty-seven to the age of fifty-five. The impact that the sex hormones had on their various target organs disappears, not without consequences. However, these days, the administration of substitute hormones enables the unpleasant consequences of this lack of sex hormones to be delayed to an increasingly later age, saving many women from a trying experience that is both mentally and physically hard to accept. In the 1950s, was this perimenopause period not referred to as "the change of life," implying that an entire chapter in a woman's life was coming to a full stop? Our better understanding of our endocrinologic world has given the menopausal woman greater quality of life on a daily basis.

But hormone substitutes may be contraindicated. They are not recommended in cases notably of breast cancer, a high-risk family background, cardiovascular pathologies, or cholesterol-related afflictions. For this reason, a medical checkup is a prerequisite for women in their fifties considering their options. Thereafter, a regular checkup should be performed.

The ovary becomes just an endocrine gland

As we've seen, the menopause spells the end of ovulation and of progesterone. The ovary, an endocrine gland, now secretes very little hormone. Its secretion has changed. Because estrogens are less present, the receptors of sex hormones receive more androgens and become more receptive to them. As a result, the vocal cord mucous membrane thickens. This is accompanied by a lack of tonicity and a deficiency of its contours. The voice becomes deeper and more masculine.

Meanwhile, the sixty-year-old woman may develop symptoms such as increased hairiness as an indirect consequence of androgens. A smear test of the cervix of the uterus indicates an atrophy of the epithelium. The same result is obtained from a smear test of the vocal cords: the parallelism is amazing.

Menopause and the vagus nerve

The larynx also is controlled by the vagus nerve. Its responsiveness is improved by estroprogestational impregnation. Therefore, at menopause, the radical drop in the secretion of estrogens and the complete halt in the secretion of progesterone induce slower nervous conduction from the brain to the larynx. As a result, vocal response slows down slightly, which can hamper rapid changes of frequencies when singing. Later, the *vibrato* (seven vibrations per second) cannot be maintained. The voice gradually gears down to the *tremolo* (four vibrations per second).

The Modigliani woman and the Rubens woman

Observation of menopausal women has led us to categorize them into two vocal types. The voice doesn't necessarily become more masculine. Why is this? Put simply, one can distinguish two types of menopausal women.

1. The first type, slim with very few fat cells, we will call the Modigliani type (as in Modigliani's paintings);
2. The second, somewhat stouter, we'll call the Rubens type (as in Rubens'paintings).

Estrogen synthesis happens on three levels: at the level of the ovaries, when these are functional, at the level of the brain (hypothalamus, tonsils, and hippocampus), and finally at the level of fat cells. These latter cells are the ones that interest us here. They are particularly active during the menopause. Since 1977, we have known that, in both men and women, fat cells can turn androgens into estrogens. The relationship between obesity and a higher secretion of estrones (estrogen derivatives) is also age-related. It's higher in menopausal women. This is the work of a specific gene in our DNA (cytochrome 19 associated with P450 aromatase) that facilitates the transformation of androgen into estrogen in our adipose cells. Thus, the lower need for hormone substitutes of our Rubens-type woman is due to the fact that her fat cells will transform her androgens into estrones.

Meanwhile, our slim Modigliani woman is more likely to need hormone substitute therapy, prescribed, of course, with due respect to contraindications.

Obese tenors have been found to have a higher level of estrogens and a slightly lower level of testosterone than those found in baritones and bass singers. Indeed, these slim, deep bass singers with their bony figures have a higher level of androgens. They have no fat cells that could help the organism to metabolize testosterone into estrogens.

With age, muscle mass diminishes; adipose mass increases; cells are redistributed differently about the body. Corticosteroids encourage the increase of fat cells. Therefore, menopausal women need to be cautious about consuming them. A carefully considered hormone substitute therapy program, associated with vitamins and minerals, can bring considerable benefits to most female voice professionals if their body can tolerate it, which is far from being a given. The work of David Elia and Henri Rozenbaum from 1985 onward gives good insight into various therapeutic programs. I have noted that women thus treated are able to avoid developing a masculine voice as they age and are able to preserve a beautiful voice for significantly longer. I have been most impressed by certain sopranos who've kept the same *tessitura* until the age of sixty-five.

Male hormones: the lower frequencies take the voice hostage

Women secrete androgens, the male hormone "par excellence," but in minute doses: on the one hand via the adrenal glands just above the kidneys, on the other hand via the internal theca, a very precise part of the ovaries themselves. Indeed, the female sex requires a touch of testosterone to ensure a satisfactory level of libido and enough low-pitched harmonics in her voice to distinguish it from a child's voice. But the level of testosterone must be around 150 μg/dl—if too low the libido disappears, if too high, masculinity sets in and excess pilosity or hirsutism can occur. This action is often irreversible. It is aggravated by steroids.

I must insist that the consumption of androgens leaves indelible marks in women. That is why voice professionals should check their medication carefully for the presence of androgenic anabolic derivatives. These elements may also be present in certain progesterone preparations and their molecular derivatives.

Female athletes from Eastern Europe

In the 1980s, I had occasion to examine female athletes from Eastern Europe. These patients had trained hard to beat records, but at great cost to themselves. Their intensive training was one of the factors that had enabled them to win medals, but there were others. Some had received injections of androgen hormones to boost their athletic performance. These "imposing" women, to put it mildly, greeted me with a man's voice that was practically devoid of higher harmonics. I examined their vocal cords; their condition comes as a surprise in a woman's larynx. The muscular hypertrophy of the vocal cords is obvious, the mucous membranes are thick and a pale, dull-looking epithelium has replaced the usual white mother-of-pearl aspect of the membrane. I also note the presence of acne and hirsutism, but no Adam's apple. The thyroid cartilage hasn't altered. These athletes hadn't had a menstrual period for three months. Given the development of their laryngeal muscles, no medical treatment could have improved their voices. Only laryngeal plastic surgery, involving microsurgery of the vocal cords, would enable them to recover their feminine voice.

A man's voice: man and his hormones

The androgens secreted by the testicles have a direct effect on the voice. They certainly act on the bony tissues, but also on the brain. They increase aggressiveness. It is no accident that yelling is often an integral aspect of male expression in combat, both in men and in animals. Androgens increase blood flow in the organism and improve oxygenation and muscle performance. Note that cortisone can have an androgenic effect and act as a euphoriant. This induces some voice professionals to overdose on it, hoping to be at their best vocally. But this is dangerous, because it can have a rebound effect. When you come off cortisone, muscle tone decreases abruptly and tiredness, possibly even a light depression, may set in.

Changing the sex of the voice

I've been consulted on occasion by transsexuals (male to female) wanting a change of voice. Voice therapy has an excellent track record in this respect. In most cases, the patient's voice can be adapted to his new personality simply by teaching him to place the larynx differently and to use efficient breathing and vocal techniques. Surgery is a last resort. No male hormones can remain in the organism, otherwise the operation is doomed to failure. It is the ultimate transformation. These men who have become women have a masculine larynx. The height of the voice depends to a large extent on the thickness and density of the vocal cords, no longer influenced by androgens. Several techniques enable us to raise the voice. Some are based on external surgery. Thus, Isshiki, from Kyoto, opens the larynx medially and pulls the vocal cords anteriorly, which makes them thinner. Another technique consists in closing the cricothyroid membrane, in other words, the muscle between the cricoid and thyroid cartilages, to allow the larynx to tip and create a falsetto voice. Laser microsurgery through the mouth allows one to diminish the mass of the vocal cords, and, therefore, their density. Some muscle is removed from one vocal cord, then six months later, from the other, thus thinning the body of both cordal muscles. These various techniques enable the patient to raise his vocal register by four to five notes. However, whichever technique is used, the results are not very satisfactory.

Does voice has a sex? a question asked since centuries

Voice has a sex, it is hormonal and genetic. It has amazing powers of seduction. The impact of hormones created exceptional voices some centuries ago! But that is another story as we shall see later with Farinelli.

$\mathscr{C}hapter\ 12$

Does the voice age?

*Our vocal age is sometimes out of step
with our legal age. Do voices wrinkle?*

$\mathcal{O}$ur voice ages, as does our body. Aging is a natural, biological evolution. It is a consequence of stress, age, maturity, and also the state of our tissues, vessels, and brain. Different theories have tried to explain aging, notably the theory of free radicals. These free radicals weaken our proteins and our cellular membranes. This increasing fragility causes cellular degradation. Other theories are based on our genetic heritage, our human print. Recently discovered genes are thought to be the "end-of-life" genes. They program our cellular death, called cellular *"apoptosis."*

Could DNA disappear?

Is life eternal? Do all living creatures on our planet have equal chances? A particle from the cosmos, perhaps deposited on Earth by comets, DNA has never stopped replicating, evolving, mutating in all sorts of ways. The amoeba, the dinosaur, the great ape, and Man all have the same DNA in their genome. Thus, DNA isn't far off immortality.

What is mortal is its carnal form, its envelope. An insect's life is very short, a few hours, a few days. Yet you'll recall that the gene of a fly's eye is the same as the gene of the eye of a mouse. They may have similar genes, but their life expectancy is very different.

The mouse lives several weeks, the tortoise two centuries, some trees survive 2,000 years, and Man's life expectancy in the West is eighty-eight to ninety-two years. Today, at the dawn of the third millennium, nearly 4 and a half billion years after the birth of the Blue Planet, according to chromosomal research, the genetic heritage of *Homo sapiens* is capable of a life expectancy of one hundred to one hundred and fifty years.

Aging is caused by life's vicissitudes: infections, diabetes, stress. Some aging factors we bring upon ourselves, like alcohol, tobacco, pollution. All contribute to our physical aging. In France, in 1980, 9% of the population was over sixty-five. By the year 2000, nearly 15% was over sixty-five. In 2030, close to 25% is expected to be over sixty-five.

The voice changes with the passing years: why?

The bones of the larynx alter

There are many reasons why our voice changes as we get older. The first alteration is mechanical and anatomical in nature: the thyroid, cricoid, and arytenoid cartilages progressively harden, lose their suppleness, ossify, and calcify. The anterior part of the arytenoid cartilage, point of insertion for the vocal cord and the epiglottic cartilage do not ossify, but they lose elasticity. As for the vocal cord joints, like any other joint they show signs of inflammation and arthritis. The cricothyroid joint also shows signs of arthritis, causing increased difficulty in the head voice and a decrease in the agility and speed of the vocal cords when practicing musical scales. Joint suppleness is affected by a loss of collagen fibers and by a degeneration brought on by dehydration.

Teeth and the aging voice

Our vocal instrument, the larynx, can't shoulder all the blame. The buccodental articulation is a key part of the vocal aging process, yet it's often ignored. Losing one's teeth causes the upper and lower lips to collapse, forming pinched lips. Our jaw is oddly designed. It is shaped like a horseshoe, with a very specific angle between the horizontal part and the two vertical parts. On the left and right sides, it articulates with the base of the cranium. This bony part is very strong. When the teeth fall out, it calcifies. The closed angle, normally forming in adults an almost 90° angle between the horizontal section and the vertical section, opens wider in the toothless person. With advancing age, lack of teeth causes the jaw to decalcify and erode; moreover, the angle between the horizontal and vertical parts becomes wider, with an angle around 120° (usually it is around 90–95°); the horizontal part of the mandible becomes slimmer, the vertical part shorter (see Plate 22). The profile of the face is changing: the mandible seems squashed under the cranium, the nose droops down to the level of the upper lip.

Paradoxically, lack of teeth means the mouth is no longer able to open fully. The joint of the jaw becomes less supple. This underscores the importance of maintaining an efficient set of teeth and resorting, when necessary, to dental implants, to ensure that the lips are able to rest against a satisfactory surface, thereby avoiding bone degeneration of the mandible. So much for the dental landscape of our voice.

Muscles and neurons must keep fit

The problem is simpler as regards muscles and ligaments. The muscles of our vocal cords and resonators are striated. With age, but especially in case of insufficient physical exercise, the myofibrils of the striated muscles degenerate and turn into fibrosis and secondary fat cells. We know of exceptional singers who are seventy-five years old; we also know of teachers who, once retired, spend considerably less time speaking, as a result of which their cordal muscles atrophy. The internal biomechanical properties of the vocal cord are no longer stimulated. The enzymatic machinery of ATP (the molecule that provides energy for our muscles), myosin (the protein muscles are made of), and mitochondria are no longer solicited. Henceforth, muscular aging is inevitable. The neuromuscular junction is also normally solicited by phonatory activity. If it isn't, muscle activity decreases. Even our nerves undergo a reduction of the myelin sheath, which affects the speed at which messages are transmitted between the brain and the muscles: the elocution of these patients slows down. This combination of muscles and ligaments receives energy from the arteries and laryngeal capillaries feeding it. A decrease in physical and sports activity reduces the suppleness of the vessels, here and in the entire organism, and accelerates the onset of arteriosclerosis. It affects oxygenation and weakens the musculature: a vicious circle is triggered. This is why it is imperative that the elderly engage in some form of sport again. The return to sports activities should be very progressive and regular. The elderly need to be very patient in their renewed quest for fitness. But the human organism is exceptional. It will nearly always return to its previous level of fitness.

What of the vibratory instrument itself?

With age, the first and second formants of professional singers become less powerful. Despite a slight decrease in muscle tone, these voice pros are able to adapt and maintain their vocal quality and performance. They are able to prevent a *vibrato* from slipping into a *tremolo*.

The vocal cord

By the age of seventy, nearly 72% of patients who have stopped being vocally active present an atrophy of the vocal cords and epithelium that they didn't have prior to their fifties. There is a loss of elastic fibers, collagen fibers, and the proteoglycan webbing. The lamina propria, an essential element under the cordal epithelium, becomes rigid and stiff. Triggering a vibration becomes more difficult. This suite of alterations, aggravated by deficient lubrication of the epithelium, often justifies supplementing the diet with substitute vitamins and minerals that have a role to play in vocal activity.

The breath: power of the voice

The energy of the voice is intimately connected with our breathing. Our lungs progressively weaken with age. In people who don't engage in physical activity, bronchial efficiency diminishes by almost

40% between the ages of forty and eighty. That's a significant drop. Our lung capacity is affected by an atrophy of the peri-bronchial muscles, a reduction in the number of alveoli in the lungs and in their elasticity. The thoracic cage loses its suppleness and, therefore, its amplitude. The stiffness of the thoracic vertebrae perturbs the elasticity of the thoracic cage. Physical activity is the antidote!

Hormones: from sex to thyroid hormones

Besides these mechanical elements, the decrease in sex hormones plays a major role. With age, there is also a frequent drop in the secretion of thyroid hormones, hormones that generate energy for the muscles and hydrate the organism. Patients with a sluggish thyroid often require appropriate therapeutic treatment to get them out of their lethargy and feeling energetic again.

Let's call a spade a spade: if you don't take proper care of yourself . . .

Your vocal register will narrow, your voice will weaken, your timbre will lose color and become metallic. You can avoid this evolution by adopting a regular and constant healthy lifestyle, by taking antioxidants, vitamins C and E, trace elements, minerals such as magnesium, and by keeping up physical and intellectual activities. Unfortunately, the impact of passing years is sometimes less forgiving as regards our hearing. We have seen that listening and audio-phonatory feedback are essential to the quality of the voice. All voice professionals should have their hearing checked regularly to test for partial deafness. If necessary, don't hesitate to correct a hearing deficiency with a hearing aid. Nowadays, these hearing aids are very well tolerated and, in most cases, they will help voice professionals to re-establish a correct balance between their vocal and auditory functions. A hearing aid keeps one in touch with the outside world, it's a safeguard against isolation, it stimulates the audiophonatory loop, and contributes to a precise control of the voice while speaking and singing.

Presbyphonia

Thirty years ago, very little was known about the aging of the voice, or presbyphonia, which begins around the age of eighty. A new medical field has opened up. As time goes by, the vocal cords lose their suppleness. The cord atrophies. There's a loss of hydration, a loss of collagen and elastin fibers. The remaining fibers are thicker. As a result, the laminar structure of the cordal tissue is less supple. Consequently, when you tighten your vocal cords, they arch and no longer make proper contact. They allow some air to slip through. If you speak for any length of time, you become breathless.

The paradox of the aging voice

In women

As the menopausal woman advances in age, her new hormonal balance, with its absence of estrogens and its very mild secretion of testosterone, the result of the atrophy of her ovaries, is no longer able to sustain the tonicity and strength of the vocal cord muscles. What are the consequences of this? The two vocal cords atrophy progressively. The mucous membrane covering them becomes thinner and dehydrates.

Initially, the voice displays a narrower register, the higher harmonics are lost, the voice is less powerful and tires faster. But a paradoxical effect sets in. Because the vocal cord has diminished in thickness and become finer, the voice, which had become a little deeper, now becomes higher, more delicate, sometimes even shrill. You often hear eighty-year-olds speaking with a very high-pitched voice. One can thicken the vocal cords again by injecting a substance into them; this ensures reasonable timbre and vocal endurance.

In men

After the age of seventy, men can present the same vocal symptoms in the male climacteric. Yet the vocal structure in this case behaves like an athlete in all respects. As with women, hormone therapy is indicated in conjunction with specific nutrition hygiene, but vocalizations are essential. Androgenic hormonal therapy is rarely advisable because of the danger of an altered prostate. For men, vocal training is the best guarantee of keeping a young voice. An example I like to quote concerns a professor of French at the Lycée Henri-IV, who also lectured at the Sorbonne and was in the habit of speaking over four hours a day. I had known him for over ten years. When he stopped his academic activities, he started writing his Memoirs and barely said a word for the next six months. He used to have an athlete's larynx. But when I saw him again a year later, I detected an impressive atrophy of his vocal cords. He was only sixty-five years old, yet he had the voice of an old man. The right treatment combined with intensive speech therapy enabled him to practically recover his normal voice. I advised him to carry on lecturing for a minimum of three hours a week. Our voice ages only if we isolate ourself from others. Regular practice and communication with others stimulates the voice and preserves its timbre.

Rejuvenating the voice

This atrophy of the vocal cords can be corrected through speech therapy and, on rare occasions, through phonosurgery (surgery of the voice). As we have seen before, this phonosurgery consists of injecting a product into the shrunken cordal muscle to increase its volume to what it used to be. The voice regains satisfactory power and tonality. The voice of these dysphonic, breathless patients once again becomes dynamic. This type of surgery is only practiced if the standard medical and speech therapy treatment has failed. This "voice lift" is often very successful.

The key to preserving a youthful voice is to be serious about physical exercise, hydration, lubrication of the vocal cords, dental hygiene, muscular activity, nutrition, vitamin and mineral supplements, possibly appropriate hormone therapy and, often, anti-reflux medication (to treat the acidity coming from the stomach to the larynx). If you take good care of the health of your vocal cords, you can most certainly retain an efficient vocal tessitura and timbre.

The voice hardly wrinkles at all

Mr. Michel Roux, a French actor, has a very distinctive voice. This comedian is just as much at home on stage as he's dubbing American actors. The ravages of time are something he doesn't suffer from. His dubbing left its mark on films and certain televised series with Tony Curtis. Thirty years later, his voice is still recognized. His talent is remarkable. His memory is exceptional, he plays with silences, and is able to punctuate his delivery with laughter or onomatopoeia. The same is true of Robert Hossein, whose vocal timbre has retained all its charm and sensuality since *Angélique, marquise des anges*, a film that marked its generation. We are able to feel his anger, his passion. He transports you into his universe. He suffuses life into his characters with his inimitable voice. His huge charm is conferred by a characteristic of his vocal cord. It's the scarring of his life. His voice does not age. Neither do his intellectual and creative capacities. Memorizing a two-hour text is child's play for him. The expression of his voice, helped by specific exercises he learned in drama school almost fifty years ago, doesn't show a single wrinkle. These comedians, these actors and singers, like Frank Sinatra or Anthony Quinn, have preserved the personality of their voice intact. It is recognizable from the first word they utter. Keeping the voice in training and actively engaging the memory is something that comes naturally to these exceptional artists.

Chapter 13

Voice injuries

*Our voice is hurt; to tend it, we dress
the wounds of our heart.*

The voice is not injured by chance

"He left me speechless," "Her words stuck in my throat," "He has got me by the throat," "I can't swallow what happened"—popular expressions of this ilk abound.

Our voice betrays our emotions. Not only our present emotions, but also those experienced since early childhood. The exceptional harmony of our vocal cords, the same harmony that enables words, sentences, languages, to be created under the control of the brain, is forged day after day, scarred by life's vicissitudes. These two cords that make voicing possible can be traumatized, injured, damaged, knocked about, and shocked in everyday life. It may seem reductionist to talk of the voice just in terms of these two little muscles, the vocal cords, and yet, we come across a surprising range of pathologies that affect these mechanical elements of the voice box. Voice injuries are all but accidental usually, just as stomach ulcers and heart attacks are all but accidental. The biographies of these voice scars depict a specific personality profile in each case.

When babies scream, as indeed they do from birth, it doesn't cause a hematoma on their vocal cords. Yet it can in an adult. Some people smoke a pack of cigarettes a day, but not all smokers end up with an edema of the vocal cords. Many people suffering from gastric reflux have to clear their throat, but few develop a cordal granuloma.

Talking in a normal voice without strain and using the appropriate technique, helps to avoid laryngeal injuries. Voice strain can cause callosities to form, known as nodules in their early stages. These small growths form on the mechanical line of force of the vibration, which, as is the case with vibrating cord, is in the middle of a vocal cord. Often characteristic of professional voice users, nodules lend a certain charm to the voice, a certain sensuous huskiness. More often than not, these nodules vibrate well, in harmony with the host vocal cord, and become an integral facet of the artist's vocal identity. There is no need whatsoever to operate on them. Is a beauty spot systematically removed?

After phonatory abuse, voice therapy is essential to prevent nodules from hardening and becoming like raw grains of rice that would need to be surgically removed.

Cysts are theoretically independent of any external aggression and are frequently of embryologic origin. Yet they only manifest themselves at certain periods of one's life. The cyst starts to grow. Its mass is formed by a small sac of liquid. Therapy has little effect on it, other than providing a stabilizing influence. Imagine a physiotherapist being asked to massage a lipoma, a fatty cyst just below the skin. It wouldn't do much good. After having been dormant for years, the cyst becomes bothersome. It can cause dysphonia, perturb the cordal vibration, and handicap professional activities. In this case, surgery (either laser microsurgery or classical surgery) becomes necessary.

Gastric reflux

Gastric and pharyngolaryngeal reflux

Gastric reflux can attack the laryngeal mucous membrane. In what ways does reflux interfere with the voice? Located behind the larynx, the esophagus often allows through acid regurgitations that lap the underside of the vocal cords. This is a pharyngolaryngeal reflux. This reflux dries the vocal cords in the same way as your hands would become dry if you were to bathe them daily in acid. Lubrication of the vocal cords is essential. When acid reflux dries them out, it causes dysphonia. The patient is not at all aware of any burning sensation.

Why is this? Suppose you were to put your hands in domestic bleach. If there's a scratch on your hand, you'll flinch because it will burn. But if your hands are free of scratches, you'll feel nothing, even if you were to hand-wash laundry in bleach for an hour. This would cause the skin on your hands to become dry and flaky, but you wouldn't feel any pain. The same goes for the throat: if you have no laryngeal lesion, the hydrochloric stomach acids won't cause any pain, they'll simply dry out the larynx and bring on secondary pathologies. This problem affects children as frequently as it does adults.

In babies

Babies spend seventeen hours a day lying down or half-sitting; therefore, reflux is common, almost normal, amongst babies. But some dairy products are more acid-forming than others, so some babies are subject to significant regurgitation, small chronic coughs, inflammations with fungi or serous otitis. Bronchiolitis with asthmatic-type coughing and rhinopharyngitis can often be avoided by administering antireflux medication. Cases of laryngeal spasm are rare. However, in case of severe regurgitation, it's best to make the baby sleep half-sitting up, otherwise acidic vapors may flow from the stomach into the throat and then up to the nasal cavities, irritating these in the same way as inhaling formaldehyde would.

The child is not a small adult

The pathology caused by gastric reflux is particularly severe in children. A child's voice, a child's larynx, is not simply a smaller version of an adult's. Its structures are different, its needs are also different. The child's cerebral environment is different. It stands to reason that the child's voice should also be different. Not only are the shape, size, density, and mucous membrane of a child's larynx a working drawing of the adult's—for example, the angle of the thyroid cartilage is 130° in the infant, 120° in men, 110° in women—but equally, the quality of the vocal mucous membrane and its hormonal impregnation are different. The esophagus and the stomach form an angle where they join up, called the angle of Hiss. This junction prevents the reverse flow of stomach acids into the esophagus, thanks to a smooth circular muscle called the cardia, the veritable sphincter of this junction. When the acid level of the stomach is too high, it causes the stomach to contract more and more violently. These gastric contractions stimulate the gastroesophageal sphincter. They cause it to open. In case of continuing hyperacidity, liquid flows upward into the esophagus and attacks the throat. This results in the need to clear the throat, coughing, pathologies specific to reflux, and sometimes laryngeal spasms because this part of the throat is not meant to receive acidic liquid. Its mucous membrane is not suited to any liquid with a pH less than 5.2, in other words, an aggressive liquid. Suppose you were to swallow some bleach: your stomach can take this sort of aggression because gastric acids assist digestion, help to break down food in the stomach, prepare it and make it aseptic. Your throat can't; consequently, the bleach would burn it.

Gastroesophageal reflux can provoke lesions of the esophagus, such as esophagitis. Children then complain of pain at the back of the lungs, which can develop into transfixing cardiac pain. Their stomach hurts, they get nauseated frequently, their voice is veiled. The gastroenterologist is then called on to treat the problem. However, more often than not, there is no pain. The acidic reflux flows upward into the larynx. This is known as pharyngolaryngeal reflux. The gastric acid doesn't burn the esophagus, it dries it out and disinfects it. This is what's known as gastric hyperacidity without ulceration, or gastritis. The motility of the stomach also increases. The first symptom that alerts one to pharyngolaryngeal reflux is a dry cough that is soon accompanied by vocal fatigue and chronic hoarseness.

In adults

One can observe a chain reaction of problems spread out over time. First, there is an inflammation and an edema at the back of the vocal cords, with pathology such as keratosal laryngitis (like a callus on the vocal cords), that produces horny plaques. Then inflamed nodules appear, followed by an edema of the vocal cords. The edema spreads to the whole larynx. The acidity continues its aggression and granuloma, fleshy growths resembling polyps, form.

Finally, and this is one of the most handicapping stages for voice professionals, the closure of the vocal cords is slowed by an inflammation of the joints. This final alteration causes voice fatigue and breathlessness within 15 minutes. Voicing is interrupted by dry coughing spells, the nature of which is immediately recognizable on the telephone. The coughing starts as soon as you try to talk. Laryngeal spasms can occur, but are more rare, and, exceptionally, the very aggressive irritation of the larynx by acid reflux can bring about secondary cancers.

Hiatal hernias and the voice

What can have provoked this chain reaction of problems? The cardia is loose, it can no longer close completely, a hiatal hernia develops often right from the start. This natural loosening of the cardia allows the gastric acids to flow back up to the throat, where, within a matter of months, they will cause this succession of pharyngolaryngeal aggressions and sometimes an asthmatic type of cough.

This is often accompanied by eructation or uncontrolled burps, bad breath, and a chronic inflammation of the tonsils, or tonsillitis. If you stand on your head or on your hands, or more likely, if you simply bend down to lace your shoes or pick up a handbag, you end up with your stomach in your mouth.

Between these two extremes, standing upright and being upside down, is the horizontal position. Here gravity is not at play. When you stand, the liquid in the stomach naturally sits low in the stomach. When you lie down, if the cardia is loose, you'll end up coughing at night. The acidity dries the back of the throat and creates a reactive edema of the uvula, a hyper-response of the nasal mucous membranes that causes unusual postnasal drip and, as a result, secretions pouring down into the throat with loud snoring. In the morning, your voice is dry, talking is difficult, you have to clear your throat of thick mucous matter to free it.

Examining the chronokinetics of the voice

Examining the laryngeal instrument, be it with mirrors as from 1854, or via dynamic vocal exploration since 1981, is the starting point for all diagnoses of vocal injury.

The introduction of a videofibroscope into the nasal fossa and down to the roof of the larynx enables one to "watch the patient's talking" or "look at the patient's singing" in real time. This was described in an earlier chapter. However, I should just add here that, to establish a complete picture of the internal structures of the vocal tract, this type of clinical analysis of the larynx provides a four-dimensional chronokinetic analysis of the laryngeal structures, which may need to be backed up by a three-dimensional CT-scan (an X-ray imaging test).

With these objective observation techniques, which are replicable and can be repeated over time, the dynamic analysis of the larynx in real time and in vivo enables one to decipher the mystery of the vocal pathology. This takes into account not only objective observations, but also posture and the emotional world of the patient's voice.

Stage fright and the voice

Destructive stage fright

It causes a funny voice: toneless in some cases, excited in others. This funk disappears once you're into your speech, your pleading, your conference, or your meeting with someone you're in awe of, but it can have unpleasant side effects in some patients and artists. Some vomit and suffer from tachycardia (a racing heart). Others find their throat is dry, in some cases so dry they can't get a word out. At times, an artist may have to resort to beta-adrenergic blocking agents to prevent an attack of nerves before a performance. When I was in medical school, colleagues and friends suffered from this very same problem just before their exams; it isn't confined to the artistic field. The causes of this fright are varied; their origin can be either mental or physical, as Drs. Alexis Wicart and Jean Tarneaud pointed out in the 1930s.

Stage fright in front of an audience

Mental causes abound. It can have a superstitious basis, an unfortunate whistle in a previous performance, strife within the performing troop, perhaps personal problems. The "magnetic" influence of the audience shouldn't be underestimated. All it takes is two or three people in the audience that you don't like, that you feel negative "vibes" from, and the timbre of your voice will be different as long as you don't succeed in blocking them out of your mind. Conversely, friends in the audience who send you positive "vibes" will galvanize your performance and enable you to surpass yourself. This is why I often advise voice professionals to have at least one friend in the audience for their presentation, or on opening night, whom they can look at regularly. The emotional transfer will help boost their performance.

Stage fright cannot be reasoned away. Only very powerful self-control can sometimes diminish its impact.

Stage fright hurts

The physical causes of stage fright before a performance are numerous and frequent. To cite but a few: an asthma attack brought on by anxiety and by allergens in the theatre, which can be very disruptive for a voice pro. The use of a spray half an hour before a performance is imperative. I advise some patients to do this systematically in order to avoid the chain reaction that may trigger an asthma attack. Use of both a laryngeal spray and a nasal spray may be necessary to avoid reactive allergic rhinitis, but the danger of addiction is real and must be avoided.

Breathlessness, premenstrual syndrome, gastroenteritis, intestinal cramp, headaches are all upsetting precursor symptoms of stage nerves. Appropriate treatment is imperative.

A faulty memory is rarely at cause, though memory can be affected by tiredness, overwork, poor quality sleep, or worrying.

One night, several singers were due to perform on stage at the Zenith in Paris when panic struck! The two main singers could not hear a thing. A third had the feeling that her ears were blocked, as in a plane. It was as if an epidemic of deafness had hit the troop. Yet the problem was easily solved. The first singer had wax blocking his ears. Once the wax was removed, he was able to hear his own voice again and tune up with the orchestra. His nerves had gone. The blockage in his ears had amplified his stage fright. The two other singers had slight colds and catarrh was partially obstructing their eustachian tubes. The smoke screens used on the stage during rehearsal had worsened their condition. It was now 5 PM, the show was due to start at 8:30 PM. Their ailments were quickly relieved with sprays and anti-inflammatories. Again, once the diagnosis was known and thanks to the reassuring presence of a doctor, the stage fright vanished. The concert was a success.

Sometimes, stage fright manifests itself through the vocal cords. The voice pro may be scared of not being able to give enough voice, not hitting the desired frequency, or his voice breaking. This is more common among singers who've already experienced a problem with their voice, like the diva S. L. (encountered in chapter 11). A singer who has already suffered a cordal hematoma knows he is at the mercy of a recurrence, of a breakdown on a high note, of difficulty with a *pianissimo*. For another, the problem will lie in producing a legato, or in passing smoothly from high frequencies to low frequencies. The *vibrato* remains feasible, the *pianissimo* is difficult, the *forte* poses no problem. Here the cause is often a nodule on the vocal cord. Yet other singers may experience a different type of problem. They may find the *forte* difficult, but singing a *pianissimo* or a *vibrato* and passing from high notes to low notes present no problem. Often, the cause is a cordal edema brought about by viral laryngitis.

More often than not, we are dealing with voice strain: after ten days of rehearsals, problems are experienced producing high notes, especially closed vowels such as *e* or *i* or *ou*. The phonatory expression becomes tight, as if muted. In an attempt to compensate for this vocal tiredness, the singer overtenses. This brings new muscles into play, which can lead to bad habits being formed. The joints of the vocal cords become inflamed, the cricothyroid muscles (between the thyroid and cricoid cartilages) become tight. The voice professional is compensating for one defect with another defect. To avoid this type of problem, I often insist on reduced singing practice and very little talk during the three days leading up to opening night.

The breakdown of the voice can be due to the presence of thick mucus between the vocal cords, caused by the air conditioning of the theater. Appropriate treatment that includes aerosol sprays can prevent this type of incident. At times we cauterize the inferior nasal turbinate preventively. This dries out the nose and stops excessive secretions of mucous matter brought on by the high levels of dust in theaters.

Stress and stage fright are important factors that the voice professional needs to take into account. Identifying mental or physical triggers enables you to treat the problem at its source and prevent the problem from happening at all. Good breathing helps with concentration. Just because the body drops its guard is no reason to become less vigilant and less focused; on the contrary, you need to dig deeper into your resources. This internal dialogue, assisted by a few vocalizations done with the mouth closed, enables the singer to build up a store of inner energy that his technical mastery will then draw on within seconds to express his present emotion. A balanced and upright posture ensures that the comedian or singer is maximally effective.

My voice has "her" proper identity

Sometimes, these mental resources depend on visual representations of the body or of the voice. Indeed, some singers confide that they consider their voice as an independent entity. They talk about it in the third person: "My voice is well"; "today, she deserted me"; "I must go easy on her"; "she betrayed me"; "I can't count on her anymore." An artistic interpreter can't merely repeat his lines. He has to recreate the opus, bring it alive, make us sense its beauty. Stress and anxiety can dry the mouth, the tongue, the larynx. All professional performers have experienced this, but after the first applause, lubrication returns to normal.

All voice professionals should isolate themselves for fifteen minutes before a performance; whatever the symptoms, it is their self-confidence that will win the battle with their nerves.

Beware of an injury before or after a performance

Restaurants strain the voice

To protect your voice from injury after a conference, a show, or a session in court, avoid going to a noisy restaurant. When you take your seat, the restaurant may still be half empty, allowing you to speak normally. As the restaurant gets busier, you'll start having to talk louder across the table, straining your voice. Tired from its earlier efforts, your voice will now be more prone to injury. In order to make yourself understood at the table, your voice has to be 5 dB above the ambient noise in the restaurant. And this is how voice professionals who go out to celebrate their success just after a performance end up with a real hematoma on their vocal cords. Imagine you have just run a marathon and have rested for 10 to 20 minutes. Then you're asked to do a 100-meter sprint. Inevitably, you would pull a calf muscle. The same goes for your vocal cords.

Indigestion and pollution

On a different register, the voice can be affected indirectly. Constipation and poor digestion can diminish vocal performance. In this case, the vibratory energy is altered. This is because thoracic amplitude and abdominal breathing are restricted. Good nutrition is essential for optimal vocal performance.

Bronchial breathing can be affected by asthmatic-type coughing. This has become more prevalent over the past 10 years. Indeed, the amount of pollution and allergens has increased dramatically over this period. Vocal energy is drained by recurring tracheitis. Suitable treatment is required to prevent these pathologies. The pneumologist and ORL specialist prescribe appropriate broncho-inhalers. But in more than one in five cases, these pathologies involving chronic coughing are associated with gastric reflux.

The voice and its environment

Man is a hardy mammal. Our health is affected by climatic and weather conditions. Our body temperature must remain between 36.4°C and 37.2°C. Our skin helps to regulate our internal temperature. But we are affected by very high and very low temperatures. Our skin envelope protects us by sweating if it is too hot, by vasoconstriction if it is too cold. The air we breathe also will be warmed up or cooled accordingly. It will come into contact first with the nasal fossae, then with the vocal cords and mucous membranes. Brutal differences in temperature are bad for us. In the middle of summer, coming in from the heat outside into a cool air-conditioned office can alter the voice. The moisture balance of the vocal cords doesn't have time to adapt. On a different subject, respiratory infections such as flu or bronchitis must also be taken seriously at all ages. Seasonal flu vaccinations are always a good idea.

If you walk in the street on a cold day while talking, you expose your vocal instrument to the rigors of the climate, to cold air that dries the breathing passages. Therefore, before a vocal performance, avoid speaking out in the cold, it makes your voice vulnerable. Also, it's a good idea to protect your throat with a scarf. Our breathing rhythm and our voice have to acclimatize to their local surroundings, to the town and country we happen to be in. You can't run the same distance in Paris as in Mexico City. When the Olympic Games were held in Mexico City, competitors arrived several weeks in advance to acclimatize. The same applies for opera singers.

In concert halls, classrooms, and offices, vocal stability is affected by parameters such as the ambient temperature and hygrometry, as well as the air conditioning. Unfortunately, all too frequently air-conditioning units are too strong. In theatres, the ventilation raises dust. Allergens make the nose run. An edema forms in the nasal fossae, the nose becomes blocked. This allergy will have two consequences. The first is difficulty in breathing that interferes with the proper humidification of the vocal cords and causes mucus to be formed and the need to blow your nose strongly and clear your throat. The second is more subtle: the mucous membrane of the nose and pharynx remains swollen. This is an allergic rhinitis that can cause vascular congestion. The use of vasoconstrictors may be necessary, but should be used sparingly to avoid becoming dependent on them. They normalize breathing in an instant. But you should systematically give up these nasal drops that unblock the nose in favor of anti-allergenic therapy and, if necessary, microsurgery of the nasal fossae to decongest the nasal turbinate. These "quick-fix" nose drops, if used regularly, can have severe consequences.

Sneezing and voice injuries

Sneezing fits are bad news. This is because each sneeze places the vocal cords under a lot of pressure. When you sneeze, the vocal cords smack up against each other: that is the noise you hear:

"atchoum!" The *a* is the inhalation, the *tch* is the noise produced by the vocal cords snapping against each other violently, and the *oum* marks the end of the exhalation. This trauma of the vocal cords can cause a cordal hematoma.

Max is in his sixties. A bass singer at the Opéra de Paris with a superb voice, he performs regularly in an opera he is fond of, *Don Giovanni*. He often has sneezing fits when he arrives at the Châtelet, but these are of little consequence. He protects himself with natural therapies, bathing his nasal passages with saline water and taking antihistamines at bedtime at the change of season. Antihistamine medication does indeed dry out the pharyngolaryngeal space for a minimum of eight hour, hence the need to take it nine hours before a vocal performance. This medication doesn't treat the allergy, it treats its consequences. It suppresses the most bothersome symptoms, the edema and the runny nose.

Max is offered a part in a Parisian theater. It is a part that requires him to both talk and to sing. In this very old theater, other unexpected guests await him: dust and acarids. They reign supreme despite all efforts to eradicate them. One spring evening, the show is going well, but in the third act, Max has such an incredible sneezing fit that the audience laughs at it. Being the professional that he is, he carries on, but his timbre is not as clear anymore. His beloved rich deep voice, which normally carries without problem to the back of the theatre, has just lost its power. Only his training as a lyrical singer enables him to carry on to the end while giving the illusion of satisfactory voice projection. I see him the very next day. He presents an allergic rhinitis, but also a slight hematoma of the right vocal cord. The cord does not vibrate as well as the left. It is thicker and has lost its pink color, it looks darker. Max is very surprised. His eyes betray a certain anxiety. He furrows his eyebrows and before he has time to ask me what vocal future awaits him, I reassure him. It is just a capillary that has burst beneath the cordal mucous membrane. But will he be able to play in two days time? It is Sunday morning. He has Sundays and Mondays off. He is lucky; this means he doesn't have to cancel any performances. And, indeed, resting his voice for three days until the Tuesday evening, combined with a decongesting treatment of the vocal cord, allows Max to get his voice back. His control over his larynx the following Tuesday evening confirms his recovery.

The hematoma of the
vocal instrument

A few months later, Max comes in for a checkup and is still perturbed by this incident. He questions me about his cordal hematoma: "Given that the vocal cord is a muscle, just like the biceps of the calf muscle, how come I didn't feel any pain? Was the hematoma caused by muscle tearing?" It's true that if you pull a muscle doing sports activities, an intramuscular hematoma forms, and this is always very painful. This is different. When Max sneezes violently, or when a singer develops a hematoma on a vocal cord after a plane trip, what has happened? In both cases, the fragility of the blood vessels in the vocal cords causes a vascular rupture. There is hemorrhaging beneath the mucous membrane. The muscle itself is intact; none of the muscle fibers of the vocal cord are injured. The muscle itself hasn't been pulled, which is why there's no muscular pain.

A sports coach yells from the edge of the swimming pool to encourage his swimmers. The chlorinated atmosphere of the indoor pool dries out his vocal cords. He is obliged to shout so loud to be heard by his athletes that it provokes an accident: his voice breaks abruptly. When he consults me, he experiences sharp one-sided pain at the level of his Adam's apple. He can describe it and locate it perfectly well. But when I examine his larynx, it's another story. The vocal cord presents a hematoma that is a purplish-blue protruding mass, with suffused hemorrhaging throughout the cord, not just on the surface (see Plate 22). The cord in this case does not vibrate, whereas Max's did. The muscle has been pulled. The coach is beside himself because his voice is broken, veiled, almost inaudible. Coughing is painful. The cordal muscle is torn. Steroids must be administered therapeutically to prevent the development of an encysted hematoma and secondary rigidity; hence, the mucosal membrane does not vibrate at all. Complete vocal rest for at least ten days is essential. It may be several weeks before his voice returns to normal.

This type of incident can also occur during a boxing match or martial arts competition, or if the larynx receives a hard blow from the safety belt, but these cases are rare.

Operating the vocal cords with laser technology

Matthew and papilloma of the vocal cords

Matthew has had his vocal cords operated on many times. I have known him for the past twenty years. He is just turned thirty-one. Since the age of eleven, he has been plagued with a rare but recurring pathology: laryngeal papilloma, caused by the *human papilloma virus*, or HPV. This disease is neither hereditary nor contagious. Small warts invade the vocal cords. The best treatment we know of today, until an antiviral vaccine is developed, is laser microsurgery. Matthew's voice is husky. The huskiness clears up after each intervention. Over the past twenty years, he has been operated on many times. The challenge in his case lies in taking out the wart and nothing but the wart. Care must be taken not to touch the cordal muscle.

The fibroscopic examination reveals small "raspberries" disseminated all over the vocal cords. The precision of the image is such that I can clearly see the sites that are infected by the virus and thus am able to determine the appropriate therapeutic strategy. These endoscopic images practiced in the consulting room give the specialist a remarkable appreciation of the problem and of the most appropriate surgical solution for it prior to surgery. In fact, inasmuch as relapses are frequent and surgical interventions are carried out at relatively short intervals, surgery is only indicated if the vibratory space has been invaded. If it hasn't, surgery can be delayed. Thus, videofibroscopic imaging of the larynx is essential. Before its invention, a papilloma was removed automatically as soon as it was spotted, without taking into consideration the functional aspects of the voice that were difficult to profile objectively then. The photographs taken today at each consultation enable the specialist to compare the lesions objectively and evaluate the evolution of a papilloma between consultations. On this September day in 2003, the lesions are numerous and interfere with Matthew's speech. Surgery is indicated.

The surgery is carried out under general anesthetic. A small tube is introduced between the vocal cords to allow Matthew to breathe during the operation. The laryngoscope that goes down to the vocal cords is placed level with his mouth. The microscope will magnify the operating field by a factor of between 15 to 20 times (remember that the lesion may be less than 1 mm). Everything is in place: the microscope coupled with a laser in the axis of the laryn-goscope, the small green compress placed under the vocal cords to protect the trachea from the laser beam. My assistant helps me position the larynx better in relation to the laser. The anesthetist ventilates the patient and monitors his cardiovascular and respira-tory condition on the screen. The surgery can begin. I grab the papilloma with microforceps. The laser beam frees it and cuts it off at its base. There is no bleeding. The precision of the cut on this 8 mm papilloma is in the order of 100 microns. The laser enables us to remove the papilloma without damaging the vocal ligament and without any bleeding. The cordal muscle is not touched.

How does the CO_2 laser function?

The sun is a multidirectional light source, its wavelengths are legion. But more than that, it is a natural light. Laser is a concept of light created by Man. In 1919, Albert Einstein presented "*Zur quan-tum Theorie der Stralung*" (the quantum theory of radiations). According to his theory, electrons, atoms, molecules, and photons interact with electromagnetic radiation by quantum units in three types of radiation transitions: absorption, spontaneous emission, and stimulated emission. These principles produced the LASER: it is the acronym for *L*ight *A*mplification by *S*timulated *E*mission of *R*adiation. The laser is a unidirectional light source. Each laser has only one wavelength, determined by its color, which defines its power. Some laser beams have a wavelength that is not visible to humans. Each type of laser interacts with tissue in a specific way, producing characteristic patterns. The properties of the CO_2 laser are particularly well suited to laryngeal surgery. The wavelength of the CO_2 laser is 10,600 nm. It emits in the infrared portion of the spectrum, which is invisible to the human eye. A helium-neon light source is required to direct the CO_2 laser beam with a precision of less than 1/10 mm. It was first introduced by Strong and Jako in 1972, in Boston. This focused beam, unidirectional, completely pre-dictable, of a determined strength, coagulates and severs at the same time. Healing is fast. It is an outstanding surgical tool. But it is only a tool! It avoids any hemorrhaging, any avoidable injury to the vocal cord (see Plates 23 and 24). It is a high-precision instru-ment that respects the nobility of the vocal ligament.

For Matthew, the future lies not in microsurgery, but in a new antiviral vaccine that international researchers are busy developing. Relapses can be spaced out by injecting a substance called Cidofovir into the submucosal base of the papilloma. For the time being, we can only hope for remission, not for a cure. When the vaccine is released, then Matthew will be cured. Preserving the voice is the number one objective of this type of microsurgery. Wanting to remove a lesion at all cost, at the risk of perturbing the vibration of the cords, is prejudicial to the voice if there is no cancerous growth. Despite numerous interventions, Matthew's voice has remained satisfactory, it has a very pleasing timbre with clear harmonics.

My thyroid was operated on, my voice broke and I'm suffocating

Nicolina was operated on for a node on the thyroid gland nearly two years ago. When she came to after surgery, she experienced breathing difficulties. "I couldn't breathe, I couldn't speak, I felt I was suffocating." An urgent tracheotomy (a hole in the trachea to allow breathing) was performed. What had happened?

Her husband was an anesthetist and had been present during the operation. He was therefore able to give me details of the surgery. The thyroid gland had been completely removed. When this thirty-six-year-old patient came to, she couldn't open her vocal cords spontaneously, which was why a tracheotomy had been necessary. Her vocal cords were no longer under her voluntary control. Four weeks later, I examined her and found that the vocal cords were moving very slightly, but not enough to open the glottis and allow air through correctly. Her breathing was weak and labored. The tracheotomy had to remain in place. Laser microsurgery would enable her to breathe better by opening up the glottic space at the back. In reality, but I am grossly oversimplifying, we speak with the two front thirds of the vocal cords and we breathe with the posterior third (the farther back you go, the wider the vocal cords open, as they are joined to a fixed point at the front.) I operated on Nicolina to ablate part of the left arytenoid and the posterior third of the vocal cord. The tracheotomy was taken out, but her voice remains veiled. Nicolina can now lead a normal life, or nearly normal, until such time as she can have a nerve graft on the larynx, a procedure that was experimented by Harvey Tucker in the United States in the 1980s and by Jean-Paul Marie in France at the turn of the 21st century.

I was operated on for multiple fractures after an accident, when I came round from the anesthetic, my voice had gone

Bernard suffered multiple fractures in a fall. This man in his forties is operated on urgently. The intervention lasts several hours. When he comes to, he can't speak properly. His voice is weak, breathy, easily tired. Examination of his vocal cords reveals that his left cord is immobile. It is fixed some way off the median line. Despite six months of voice therapy, his voice remains altered. For him to speak correctly, his vocal cords need to come into contact, which is not the case. Surgery is envisioned to bring the left vocal cord as close as possible to the median line to enable the right cord, which is mobile, to come into contact with it during phonation. Presently, this is not the case, the left cord is too far away. This procedure, known as cordal medialization, involves injecting a product into the left vocal cord to medialize it.

I operate and first inject collagen. The result is very encouraging, his voice is pleasant. The collagen is reabsorbed within a few months, "cannibalized" by his own organism, as happens in one-third of cases. We decide to try again, this time injecting an inert substance that can't be reabsorbed by the vocal cord. The result is satisfactory. Yet this left vocal cord remains immobile. It neither lengthens nor shortens. Only the right vocal cord does this. Little by little his voice improves, but though his spoken voice is correct, his singing voice is limited by the length of the immobile vocal cord. The laryngeal endoscopic surgery has avoided voice strain and has re-established a very satisfactory spoken voice, as well as avoided any danger of swallowing the wrong way or choking. Other surgical options include open surgery of the neck to place a prosthesis. Several techniques exist, but none has given sufficiently good results to outclass the others. Bernard has his social voice back. Talking no longer tires him, his timbre is once more recognized by his close family.

The brain can be the cause of language disorders

The voice is halting

Sometimes voice problems result not from lesions of the vocal cords, but from neurologic lesions, whose consequences can sometimes be treated through phonosurgery. You'll recall the case of Paul, who was reticent to answer the phone because he suffered from laryngeal spasms.

In spasmodic dysphonia, the voice is halting and trembles. "The ppa . . . tient ttalks li . . . kkke thhhis." There are two types of spasmodic dysphonia: in adduction (or closed) and in abduction (or open).

Spasmodic dysphonia in adduction (the vocal cords hypercontract as they close) is akin to speaking with a tight throat. The vocal cords are so tense they can barely vibrate. This produces laryngeal trembling. Observation of the cords with a fibroscope reveals anarchic movements, constriction of the pharynx, the tongue, the lips, shaking of the head. In this case, one must put an end to this hypercontraction by creating a pseudoparalysis.

Dysphonia in abduction (the vocal cords are bowed) is accompanied by breathy and halting speech. Fibroscopic examination of the larynx reveals tetany-induced movements of the vocal cords, which shake without apparent reason. In all these cases, spasmodic dysphonia is considerably aggravated by an emotional component and voice therapy can make an essential contribution here.

Aside from voice therapy, nowadays this disease is treated with injections of botulinum toxin repeated every four months. This injection partially paralyzes the vocal cord and prevents spasm. It normalizes vocal cadence and speech flow. The voice becomes audible, sociable, almost normal. The paralysis thus induced is temporary, but effective. It acts on the junction between muscle and nerve, and blocks the nervous impulse from the brain.

Another technique involving microsurgery consists in removing a part of the vocal muscle, at the same time using the laser to coagulate the terminal ramifications of the vocal cord nerve. The objective is the same, namely a diminution of the muscle tension of the cord, but the remission time is much longer in this case.

Mister Parkinson

Since Parkinson's disease was first described by James Parkinson in 1817, voice problems involved in this pathology combine trembling, a breathless voice, and difficulty in beginning a sentence. The treatment in this case is none other than the treatment of the disease itself. This type of dysphonia is defined as a hypokinetic dysphonia. It results from a lesion of the gray matter of the central nervous system. These vocal problems induce a monochord voice that is uniform and weak, difficult to understand. The resonance seems normal, but the musicality and consonants are imprecise. Often there is a rush of words, followed by brutal silence. Sometimes, quite involuntarily, the patient repeats certain syllables. Yet the intellect is intact. The vocal cords move symmetrically, but they are slightly atrophied. This is why when the disease is stable; some specialists propose an injection of collagen, or inert matter, to shape the body of the vocal cord. This remains a fairly polemic procedure and one that has limited applicability.

The muscles tire

Often misunderstood, myasthenia and its derivatives cause a weakening of the vocal muscles, vocal fatigue during speech, and a pinched vocal register while singing. The cause is a lesion of the neuromuscular junction. The lesion is induced by a decrease in acetylcholine, the neurotransmitter that is indispensable to connect muscles to nerve synapses. This results in a slight paralysis of the vocal cord. Its closure or adduction remains incomplete, hence the dysphonia. Sometimes, the abduction, or opening, is also perturbed. The vocal cords are unable to open correctly. There are breathing difficulties. Other symptoms of myasthenia are a droopy eyelid, a relatively lazy soft palate, a slightly nasal voice. The voice may be shaky. Medical treatment is required. The psychologist, the voice therapist, and the doctor form an important team in the treatment of this complex pathology.

Treating the larynx is necessary, but often it only represents the surface of the vocal injury. Science is nothing without a compassionate ear for the patient's feelings, experiences, and personality.

Chapter 14

Your voice:
a vulnerable instrument

Your voice travels with you, take good care of it.
If you don't protect it, no one else will.

A thorough understanding of our musical instrument, the larynx, enables us to avoid any violent efforts that might irreversibly damage it.

This chapter should be of interest to all voice professionals, especially singers, actors, lawyers, politicians, teachers, secretaries, hostesses, or sport coaches. The anatomic aspects of our vocal instrument that need to be taken into account are but the tip of the iceberg. Indeed, psychological aspects play just as important a role in our voicing.

Voice hypochondriacs are rare, but they exist! "Always consulting, never cured." These hypochondriacs are convinced that their vocal tone is affected by a passing hoarseness, excessive mucus, or a microbe on the vocal cords. Sometimes there's a grain of truth in what they say, but mostly, their problem is allergenic. The slightest ailment affecting any part of the anatomy between the lungs and the sinuses, the vocal cords and the lips, can alter our vocal timbre, the color, frequency, and power of our voice.

My voice is unstable

My voice betrays me at any time

This Tuesday afternoon in February 2003, a reputed lawyer, Sir M., consults me. His "Hello doctor" reveals a serious case of dysphonia. I ask: "How I can help?" His answer is eloquent. "My voice is unstable, I can no longer plead. I'm anxious, because instead of concentrating on what I'm going to say, I find myself worrying about my voice. I'm concerned that it's going to betray me at any moment." Sir M., fifty-nine years old and a smoker, continues: "Four months ago, I had an asthmatic type of cough. I coughed until I almost choked. Cortisone sprays were prescribed to me several times to treat my nose, since I also suffered from allergic rhinitis. In spite of this, my voice problems persisted. Instead of recurring, they became permanent. Presently, my voice misbehaves mostly at the end of the day. My cough is worse at night. I can hardly plead at all. I've had to delay all my cases this past month. You can appreciate that, if I'm paying attention to my voice, I'm not paying attention to the message it's delivering. I no longer control my voice. I'm not convincing. It's not me talking, it's my shadow. My voice is not in tune with my thoughts, therefore, I can't think. How can I explain this: my thoughts are killing me; I think so fast that my voice doesn't have time to express what I'm thinking, my thoughts are consuming me."

Listening to his tragic plea, I was very conscious of Sir M.'s distress. A pianist unable to move his fingers would feel the same distress. Faced with this broken, hoarse voice, sometimes inaudible and interrupted by coughing fits, I wondered what I was going to find.

"Before this episode, had you already suffered from any throat infection?" The answer was a categorical "No." "Are you allergic to anything? Have you been asthmatic? Are you on any medication?" (Asthmatic types of coughs can be induced by certain types of medication.) Again the answer was negative. Apart from this broken voice, his only other complaint concerns thick mucus that slides down into his throat and that he's forced to swallow. Until this point, I hadn't picked up on anything significant. There was little for me to go on. Before examining him, I question him further.

"Come to think of it, now that you mention it, Doctor, I do believe that in between meals I regurgitate and burp, I feel some burning, but it's nothing much. I've had cortisone, antibiotics, anti-inflammatories, nothing has worked." There's still nothing concrete for me to base a diagnosis on. I examine him, and a surprise is in store for me: the larynx is inflamed, red and covered in small white spots, as if covered with a sprinkling of snow. The appearance of the vocal cords, the epiglottis, the tonsils, the velum, and the back of the tongue remind me of something we see in babies: thrush. These little white spots are a fungal infection. There seems to be considerable swelling at the back of the throat. He has thrush, but there's more.

Why the voice has been hoarse for so long?

1. Now why would this thrush have settled in so long ago? Why has he had a burning sensation for the past two months? Two elements brought about this severe case of dysphonia. The first was gastric reflux, which opened the way for the second, the fungal infection in his throat, probably induced by the aggressive cortisone and antibiotic treatment he'd been on for several weeks.

2. My hypothesis is this: probably the gastric reflux bothers him first. It flows up from the stomach into the trachea, making him cough. The contractions of the abdominal wall caused by the coughing aggravate the reflux, which aggravates the coughing, and so on. A few weeks later, he's given cortisone sprays that he applies without protecting his mucous membranes from the acid reflux. The flora of the throat is now destabilized by the gastric acids and by the cortisone spray. It's a hotbed for thrush. Coughing involves a mechanical movement that brings the two vocal cords into brutal contact, as when you clap your hands together. No wonder the laryngeal instrument suffers if you cough twenty or more times a day.

3. The clues are now lined up, a therapeutic strategy can be devised for him: I must treat, on the one hand, the thrush and, on the other, his gastric reflux and cough, avoiding all use of

cortisone sprays. This treatment must be backed by an appropriate diet.

Ten days later: "Doctor, my voice is free again it's as if it had been taken hostage by the disease. I'm thinking again as I used to. I can plead without thinking about how I sound, I'm able to concentrate on what I must say to be convincing."

The power of the melody of the voice must be protected

Sir M.'s case is fascinating. It reveals the intricate ties between voice and personality, between thought and expression. Hurt the voice and you hurt the person's psyche. Gastric reflux must be treated, especially in voice professionals, and more importantly, its early diagnosis will ensure that the reflux is caught before it triggers other ailments that may mask the original problem.

An appropriate diet is the key for a healthy voice. Fruit, vegetables, pasta, and fish are all essential. We know from experience that dairy products, sauces, and cheese create and thicken mucous matter, which alters the vocal cords and affects their performance. Two hours before a lawyer is due in court to plead a case, he should restrict himself to a light, simple meal that provides him with slow-burning sugars—for example, pasta, certain fruit containing vitamin C, dried fruit. Avoid cassoulet (broad beans with fatty meat) and beer. In moderate doses, tea, and coffee are unlikely to cause any discomfort, in my experience. I suggest to Sir M. that he adopt suspenders. Indeed, his belt is too tight and this is propitious to reflux. I also advise him to drink frequently (water, of course!), which is not to say he must gulp down half a liter of water in twenty seconds, as this would cause violent gastric dilation; he must drink a glass at a time and drink more frequently. The known brands of energy drinks on the market can also be consumed, mixed in equal proportion with water.

But that is not all there is to a healthy diet. Green vegetables, broccoli are important for good abdominal transit. Stubborn constipation or excessive diarrhea perturb the diaphragm and, therefore, controlled breathing. Our vocal art forms a complex whole, yet protecting it is simple enough.

Athletes of the voice

Voice professionals are real athletes. Singers, comedians, speakers of all sorts, all need to associate their vocal activity with some form of sport. They owe it to themselves to improve and entertain their abdominal and thoracic respiratory muscles, as well as find inner harmony and balance. This is essential.

The first step to protecting your voice is to protect your breathing: the outward air stream is your vocal energy. Inhalation is mainly nasal. The nose acts as a filter that also humidifies and warms the incoming air stream.

When you speak or sing in public, the sentence, prosody, or melody often require you to take a brief inhalation, with the vocal cords fully open, followed by a long, well-controlled exhalation, with the vibrating surfaces of the vocal cords in contact. Lubrication is essential here. These incessant "ins and outs" are relatively dehydrating and the vocal cords can quickly dry out; hence, the increasing use of humidifiers in the dressing rooms of some singers and actors, in the homes of lawyers, lecturers and teachers.

These same voice professionals must watch their diet before an important performance in order not to ask too great an effort of their respiratory tract: after a copious meal, the digestive tract is heavily solicited and, therefore, requires more oxygen than usual. Finally, voice professionals are perfectly aware that the voice is affected by a humid house with fungi, as by a house that is over-heated and too dry.

Knowing how to dress

How you dress is also important. The lungs must be free to breathe. Constricting trousers or a corset, unfortunately often required in musical works from the 18th and 19th centuries, should never be worn. Within the thoracic cage, the lowest ribs or floating ribs are, as their name suggests, mobile anteriorly. Instead of being anchored to the sternum like the other ribs, they are fixed only posteriorly, to the spinal column. These floating ribs play a primordial role in respiratory amplitude during inhalation. Watch the maestro tenors as they prepare to emit a counter *C*! The amplitude they gain in this part of their body is impressive. It's important never to interfere with this amplitude between the inhalation and the exhalation. The symbiosis of the abdominal and thoracic breathing must be respected.

Talking of suspenders, two comments: their use gives certain voice professionals complete freedom of their diaphragmatic and thoracic breathing; the trousers must be ample. Braces have an added benefit: their pressure on the clavicles reminds professional singers not to lift their shoulders while they perform.

Voice, tobacco, and personality

A fine layer of mucus in the nasal fossae, at the level of the inferior turbinate, provides a protective covering. It traps dust particles, microparticles of pollution, it stops germs, humidifies, warms, or cools the air you breathe. When thick mucus is evacuated from the back of the throat, it causes significant scraping, on allergenic ground. This abundant posterior mucosal discharge is swallowed. The consequences of swallowing it are multiple: when it reaches the stomach, it provokes gastric contractions and reactive hyperacidity, which in turn attacks the posterior part of the larynx. This posterior discharge is, therefore, harmful on two counts: because of the scraping it causes and the gastric reflux it provokes.

Your lips and mouth must be moist at all times. Dry lips don't allow satisfactory vocal activity. This is where the salivary glands come in, the parotid gland on either side of your cheeks and the submaxillary gland on either side of the jaw. When you eat, it triggers a Pavlovian reflex: the mere fact of bringing food to your mouth causes secretions from your salivary glands and moistens the buccopharyngeal cavity. This saliva predigests food. It's also essential for the lubrication of the buccal cavity. When your mouth is dry, chewing gum can be a precious help as it stimulates the salivary glands and increases their secretion. However, don't chew gum that contains nicotine on the pretext that you are trying to give up smoking. It dries the salivary glands, irritates the base of the tongue, and dries out the vocal cords.

Muriel and Lauren Bacall Voice

Muriel, barely fifty, elegant, with a deep voice, is bothered by the raucous quality of her voice. For some months now, she hasn't dared to talk on the telephone. Her high notes have gone, and after a few minutes of conversation her speech is hardly intelligible. She can only talk for five to six minutes on the telephone, which is of hardly any help to her! She's become used to people greeting her with a "Hello Sir" on the phone. Her frequent coughing throughout the day, and sometimes at night, doesn't bother her. What bothers her is her voice. Muriel smokes nearly forty cigarettes a day, Gitanes (very strong cigarettes); what is more, she has done so for thirty years, since the age of twenty.

Her voice problems have perturbed her peace of mind. She is beginning to worry about cancer. Her voice is broken, gravelly, irregular. Examining her larynx, I notice significant swelling of the left vocal cord that looks pudgy, but shows no signs of a malignant tumor. The right vocal cord is slightly swollen and puffy looking, with a huge edema on each vocal cord . A personality such as hers, though not suited to a very high timbre, is out of kilter with her present voice. Surgery is necessary. In this case, cancer is not the issue, it's her communication with others.

Operating on Muriel and removing the two edemas from her vocal cords is going to change her voice. She will have a soprano voice. How dreadful! she exclaims. It's true that it would alter her personality significantly. This woman, who is an artist and a painter, couldn't abide this. I have to find a way of operating that will preserve her vocal identity while eliminating its raucous quality. Our challenge is to restore the voice she had when she was thirty, without removing the lower harmonics.

Both the body of the muscle and the quality of the cordal mucous membrane play a role in the timbre of the voice. An epithelial edema imparts a deep tonality and often unusual vocal sensuality. The procedure must take away enough of the edema, but not too much if she's to keep her Lauren Bacall voice. Having explained this technical approach to Muriel, we set a date for the surgery, four weeks later. I operate on her under general anesthesia. The laryngoscope is in place, I can begin the laser microsurgery of the larynx. Eyes riveted to the microscope, I observe her vocal cords. My assistant Jimmy and my son Patrick provide me with a better view of them by applying pressure to the larynx through the neck.

Here is the procedure followed:

1. On the left cord, there is an irregular-looking swelling, a polypoid cord. The laser, with its high precision of 120 microns,

enables me to remove the lesion while leaving part of the edema in situ.

2. On the right vocal cord, the edema is minimal; if I were to operate on it, her vocal register would go up by four notes (too high for such a personality). I decide to leave it alone. In her room, she utters her first voicing with her new voice, although I had asked her not to talk for a week. She's surprised by her voice. I insist: she must rest her voice until we meet in a week's time.

3. Three weeks have elapsed. Her voice has stabilized, regained its clarity, the timbre has retained its deep harmonics and its sensuality, but is now free of hoarseness and crackling. Her voice problems had stemmed from the passing years and from her smoking.

4. Six weeks after the operation, her vocal cords look satisfactory at her checkup visit. Her voice is clear, but Muriel tells me that by the end of the day, her voice is tired. Indeed, the vocal cords look dry to me. I ask her if she's still smoking on the sly. She answers immediately, a categorical "No" that allows no comeback. "But," she admits, "I chew between ten and fifteen nicotine gums a day." True, she has eliminated the tar that is carcinogenic. But nicotine chewing gum interferes with vocal suppleness, dries the mouth, perturbs the secretion of saliva, and alters the lubrication of the vocal cords. In Muriel's case, a patch will be more efficient and avoid this dehydration of the vocal cords. Three months later, she still hasn't smoked. The postsurgical scar on her vocal cords is no longer visible, and her voice has recovered the timbre she had in her thirties.

Voice and cigarettes

A real drug

Mr. L. B., an author with a number of books to his name, consults me about his broken voice. "This is not a recent problem, my voice has been hoarse for over a year. I started having a few problems with my voice in December '87." We were now in January 1989. "I have too much work on, I don't have time to go to the doctor." I examine him and find a small whitish mass that protrudes like a small cancerous growth in the middle of the right vocal cord. Aside from this, the larynx is mobile, which is an excellent sign; it means that the tumor hasn't invaded the vocal cord joint, the front part of the larynx, or the ganglions. In cases like this, in which the tumor is very localized, the success rate is 98%, performed under general anesthetic, for microsurgery with CO_2 laser, going in through the mouth without any incision of the skin, as described previously with a laryngoscope. During surgery, the pathologist informs me that the sample is cancerous, but that the surrounding tissue is healthy. As a result the cancer is completely removed.

A few days after his operation, I inform Mr. L. B. that the growth was cancerous, that it was completely excised, and that his chances of being cured are excellent. I ask the impossible of this writer who smokes sixty cigarettes a day: he must give up smoking! Passing from sixty cigarettes a day to none is a brutal shock for the organism, one that requires admirable willpower. What I asked, I got. He stopped smoking. The follow-up was regular, every two months. But something happens eighteen months later.

When he comes in for his scheduled checkup (a year and a half later), Mr. L. B. enters my consulting room with a good sonorous voice. Everything seems hunky-dory. And yet!

He sits in the armchair opposite me, having first deposited his hat and coat. He looks at me with upsetting anguish and says to me in his deep voice: "Doctor, I'm well, I have a good voice, I don't smoke, but that's all I can say that's positive." I must admit I wasn't quite following. The cancer was in complete remission, the vocal cords were vibrating perfectly. He then asks me for a blank sheet of paper. He places it on the desk in front of me. He takes out his pen. He leans on his elbow, his left hand to his forehead, his right hand poised, ready to write. A few minutes go by. He remains silent, his hand isn't moving, the sheet remains blank, the nib of the pen remains fixed to the same spot on the paper for two minutes. Two minutes seem very long when you are not talking, not moving, almost not breathing! At this point, a tear rolls down his left cheek, falls onto the paper and wets it. He looks up at me, takes his glasses off, puts them down, and says to me: "That is how it's been for a year and half. My Muses have abandoned me. I can no longer write. If I don't smoke, I have no imagination."

Life can be cruel. How terrible is this deprivation that he accuses of murdering his imagination. This man, this artist of the written word, is not a vocal cord, he's a human being. Tobacco was his drug. It seems it was indispensable to his creative flow. I suggested he smoke a pipe, with moderation; this way he could resume the familiar gestures and maintain a modest consumption of tobacco. Back then, nicotine substitutes weren't what they are today.

Since then, I see him regularly, two to three times a year. He has found his Muses again, his larynx is fine, his creative juices are flowing again

The dangers of tobacco: tar and nicotine

Tar or benzopyrene is carcinogenic. It forms deposits on the mucous membrane of the vocal cords, and also on the pulmonary epithelium. It is responsible for 97% of all cancers of the larynx. In the initial stages, it's just a simple white plaque that causes the voice to break periodically. Mr. L. B. allowed the tar to pursue its deadly course unperturbed. First, it provoked laryngitis, associated with gastric reflux. Smoking weakened the immune defenses of the laryngeal mucous membrane and opened the door, first to the laryngitis and secondarily to the cancer.

Nicotine works in a different and far more subtle way. It is a long-term process. Nicotinic acid operates on a vascular level. It provokes and even aggravates arteriosclerosis.

Tobacco is a drug. Mr. L. B. is a case in point of the consequences of tobacco addiction. Nicotine acts on the brain, more specifically on the hypothalamus. It can have an excitatory action and often creates dependency. In effect, your own organism begins to secrete nicotinic acid. It also acts on the regulating center of your base metabolism. When you stop smoking, the nicotinic acid no longer acts on the hypothalamus. It no longer has a braking influence. This is why there is a risk of putting on weight. Many heavy smokers who give up smoking from one day to the next without taking any nicotinic substitutes, find themselves putting on 5 to 10 kg in a few months.

Smoking with the vocal cords open or closed

Voice professionals who smoke during their phonatory activity are more subject to laryngeal lesions than someone who smokes at his computer without talking. When you talk, you exhale and the vocal cords move inward. They vibrate, they join up, the edges of the left and right cordal mucous membranes come into contact. This allows the nicotine and tar to infiltrate the mucous membrane of the vibrating cord. Little by little, microtraumatisms affect the epithelium. Lesions gain a foothold. When you exhale without speaking, the vocal cords are open, almost absent from the glottic space, as during the inhalation. They don't form an obstacle in the pathway of the outward air stream. The nicotine and tar still have an impact, but it's much reduced at the level of the vocal cords, because they're wide open.

As for alcohol, when imbibed in great quantity, it causes vascular lesions as well as hepatic, venous, and gastric disturbances. It aggravates the impact of smoking, increasing by a factor of 3 the complications caused by tobacco consumption.

"Hello, good morning, Sir.—Actually, it's Madam."

Tobacco doesn't just have a carcinogenic impact, it can also provoke an edema of the vocal cords. This edema is the result of gelatin or glue forms located between the muscle and the mucous membrane of the vocal cords, just under the surface. This gelatinous oozing weighs down the vibratory organ. But how does it form in the first place? In nearly 99% of cases, it afflicts smokers, especially female smokers who smoke more than 15 cigarettes a day. It seems that inhaling cigarette smoke provokes a double aggression, vascular and keratosic, due to the nicotine and tar contents of tobacco. Keratosis is none other than a fine horny layer that forms on the cordal mucous membrane as a result of a chronic irritation induced by the smoke; this is associated with voice strain and frequently with gastric reflux. This polypoid edema of the vocal cords gives women a deep, masculine voice, which is not necessarily bothersome. It need only be operated on if cancer is suspected or if the voice jars with the rest of the smoker's personality.

It's not always the fault of the cigarette

Air conditioning

But smoking is not the only guilty party causing alterations of the larynx. Pollution and allergenic substances that perturb the nasal cavities can provoke an inflammation of the vocal cords. The same is true of very dry environments. Proper lubrication of the pharyngo-laryngeal structures should be of concern to us not only in the work-place, but equally in our everyday lives. In an air-conditioned car, the level of moisture in the air is too low. If you speak in the car, you'll strain your voice. This is because you'll be raising your voice above the noise of the engine, in an atmosphere that is dry because of the air conditioning. The same applies if you take a train or plane. During a relatively long trip, you are well advised to drink often, speak little, and avoid alcohol and aspirin. Alcohol provokes vascular dilation, aspirin thins the blood, and this weakens the vocal cords. In a dehydrated atmosphere, the microvessels on the vocal cords are less resistant. All it takes is a violent sneeze or a cough, or having to raise your voice during a discussion, and the weakened vessels won't resist. Aspirin can also provoke a microhematoma of the vocal cords.

Airplanes and the voice

Mrs. C. B., a singer in her thirties, arrives from foreign parts after a long plane trip. When she lands, her voice is hoarse. I receive her a few hours after her arrival in Paris, in the afternoon. "My voice is hoarse, Doctor; it's true I talked nonstop on the plane. I drank two glasses of champagne. Within a few hours, I felt my voice deteriorate."

What happened? In the plane, the degree of moisture in the air is 3%, compared to 40% in Paris. The noise of the engines is 60 to 70 dB, whereas ambient noise in normal surroundings is 15 dB. Drinking champagne causes the capillaries of the larynx to constrict and dehydrates the vocal cords. The flight lasted eight hours. These elements combined to alter the vibration of her vocal cords. In order to be heard, she had to speak louder over the engine noise in a dry atmosphere, but that is not all! Mrs. C.B. was in her premenstrual phase. We've seen that in this phase, capillaries are more fragile, frequently the vocal cords may present an edema. Worse still, she'd had a headache the night before and had taken aspirin. On landing at Roissy, she was interviewed. At first, her hoarse voice didn't bother her. But a few hours later, her voice changed. She began to panic. The stroboscopic dynamic vocal exploration reveals a slight hematoma of the right vocal cord. It's benign, but requires vocal rest for ten days.

This revealing anecdote shows the important consequences that these lesions of the voice can have due to our environment. Thus, the voice professional who wants to avoid this type of incident is well advised to maintain complete silence during a flight, especially in the premenstrual phase.

Allergy and chronic dysphonia

In another register, Mrs. A. G. consults me for excessive vocal fatigue and a frequent complete break in her voice. In her childhood, she suffered a few asthma attacks. Her carpet was changed a few months ago, which is when her dysphonia started. This thirty-nine-year-old woman doesn't seem to be at all psychologically dependent on her broken voice. Examination of her larynx reveals a swelling of the vocal cords, associated with an inflammation. Besides this, the nasal fossae reveal the presence of a few small growths, small allergic polyps. Because of the swollen vocal cords and because breathing through the nose is difficult, Mrs. A. G., who is a nursery school teacher, had to raise her voice. Within a matter of weeks, the vocal strain caused tiny nodules to appear. The problem has to be treated at its source. The trigger was allergens. They provoked a chain reaction: altered nasal breathing, nasal polyposis, asthmatic type tracheitis with coughing that is traumatic for the vocal cords, cordal nodules. An allergy test establishes her sensitivity to acarids and dust. Acarids are tiny living creatures that eat our dead skin and can provoke allergic reactions. A desensitization program associated with her medical treatment enabled Mrs. A. G. to recover from her allergic dysphonia in a matter of months.

What is an allergy? Why is our larynx so sensitive to allergens? An allergy is a hyperreaction of the organism that overreacts when aggravated by an external molecule such as dust, acarid, pollen, animal hair, and so forth. This reactive phenomenon is an immune response from cells called "macrophages." Instead of neutralizing the molecule, these large phagocytes make a whole song and dance over it and alert the entire organism. They create an edema, a disproportionate inflammatory reaction such as an asthma attack, for example, or a sneezing fit.

Around the vocal cords

However, many things can cause a vocal disturbance. A serous otitis, an inflammation of the middle ear can be bothersome for the voice: the retro-control "voice-ear" does not function correctly anymore. An appropriate treatment is essential, not for the larynx, but for the person's hearing.

Singing or talking for too long, too loudly, overtraining the voice can also be bad news for the voice. It's as if an athlete at the Olympic Games were to run 100 meters in 10 seconds, an hour before a competition. He would have exhausted his reserves, both energetic and mental, before the race.

The nursery school teacher

Whenever you talk, sing, laugh, or shout, your voice should never hurt. It can feel weak, but if you feel pain, you have just been put on alert. You may be reacting to a minor muscle tear, tightness of the larynx, or simply general fatigue. You can shout, but you must know how to shout.

Recognizing that you are entitled to feel tired is a strength. You must not systematically want to palliate this tiredness with medication. However, occasionally rehearsals do impose a forced rhythm on voice professionals. Annoyance can affect your vocal vibration. This is where professionalism enters the picture; your experience protects you., You must be able to isolate yourself from the outside world during your rehearsals, and know when to stop. As the proverb says: "Better is the enemy of good."

Training, not overtraining

If you are just starting a singing career or another career that requires you to speak in front of an audience, beware of bad habits and inappropriate vocal techniques. Your singing teacher, who has your best interests at heart, is your best insurance if you want to take good care of your voice and avoid abusing your vocal cords. Rehearsals are essential: they focus on precise exercises that help to assimilate the technique.

Professional singers normally do between one and three hours of singing practice a day. This enables them to keep their muscles supple and preserve their acoustic training. However, a word of advice, never start singing straight off. You should never stretch your muscles without first giving them a warm-up, for example, by voicing with your mouth closed. Otherwise you risk microslashes in the cordal muscles, which would cause you to lose the high notes of your register. Obviously, you should never rehearse an opera or a play six to eight hours a day, yet I have seen this happen all too often. It's hardly surprising that this can bring about a nodule or a hematoma of a vocal cord. Do you see marathon runners training eight hours a day? Even when training for the gruelling Tour de France, cyclists never practice for more than seven hours a day, and that is considered to be a real feat.

School teachers must learn to place their voice. They too are marathon competitors, of the voice. They would be well advised to take six to eight voice therapy lessons once or twice a year.

Fans shout their support at a tennis or a football match, a mother yells at her children in the street, but their voices haven't first been properly warmed up. If a hematoma appears and is not treated, the pathology evolves. The small pocket of blood pools and forms a reddish angiomatous polyp. The voice becomes increasingly hoarse, but not so much that it worries the fan or the mother. The polyp grows bigger over the years, alters the voice, and creates hoarseness and voice strain.

My voice breaks in the afternoon

"My voice breaks in the afternoon. It's slow getting going in the morning." Mrs. E. S. is a teacher at a nursery school. She's forty-four. She doesn't smoke, but the little ones take a heavy toll on her voice: she has to sing, speak, imitate animals. Voice strain is inevitable. By the end of the term, teaching her class poses a real problem to her. About a year ago, she became very hoarse during singing practice with the children at the end of a school day, but her speech was not particularly affected. The next day, when class started, her larynx was painful on the left side. She could no longer sing. She's slightly hoarse when she speaks. "I was tired, my problem persisted, but my voice was intelligible."

Time passes. The pain disappears, but her voice worsens. She has two problems: her voice tires easily, and she's lost all the high notes of her singing register, with the result that she hasn't been able to sing for some months. On examination, her left vocal cord presents microvaricose veins and a hemorrhaging polyp hangs on the edge of the cord, preventing it from making proper contact with the right vocal cord. This alters the cord's vibration. The ill treatment of her voice over the past year caused the polyp to form.

The more Mrs. E. S. talks, the more she forces her voice in order to speak, the worse the polyp gets. This is what happened: the hematoma that appeared when her voice got hoarse while singing in class a year ago was not treated. Under the influence of constant vibratory traumatism and because she didn't rest her voice, a pocket of blood collected. The hemorrhage liquid formed a polyp on the part of the membrane that is most solicited during the vibration, words the medial third of the vocal cord. The hematoma was the guilty party. The polyp is its manifestation.

The health of your voice, its efficiency, and its characteristics depend on three factors that we have already seen—*closure*, *vibration*, and *lubrication* of the vocal cords. At least one of these three factors is implicated in all pathologies, all alterations, all ailments, or accidents of the voice.

An example: open your fingers and spread your index and middle finger apart. Imagine they are your vocal cords. Close the fingers, so they are now touching. That is when the vocal onset happens, while the vocal cords are closed. This closure activates and enables the vibration through contact. Lubrication, or proper hydration of the vocal cords, is essential to prevent the cords from overheating and allows them to make contact, for example, 440 times per second for the *A* note, which amounts to 4,400 vibrations in ten seconds. Rub your hands just ten times in two seconds, they'll begin to burn if they are not hydrated.

Coming back to your two index and middle fingers. Place a pencil between them: they don't touch anymore, just as your vocal cords wouldn't if there were an obstacle between them. When a vocal cord is in spasm, it's paralyzed and this prevents the two cords from coming into contact. No voicing is possible, because there is no contact; contact is our first key word.

If the cords are in contact, but the vibration is perturbed, the voice sounds raucous, as in the case of Mrs. E.S. with her angiomatous polyp. The same happens with a hard nodule, a granuloma, or a severe edema forming a cordal mass. Sometimes the hoarseness is caused by an inflammation, laryngitis for instance. Or it can result from tired laryngeal muscles. Muscle fatigue changes the vibration of the vocal cords: *vibration* is the second key word.

Close your fingers and pour bleach over them. The skin becomes less supple, harsher. Its vibration is altered. The voice is raucous. It is not properly lubricated. Overheating of the vocal cords is an aggravating factor in laryngeal pathologies. Gastric reflux perturbs the lubrication of the vocal cords: *lubrication* is our third key word.

Any mass on the vocal cords results in bad vocal habits

Mrs. E. S. has a well-defined polyp that needs to be removed if she is to recover her normal voice. But surgery alone won't do it. She's acquired bad vocal habits. She needs to rebalance her pneumophonic efforts to harmonize her voicing with her breathing. This teacher has been straining her voice for several months now. Voice therapy is essential in her case, both before and after her surgery, to help her regain the harmonious vocal movements her work requires. To understand the role of the symmetry of the vocal cords during phonation, imagine yourself extending both arms straight out, nice and solid. On your right arm, I hang a 1.5 kg weight. This flexes the arm slightly. You now use your muscles to re-establish the symmetry between the two arms and have them both level with each other again. When I remove the weight, your right arm lifts a little, because the extra muscular effort that was solicited is still memorized. There's a slight delay before it readjusts itself once more level with the left arm. The same happens in the larynx, the polyp being the weight on one vocal cord. After its removal, a new balance has to be found between the two cords.

Dental hygiene

The bite, the structure of our teeth, can also be responsible for voice problems.

We saw earlier that the articulation of the jaw is unique in the human body. Remember that the jaw has two joints with the cranium. Indeed, it forms a veritable arc with its two associated joints, one on the left and one on the right, both perfectly mobile in the vertical axis. An impressive mass of muscles allows this mobility. Together, these muscles enable us to speak, to create vowels, to sing, to eat, to swallow, to yawn. A grain of sand in this perfectly oiled mechanism can trigger serious secondary effects. Of course, the teeth themselves have a role to play in this; thus, a defective bite can cause an asymmetry of the mandible joints and affect the cervical muscles. The voice changes progressively if the bite is defective. The importance of proper buccal and dental hygiene is too often neglected. This complex mechanism must be cared for properly, as it's an essential element in structuring the voice. Dentition plays a role in our vocal expression. In their first year, babies acquire milk teeth that enable them to pronounce their first words, switch to solid nutrition, and perfect their vocal expression. This dentin barrier between the outside world and our inner pharyngeal world puts in place the internal buccopharyngeal architecture required to communicate with others. The first teeth appear around six months. Some of us will lose our teeth around the age of seventy. Technological and surgical advances in the dental field point to an undeniable trend to healthier teeth and gums in old age, with the help of prostheses and dental implants that ensure a tonic and satisfactory voice.

Voice and posture

Hunching and the voice

Mr. S. R. is a comedian and singer. For some months now, his voice has been breathy. He lives in Sri Lanka and is unable to pursue his livelihood. His voice deteriorated initially after a bout of flu that brought on coughing and a bronchial infection. "This isn't the first time I have had bronchitis, but usually I can carry on acting and singing. This time around, my voice abandoned me after ten days. They want to operate, they say my right cord is paralyzed. What is your opinion?"

I examine him and notice that the right vocal cord is immobile. Note that I didn't say it was paralyzed, just that it wasn't possible to move the cord on the right side—there's an important difference. The elasticity of his vocal muscles is satisfactory and the body of the muscle shows the same bulk on both cords. This means there's no paralysis. Indeed, when a nerve is affected, the vocal cord becomes thinner and atrophies. His mucous membrane vibrates harmoniously and correctly, but only in the medium frequencies. High notes are impossible, deep notes are tricky. In effect, because the right cord is not moving, the left cord has to work harder to make contact and allow some form of vibration. Looking through a magnifying glass associated with a video camera, the diagnosis becomes evident. There is significant inflammation of the right cordal joint. It's a case of arthritis of the vocal joint (this formation is also called the cricoarytenoid joint: between the cricoid and arytenoid cartilages, the vocal cord is fixed on the arytenoid cartilage and can move thanks to this joint). This chronic cricoarytenoid inflammation on the right followed an acute inflammation that blocked the mobility of the vocal cord.

But I'm not entirely satisfied. It is not customary for arthritis to develop like this without some sort of trigger. I try to ferret out more information: "What exactly does your work consist of? How do you perform your roles, your songs on stage? What is your posture, what movements are required?" I ask this because Mr. S. R's posture is odd. He holds his head slightly inclined to the left. This indicates a defective cervical alignment. His answer provides me with all the clues I need to understand his pathology, which is an unusual one. He explains: "I'm a puppet-show actor and singer. I always hold my right arm up in the air to control the puppet. I'm standing, and my hand is wrapped in a piece of cloth that is supposed to talk." As his left arm is alongside his body and inactive, this significant extension forces him to incline his head to the left when he wants to speak, so that he can extend the right arm better. The right cervical muscles are in hyperextension. But he's been holding this position for over fifteen years. Why did this crippling arthritis of the right vocal cord only materialized three months ago? This prompted my next question: "Have you changed the setup of the puppets?" "Ah! he answers, I forgot to tell you that for technical reasons, the curtain that hides my hand is now 7 cm higher. It was altered three weeks before my voice broke."

The guilty party has been unmasked. This alteration brought the right arm into maximal hyperextension; this created an imbalance between the pectoral and laryngeal muscles and overtensed the cricothyroid joint, causing it to be jammed by the neck muscles and cartilages (this joint between the thyroid and the cricoid cartilages allowed the larynx to rise in the neck and to produce a head voice).

The flu episode and the cough were only aggravating factors. My diagnosis was, therefore, fixation of the right vocal cord, brought on by arthritis of the joint induced by defective posture of the neck during phonation! The appropriate treatment wasn't surgery, but medication, in the form of a cortisone infiltration into the joint, as well as cervical massages and anti-inflammatory treatment. Within a few weeks all was back to normal. The right vocal cord recovered its mobility, and the puppets recovered their voice. Mr. S. R. is no longer allowed to hunch while he talks on stage. Awareness of the importance of good posture for vocal health is essential.

A singing and piano teacher: a badly positioned head, a broken voice

Mrs. C. G. is a singing and piano teacher. She teaches eight hours a day. This has been her line of work for the past forty years. She has her habits. Her pupil sits on her right. He practices his scales, one after the other, and she accompanies the vocalizations of the young singer both at the piano and with her own voice. For some time now, her voice has been tiring. She has to pause for almost twenty minutes between lessons, massage her neck, and relax her cervical vertebrae. "I can speak all right, but I can't sing for longer than twenty or thirty minutes at a time. My voice tires."

I examine her and find her larynx is normal. The vocal cords are symmetrical. "Madam, everything looks fine. The vocal cords are white and pearly. The vibration is harmonious, there's no visible inflammation." I then ask her to sing while mimicking the position she normally adopts in her lessons. The outcome is surprising. I study her larynx as she sings: her head is turned 90°, the vocal cords are asymmetric. The right vocal cord now seems bulkier than the left and the joint of the left vocal cord swells within a few minutes, as if turning her neck were constricting the joint's mobility. The head is turned, but not the torso, and the head is slightly inclined to face her virtual pupil. She mimes for me with her hands, as if she were accompanying the pupil on the piano. She explains that, to maximize her influence over her pupil, she moves in closer to him. Because the piano doesn't move with her, she's forced to extend her arms in tension farther and farther in the opposite direction to her head.

What is happening here? Her thoracic amplitude and pulmonary breathing are constricted. The body is no longer in its customary physiologic position. The angle of the neck relative to the thorax strains the spinal muscles. Her vocal fatigue is strictly mechanical. In no way is the teacher's singing technique implicated. One could have supposed that the menopause could have been partly responsible; but this wasn't the case. The treatment boiled down to some eminently practical advice: move the piano or position your pupil differently. Now the pupil sits in front of Mrs. C. G. Physiotherapy on her cervical muscles and spine enabled her to correct her defective posture.

Craning the neck like a tortoise

An English judge has suffered badly from voice fatigue for nearly a year. In his sixties, Mr. W. R. loses his voice after speaking for barely ten minutes. He also complains of being slightly deaf. His explanation is highly theatrical. Seated in the examination chair, he sits bolt-upright and mimes a court case for me. I feel I'm right there in court with him. He tells me about a verdict he rendered last week. His whole upper body now leans forward, chin up, head turned slightly to the left. He informs me that this is the posture he assumes when listening to the defense lawyer. His neck is taut and sticks out, reminding me of the way a tortoise sticks its neck out of its shell. His back is under maximal tension, buttressed in the chair. In fact, he has to lean forward in this position to hear what's being said in the courtroom, compensating for the defective hearing of his left ear. He cranes his neck to hear better. The abnormal tension exerted on the muscles between his chin and his trachea causes excessive muscle strain and tires his voice. This dynamic distortion alters the symmetrical movement of the vocal cords, as became evident from examining his larynx. Judge W. R. needs appropriate physiotherapy for his cervical vertebrae, a course of anti-inflammatory medication for a few weeks, and a hearing aid for his left ear.

Maintaining the correct posture avoids distortions of the larynx. Speaking in a contorted position can alter the voice as much as a polyp can, in spite of being external to the laryngeal music instrument. Daily breathing and stretching exercises would be an additional bonus for the vocal health of the judge.

The voice, clearing one's throat and halitosis

This actor, a member of the Comédie Française and a nonsmoker, complained of episodic bad breath, a chronic need to clear his throat, and more frequent breaking of the voice at the change of season. On examination, the larynx is ruled out. His vocal cords are fine. But I detect small spongy-looking crypts, or holes, near the tonsils. Whitish deposits stagnate in these cavities. They look like curdled milk; this is known as caseous tonsillitis. Moreover, the nasal fibroscopy reveals another surprise: an inflammation of the nasal vegetations. His voice problems arose not from his vocal instrument, but from its environment, as when the resonating box of a violin is humid, but its cords are dry. The solution in his case was to medically treat the nose and tonsils with a local disinfectant, carry out a simple microsurgical procedure under local anesthetic to remove the vegetations, and vaporize the tonsils with the laser to make them smooth again and avoid a return of the caseum.

This anecdote is interesting on several counts. The vocal cords were normal, yet the patient complained of voice fatigue. The cause of his problem was an indirect one. This is why we specialists can't just check out the vocal cords. We have to be on the look out for tonsillitis, an inflammation of the vegetations, or gastric reflux. Removing the tonsils completely could have had dramatic consequences for this actor. It would have changed the harmony of his vocal resonance chamber. However, it's worth noting that the removal of the tonsils is sometimes indicated for voice professionals suffering from hypertrophied tonsils complicated by frequent infections.

The voice catches a cold: it can be bad news, just as it can be nothing

When you catch a cold, your voice commonly becomes hoarse. Your voice breaks, you have a moderate temperature and your throat burns.

The clinical examination usually begins with the ears. Patients can present a serous otitis (an inflammation of the middle ear, with liquid trapped behind the tympanum, with no pain). This serous otitis would give the patient the impression that his hearing is distorted and damped. He hears himself faintly. This makes it difficult for him to balance his voice. Next we examine the nasal fossae, to see whether a possible deviation of the septum could be making breathing chronically difficult. We check for sinusitis and for any purulent discharge at the back of the nose. We examine the appearance of the tonsils. If the vocal cords are red and inflamed, this signifies some sort of infection, bacterial or viral, or both. A cough aggravates the inflammation of the vocal cords and can trigger gastric reflux. To avoid a secondary bacterial infection in voice professionals afflicted with a viral infection, we prescribe antibiotics, as well as acetaminophen. A treatment including inhalations (eucalyptus, sulfur) and throat gargles (water and sea salt)—these two therapies have existed since Aristotle and Socrates—cough mixtures, essential oils, vitamin C, and sometimes vasoconstrictors for the nose, accelerates the recovery and return to health of both the organism generally and the laryngeal instrument specifically.

An altered voice and a normal larynx

Some children experience difficulties placing their voice. If boys experience problems stabilizing the lower frequencies naturally, a pneumophonatory imbalance is normally involved. The adolescent then speaks in a falsetto voice. This seems to happen when the exhalation is excessively powerful in relation to the muscles of the larynx. But the emotional element of this problem should not be passed over. The specialist is often forced to conclude that his young patient doesn't want to face up to his adult responsibilities but wants to remain mama's little boy. I'm simplifying again, but the psychological component is certainly fundamental, and it is often associated with a mechanical problem of the larynx. This pneumophonatory alteration normally responds well to voice therapy. Of interest here is the fact that some sixteen-year-old boys whose voices haven't broken in the mother tongue, nevertheless have a deep voice when speaking in a foreign language. The psycho-affective barrier is perfectly obvious in these cases.

This same barrier is operative in psychogenic aphonia; here the person, often a woman, suddenly decides subconsciously not to talk anymore, instead, she whispers. But this unconscious masquerade is soon exposed when the doctor or specialist asks the patient to cough. The cough comes out loud, deep, natural; coughing is a reflex, therefore it can't be controlled and the natural voice is revealed, undampened.

To protect your voice is to protect yourself.

Protecting your voice requires more than knowledge of the vocal mechanism and its mechanics; it requires knowing yourself well. Sometimes resorting to a foreign language that you can hide behind can be a great psychological shield. Indeed, you can always pretend that you used a word mistakenly.

Chapter 15

The voice's health

We all have an internal clock that regulates our life style, our daily activities, our sleep. It's important to respect it.

Hippocrates: "Your diet is your first medicine."

The voice professional is a vocal athlete

Masters in communication, athletes of vocal expression, teachers, singers, lawyers, diplomats, or lecturers all use the same working tool. A working tool that isn't sheltered from the outside world, bad weather, allergies, pollution, and hygrometry. It's closely related to our intimate thoughts and emotions. To preserve this irreplaceable musical instrument of yours that is the larynx, you need to observe some simple rules of vocal hygiene. Your brain has to be suitably oxygenated and nourished to give others, but also yourself, the benefit of its best performance.

Your voice derives its energy from its outward airflow. This presupposes a healthy respiratory tree. Your voice is born from the vibration of your tensed vocal cords, striated muscles covered by a mucous membrane. These muscles require seven times more energy than your biceps. Your resonators are also made of striated muscle hungry for energy. Thus, if this multifactorial system (oxygen, energy for your muscles and joints) is to endure, voice professionals must behave as athletes.

Are there any specific requirements? The answer is a most definite "yes." However, voice professionals should adapt these recommendations to suit their specific line of work and their personality.

Your voice and medication

Appropriate dosages

The response to a given medication and to a given dose is individual, whether the medication is allopathic, homeopathic, or composed of vitamins, minerals, or essential oils.

For instance, 0.5 g of aspirin may suffice to clear your headache, whereas a friend may have to take 1 g. The response is individual, as is the time of day for the medication, which influences how much needs to be taken for the medication to be effective. We call this the "chronobiological" factor.

Our medical reference books suggest an average dose, never intending to be a bible of invariable dosages. Numerous variables can influence and determine the efficacy of a medical treatment: the patient's age, weight, degree of tiredness, stress, and, in a woman, the phase of her hormonal cycle. Age is the most obvious variable. The metabolism, digestion, and capacity for absorbing medication of a man in his thirties are faster and more efficient than those of a man in his sixties. Height, ratio of fat to lean tissue, or simply degree of overweight and muscle mass will influence the diffusion of the molecules contained in the capsule you are about to take.

If you are obese, fat cells will trap certain medicines. In this case, the dosage must be increased to obtain a maximal effect on the larynx. For example, let's say an overweight patient takes 2 g of a substance we'll call X: if 1.5 g are trapped by his fat cells, only 0.5 g will get through to the part needing treatment. If the patient is thin, only 0.5 g of the 2 g ingested will be trapped by his fat cells, so that 1.5 g will get through to the vocal cords. Thus it is that the same dose can be of variable efficacy. Prescriptions must take these factors into account if the medicine is to be effective without overdosing the patient. What happens to molecules that are trapped by fat cells? They are either destroyed by the same cells or released later on into the bloodstream, which isn't without consequences.

Indeed, this new molecular release may cause the medicine's action to reach a peak in the patient's organism 24 to 48 hours later.

The kidneys must function well. They eliminate the remains of the medication into the urine. They also eliminate harmful ingested substances after these have been detoxified by the liver.

The threshold effect of medication: "The medicine cured me, but it made me ill."

Having said this, and to avoid any confusion, it is important to specify that an effective dose, called the threshold dose, is primordial in the treatment of any ailment. If the dose is below this threshold, the patient will not have been treated, but simply will have taken in medication, the sole "advantages" of which will boil down to its harmful consequences. These side effects, such as diarrhea, allergies, intolerance, they bring no benefits.

On the other hand, if the dose taken is above the threshold dose and significantly above it, such an overdose can also have negative side effects: the patient may be cured of his original ailment, but the capsule may now make him ill. These secondary side effects can be worse for the patient than the original ailment. As the elderly often say, "Doctor, the medicine cured me, but it made me ill."

The subtlety consists in adjusting the dose so as to be somewhere between the threshold dose and the patient's maximum tolerance dose. This is where good knowledge of one's patients, their environment, and their illness, combined with the doctor's own experience, helps to determine the optimal dose in each individual case, something the country doctor, who has one of the most enviable professions in the world, does remarkably well.

What is the action of certain medicines on the voice and what are their side effects?

Any medication can have an impact that improves the vocal tract, yet also penalizes it.

A well-known example of this is aspirin, which even in low doses can liquefy the blood significantly and cause capillary fragility; aspirin is, therefore, not recommended for female voice professionals just before their periods, as it could cause excessive bleeding and considerable tiredness.

Allergies and asthma require specific treatments, some of which dry out the vocal cords. The best known are antihistamines. These molecules inhibit histamine receptors and diminish edematous reactions and liquid discharges. But their advantages have disadvantages. They dry out the resonators and the larynx and can cause slight drowsiness (an anticholinergic reaction). They must, therefore, be taken at least eight hours before a vocal performance, or the night before, in order to avoid drying out the vocal cords. Also, they should be associated with a significant increase in liquid intake: 2 to 3 liters a day.

Cortisone or steroid inhalators are another type of medication that is particularly effective in the treatment of asthma and some forms of allergic rhinitis. They have the advantage of acting directly on the respiratory mucous membrane. A few micrograms might be absorbed into the bloodstream, but the most recent molecules released on the market have a minimal systemic or circulatory impact.

However, three precautions are primordial. First, after inhaling corticosteroids, patients should systematically rinse out their mouth to avoid a serious complication: buccopharyngeal fungi. The second precaution relates to a more perverse reaction: it concerns a side effect of corticosteroids that affects the cordal muscle. Months later, possibly even years later, the vocal cords begin to lose muscle strength. The cordal muscle atrophies slightly. The cords lose some of their agility. Their response time is slightly longer, especially in relation to short, sharp staccato notes. To palliate this type of side effect, which I have observed in about 10% of my asthmatic patients, an adjuvant polyvitamin treatment should be prescribed to maintain a satisfactory and efficient musculature. The third precaution is to avoid the appearance or recurrence of gastric reflux. The inhalation of corticosteroids triggers ipso facto, within the minute, a swallowing reflex; hence, repeated inhalations irritate the esophagus and cardia (the superior level of the stomach) and induce gastric reflux. The reflux must be treated, but it can be prevented by drinking a glass of water after each inhalation.

The inhalation of corticosteroids associated with a bronchodilator is a therapeutic modality asthmatics are very familiar with. It improves their quality of life significantly. Many singers and actors,

30 to 40 minutes before a show, have to resort to inhalations of corticosteroids and bronchodilators, or sympatomimetics, in order to be in top breathing form for the performance.

What role can cortisone play, so rejected by some, so appreciated by others?

Cortisone is by far the most efficient anti-inflammatory. It's also the treatment of choice for acute allergic crises. It reduces the reactive edema brought on by the allergy. It diminishes the inflammation secondary to an infection. It re-establishes the muscle structure after a problem caused by muscle tearing, avoiding prejudicial inflammatory and fibrous scarring. This tricky medicine remains a more than satisfactory weapon against certain throat and lung diseases; nevertheless, its prescription for voice professionals should be carefully weighed.

Appreciated by some for its truly doping effect before a show, such usage is to be proscribed to protect the long-term health of the organism and vocal cords, given the negative side effects that cortisone can have in the long term if taken over a period of years (insomnia, gastritis, muscular weakness and atrophy, sometimes edemas; more rarely, a diabetic reaction or decalcification that can provoke bone fractures).

This being said, if you are suffering from a serious infection or an acute inflammation, corticosteroids are spectacularly efficient. They should be taken over a short period of three to four days, with no requirement for progressively lowering the dose. Moreover, in order not to gain weight while on the medication, and for the next two days, the patient should be on a strict diet that excludes salt and alcohol: cortisone can be trapped by fat cells and released later. Some patients present a mycosis after taking cortisone, especially if the cortisone is taken with antibiotics and the patient suffers from gastric reflux. These patients should systematically start a suitable antimycosis treatment.

But remember the need to be above the threshold level. Taking too little medication is of no use and just delivers its negative side effects. That is why only doctors and specialists are fit to judge whether a molecule is required and what the effective dosage for you is. Auto-medication should be proscribed.

Reflux: an ailment of the 21st century

These days, nearly half the patients suffering from laryngitis associated with a chronic cough also present pharyngolaryngeal reflux. Treatment for this is relatively straightforward, provided a healthy lifestyle is adopted.

Reflux is a consequence of a reverse flow of liquid from the stomach toward the esophagus. (The acidity level of this reflux, even if the reflux is minimal, is such that it provokes laryngitis and chronic coughing and dries out the vocal cords. The gastric acid is not abundant enough to cause pain, but it's sufficient to make the surface of the vocal cords rough.)

The appropriate hygiene and dietary advice in this case is simple enough and brings to account gastroesophageal mechanics. Sleep with your head raised, using two pillows: avoid lying flat as this increases the risk of reflux. Avoid going to bed on a full stomach, that is, straight after a copious meal. It's best to wait an hour or two. If you are a bit paunchy, don't constrict your stomach with a tight belt. As regards diet, reduce your intake of alcohol, beer, fizzy drinks, tea, and certain fatty foods, and avoid copious meals. Tobacco aggravates the esophagus. Finally, stress is an exacerbating factor, and one that is difficult to avoid in this day and age.

In point of fact, a healthy diet, an acceptable weight, and a healthy level of physical activity are often all it takes to cure reflux, without recourse to allopathic medicines or a medical solution.

If treatment is required, four families of antireflux medication are efficient. They act on the gastric hyperacidity and the excessive peristalsis of the stomach and esophagus. The first includes proton pump inhibitors that get to work inside the cells and stomach. They decrease the acidity at its source. They work remarkably well for ulcers and esophagitis, which today very rarely call for surgery. The second family includes anti-H2 medicines. They act on the acid molecule itself, as it emerges from the gastric cell. They do have one disadvantage: they can dry the vocal cords. The third family includes peristaltic medicines. They calm gastric and esophageal contractions and, therefore, reduce the reflux on a mechanical level. The fourth family is composed of gastric balms such as gels, syrups, or antacid pills.

If a gastric ulcer or esophagitis is suspected, the gastroenterologist will inevitably test for the *Helicobacter*—not "helicopter," as a patient of mine called it!—germ. To do so, he will practice a gastric fibroscopy.

Hormonal treatments

It isn't necessary to underscore again the importance of the female hormonal cycle or the impact of androgens. Sex hormones, notably androgens, aren't an appropriate solution for women. An injection of testosterone can cause permanent masculinity. If a woman is taking a contraceptive pill containing progesterone, her medication should not contain any derivative of androgen molecules (which exist in some pills with progesterone). The same applies if the woman is on hormone replacement therapy at menopause. One should also look out for hypothyroidism, as many menopausal women are deficient in this respect. They're excessively tired, are slightly overweight, and have a duller tone of voice. A thyroid substitute hormonal treatment is indicated and is adapted to each woman by the endocrinologist according to her clinical and biological medical profile.

Anti-stage fright medication

Highly anxious voice professionals sometimes use beta-blockers. These succeed in damping extreme stress. Artists are under a lot of pressure from their public, and beta-blockers overcome the dry mouth syndrome by increasing the secretion of saliva, reduce other stress symptoms such as anxiety, a knotted stomach, shallow breathing, and tachycardia (a racing heart), and overcome the dreaded toneless voice of the first few seconds on stage on opening night. But beware of beta blockers' undesirable side effects: they can aggravate an asthma attack, slow down the cardiac rhythm, or induce a state that's too relaxed, bearing in mind that stress has a galvanizing effect.

Relaxants and psychotropics act on the central nervous system and can lower alertness, as well as induce pharyngolaryngeal dryness and a drop in vocal performance.

On a day-to-day basis

- Aspirin liquefies the blood. It can induce subepithelial hemorrhaging of the vocal cords. It causes gastritis in people predisposed to it. When pain or a low fever is present, acetominophen is preferable to aspirin.

- Antibiotics don't influence the voice. However, they can bring on a secondary fungal infection.

- Medication for arterial hypertension is often contraindicated for voice professionals. It dries out the vocal tract, thickens mucus and, in some people, provokes a dry cough.

- Cough medication should be administered prudently. It can contain codeine that dries the respiratory tree and can cause constipation. Lubricating syrups are preferable.

- Sleeping pills, if wisely taken, are sometimes indispensable to ensure a good night's sleep. A voice professional who sleeps badly is more limited and less effective in his artistic expression. Sleeping pills should not contain antihistamines or neuroleptics, as these dry out the pharynx excessively.

- Sprays are controversial. My opinion is that if they contain a local anesthetic, they should be proscribed. They dull pain, and pain is a critical element insofar as it enables voice professionals to know their limits. Therefore, they do more harm than good. Teachers, singers, or actors who use these sprays repeatedly, anesthetizing pain, end up damaging their laryngeal muscles and create a complication that will have to be treated in the long term. Pain is a natural and highly important signal that avoids irreversible vocal injury.

- Cortisone-based sprays, whether for treating the nose, the larynx, or the trachea, have a drying effect, but their efficacy is almost instantaneous.

- For a blocked nose, vasoconstrictors are of interest. They unblock the nose and normalize the nasopharyngeal airflow satisfactorily. However, they should only be used for a short time, because they treat the symptoms of the blockage, not its cause, and they can be habit forming.

• One should treat the voice and medication with the utmost rigor and respect.

Vitamins

Liver juice in the eyes to see better!

Beriberi (a vitamin B1 deficiency) was described already in 2600 BC in China. More recently, scurvy (a vitamin C deficiency) was described in the papyrus writings of Eber in 1150 BC. Under the Pharaohs in Egypt, subjects with sight problems, especially if they had vision problems at dusk, were advised to bathe their eyes with fresh liver juice: a strange custom, indeed, but it did improve their sight! Today we know that hepatic cells are a vitamin pantry and that they're bursting with vitamin A.

Sailors and vitamins

In 1497, Vasco de Gama embarks in a port in Portugal and sets sail for India via the Cape of Good Hope. One hundred and sixty sailors are onboard. During the voyage, many tire quickly, are weak or depressed. They can't eat because their gums hurt. Their muscles don't respond. Their calves waste away. Their biceps vanish. As the weeks pass by, the sailors are increasingly covered in bruises all over their bodies; they cough and have diarrhea. Only sixty sailors survive this terrible ordeal and arrive in India. Vasco de Gama is unable to explain this dramatic outcome. Was the crew so fragile? Was he not sufficiently well prepared for this adventure?

In 1530, Jacques Cartier reaches Quebec on his ship, the Saint Laurent. This French navigator has also sustained terrible loss of lives. Most of his crew died during the voyage. Others are ill, weak, but still alive. The indigenous Indians of this region observe the invaders disembarking. They take pity on them. The survivors are at death's door. Their gums are swollen, their arms and legs are ulcerated, they are covered in bruises. Some bleed from the nose.

The Indians give them some shrub leaves to chew on. Within weeks, the sailors are cured.

We have to wait two centuries before James Lind, a Scottish doctor of the 18th century, pierces the mystery. He evokes the possibility of a diet that wasn't adapted to such long voyages to new worlds.

He reaches this conclusion with the help of the diaries kept by the explorers whose sailors suffered from scurvy. In 1753, he publishes the first work on vitamin C deficiency. He hits on the idea of treating twelve sailors suffering from this illness with a simple diet. Two of them are made to drink cider, two others drink sulfuric acid, two more drink orange juice, lemon juice, and decoctions of pine needles, yet others drink a little sea water or vinegar. Who do you suppose survived? Of course, only the two who had drunk orange juice and lemon juice, with their vitamin C content. They recovered fully. The impact of vitamins is seeing the light of day. This discovery incited captains, henceforth, to include fresh foods, and especially citrus fruit, in their crew's rations. Everyone supposed that scurvy would be a thing of the past.

Yet in the 19th century, some babies presented the same symptoms, due in fact to the way milk was being heated to be preserved, a recent discovery. This pasteurization process left intact the carbohydrates, lipids, and proteins contained in milk, but destroyed its vitamin C content.

Vitamin C: the combating vitamin

Vitamin C, or ascorbic acid, owes its name to the illness it prevents, namely scurvy. This vitamin is sensitive to excessive heat and to light. It is a crystalline, whitish substance that is water soluble. It plays a primordial role relative to collagen (fibers that intervene in scarring and the suppleness of mucous membranes, notably the vocal cords), histamine (the molecule that intervenes in allergies), and the organism's immune defense system (well-known to all in the context of a viral attack). Vitamin C also interacts with numerous molecules that intervene in cell regeneration, with the adrenals, and with iron recovery. It solidifies the gel that binds cells together and prevents the formation of small hematomas thanks to its reinforcing effect on capillary walls. This effect also ensures the nourishment of dental and bone tissue. It accelerates scarring. It has an antioxidant effect on cell aging and the prevention of chronic inflammations of the respiratory tree. Its action is often coupled with that of vitamins D and E. Its impact is multifactorial: it helps fight fatigue and allows better mental, vascular, bony, and muscular recuperation. Practically all fruit contain vitamin C, especially oranges, grapefruit, and kiwis, but also certain vegetables, such as cabbage and broccoli. It may come as a surprise, but today, we still come across deficiencies in vitamin C. It is especially prevalent in population groups whose diet consists essentially of cooked foods with few fruit or fresh vegetables. They complain of tiredness, bleeding gums, fragile skin. Thus, taking vitamin C can boost intellectual, physical, and vocal performances remarkably. An excess of vitamin C can cause hyperexcitation, sometimes a racing heart and, more rarely, intestinal trouble.

What is a vitamin?

"Vitamin" is the name given by C. Funk in 1911 to nutritive elements that are essential to human life. This revolutionary concept brought him no less than fifteen Nobel prizes between 1910 and 1950. The first vitamin to be isolated was vitamin C, by Reichstein, in 1933.

Vitamins are organic substances, some with an amino acid base, found in plants, vegetables, and fruit, that humans are unable to synthesize. For centuries, many people suffered from nutritional and vitamin deficiencies. Today, the chances of a dietary imbalance in our organism are increased by the poor dietary habits of many people; by the insults caused by pollution, alcohol abuse, poisoning from the nicotine and tar content of tobacco; the significant consumption of prepared foods that aren't fresh; the decreasing consumption of natural foods, fiber, and fruit; and, incredible though this may seem, this modern dietary imbalance represents a step backward in our dietary balance.

Vitamins: so often ignored in prescriptions, yet so essential

Vitamins, essential molecules for all living cells, for your body's metabolism, are micronutrients that Man can't synthesize. They provide energy, but provide zero calories, something many dieters tend to forget.

They are essential for immune balance and have no negative effects when taken in recommended doses. It's a real pity that this therapeutic approach is considered by some to be accessory because it doesn't treat the acute symptom. This view fails to take into account a factor essential to the preservation of our health: prevention!

In an era in which the medical imbalance is turning toward aggressive therapies that are unfortunately necessary and essential in emergencies, it seems equally essential to balance your organism with a suitable diet and to avoid general tiredness, voice strain, infections, or inflammations. Indeed, vitamin complexes are required by the incredible energy factory in your organism that is the cell, by your enzymes and also by your struggle with precocious aging due to free radicals. The prevention of numerous accidents of the voice depends upon a balanced diet.

We should emphasize once more the deleterious effects of tobacco and alcohol on the voice. Tobacco, and more specifically cigarette smoke, contains two harmful agents: tar, which is carcinogenic, and nicotine, which provokes a deterioration of the mucous membranes and vessels. Alcohol causes a thickening of the larynx, as well as an edema.

The elongation of the vocal cord with hematoma, laryngitis with its bacterial or viral infection tied to a reduced immune efficiency, excessive tiredness with cramps due to a deficiency in magnesium, calcium, and vitamin C, these ailments all depend on your dietary habits and on how you warm up your muscles. Thus, an unbalanced diet, one, for example, rich in saturated fats, will put weight on without allowing the body to put in place the sentinels of its immune defense system, guardians of muscular and cerebral health.

Vitamins: essential for good cerebral function

Vitamins, essential to life, are devoid of calories, just like the water you drink, yet your organism cannot do without them. The minimum requirement for each vitamin may seem minute, but 1.2% of our DNA differs from that of the monkey, and that difference is sufficient to enable us to speak. The human voice is complex. It brings into play the brain, the musical instrument that is our larynx, our resonators, all the striated muscles of the body, and our respiratory rhythm.

Bear in mind that if we can talk, it means we can hear. But also, we can talk because of what we have in our brain, the evolution of mankind.

Remember: we have three brains that are superposed, but one of them consumes a lot of vitamins:

- The reptilian brain, called the encephalon, which regulates vital elements such as breathing and cardiac rhythm;

- The limbic brain or rhinencephalon, unique to mammals, devoted mainly to our sense of smell, to emotions, affect, seduction, and sexuality. It receives information from the right brain;

- And our "third brain," also called the neocortex. It comprises two hemispheres, with the most developed gyri in the primate world. The left hemisphere is the seat of reason, of logic, but especially of language and solfeggio. Here too we find Broca's area and Wernicke's area. The right hemisphere is the seat of emotion, harmony, musical melody, art, affect. The third brain is the greediest when it comes to vitamins; it also consumes the most energy as compared with the reptilian and limbic brains.

Your neuronal heritage is practically defined from birth. It does not renew itself. Worse still, we regularly lose neurons, especially if neuronal connections aren't stimulated and used regularly. The brain's energetic requirements are considerable. It represents nearly 20% of our entire organism's energetic consumption, and yet represents only 1,500 g in a person weighing 70 kg, or 2% of body weight.

Thus, 20% of our oxygen is required by 2% of the body. Vitamins, mineral salts, and certain lipids are absolutely essential to cerebral activity. We can foresee its fragility. To memorize words and musicality when they speak or sing, voice professionals have to be in remarkable health, both physical and mental. This memory has its seat primarily in the limbic brain, an area of the brain particularly well developed in artists. Muscular and mental recuperation are indispensable to the full exploitation of the professional's vocal expression. Paradoxical sleep, with its dreams, is the cornerstone of our health; combined with an optimal diet, it enables voice professionals to be in full possession of their means. Without wanting to be pessimistic, we should point out that, in France, alcoholism in women is responsible for nearly 10% of the cases of mental backwardness in children, and that tobacco abuse causes a significant number of premature births, as well as immune deficiencies in numerous infants.

Vocal hygiene and good cerebral function go hand in hand. The B group of vitamins is one of the elements essential to the development and maintenance of memory. You find them in cereals. The unsaturated fatty acids contained in vegetable oils reinforce the cellular membrane, notably in the brain. Experience has shown that cerebral aging is less pronounced in populations who eat a lot of fish.

In order to understand dietary hygiene better, let's look at the role of each vitamin. Vitamins are necessary for growth, balance, evolution, and the protection of our organism. Eating copiously is bad for you, eating healthily fortifies you and keeps you in good health.

All foods don't contain a sufficient quantity of vitamins. We know of 15 vitamins: A, D, E, F, K, C, and B1, B2, B3, B4, B5, B6, B8, B9, and B12. Their molecular structure is very heterogeneous. Absorbed with food, they are digested once in the stomach where gastric juices free them. The course they take differs according to the nature of the vitamin. They enter through the small intestine; therefore, the organism must be capable of isolating the vitamin from the food ingested. Your enzymes must be capable of extracting vitamin C from oranges, vitamin A from carrots. These vitamins must then be ferried inside the body to your cells.

Vitamins and aging

Beyond a certain age, our impressive digestive structure composed of the stomach, the duodenum, the small intestine, and the colon lose their capacity to extract vitamins; their enzymes aren't as efficient as before and fail in this task. So what can be done? The answer is simply to take a vitamin complex regularly, in the shape of pure vitamin pills ready for use. Nowadays, tobacco and pollution foster the development of free radicals and this increases the body's need for protective vitamins such as vitamins A, C, E, and beta carotenes.

Stress and alcohol consumption also create an additional requirement for the B group of vitamins. But we mustn't forget certain minerals such as calcium, iron, zinc, and iodine. If these simple facts were taken into account, the dosage of allopathic medicines such as anti-inflammatories, antibiotics, and antihistamines, as well as antireflux medicines, could be significantly reduced and the natural balance between health and diet would be respected.

Vitamin A

This vitamin ensures the rejuvenation of skin cells and also mucous membranes and, therefore, vocal mucous membranes. This vitamin has to do with growth and eyesight. It helps form and increases the light-sensitive pigments of the retina and, therefore, improves nocturnal vision. It significantly improves resistance to allergens. It intervenes in the lubrication of mucous membranes. It intervenes also in the synthesis of sex hormones and cartilage suppleness, notably the larynx. Its multifactorial impact acts on your respiratory tree, on the one hand, and on the speed of nervous impulses on the other. How does it influence nerves and improve their conductivity? Quite simply, it improves the protective layer that covers nerves, the myelin sheath. This sheath isolates the conduction of nervous impulse and protects the nerve from all external parasitic influences.

Vitamin A, or retinol, was discovered in 1913, when scientists noticed unusual occurrences in the growth of rats. On a purely lipid diet, fed exclusively pork fat, they don't grow. When fed butter, they start growing again. Retinol was isolated later and found to exist also in egg yolks and cod liver oil. Vitamin A, yellowish in color, is often masked by chlorophyll, which is green. It's associated with carotene.

Together with vitamin C, it plays a role in preventing aging and in helping a number of cells fight certain degenerative phenomena. It's ingested through the digestive system, then diffused in the bloodstream, and reaches the liver, where it is stored. The liver then regularly dips into its stock of vitamin A to distribute this molecule around the body, where it helps fight dryness of the skin or mucous membranes.

Cheese, butter, egg yolks, fatty fish, and calf liver are all rich in vitamin A. It's also found in numerous plants, such as spinach or sweet potato, lettuce, and cabbage. Colored fruit contain it, mangoes, papayas, tomatoes, and, of course, carrots. Of the cereals, only maize contains beta carotene. Vitamin A is altered by cooking. Also, in nature, the drying effect of the sun on green leaves reduces their concentration of beta carotene. During the digestive process, for every 6 mg of beta carotene ingested, only 1 mg of retinol will be effective. Indeed, your organism can produce vitamin A from beta-carotene, which is called provitamin A. This provitamin A can't be consumed in excess; in other words, there's no hypervitaminosis (overdose) associated with beta carotene. Its antioxidant and anti-carcinogenic action is more efficient than that of vitamin A. It traps free radicals, notably in mucous membrane and skin. Your body's daily requirement of beta carotene is 10 to 20 mg.

Too high a consumption of vitamin A can be toxic, causing headaches, vomiting, and in extreme cases, hair loss. It is not recommended for pregnant women. The symptoms of vitamin A deficiency are dry eyes and inelastic skin. These days, supplementing vitamin A is essential, as our diet doesn't satisfy the minimal requirement to allow any significant antioxidant action. From the age of fifty, a daily supplement of 20 mg is recommended.

Vitamin D

It is essential for the newborn infant. Sir Edward Mellamby demonstrated its action in puppies in 1919. He proved that a deficiency in vitamin D causes rickets. Thanks to him, cod liver oil, rich in vitamin D, was prescribed to prevent rickets, then very prevalent. Vitamin D helps with bone development, assists in the body's absorption of calcium and phosphorus, and fixes calcium in teeth and bone. It is the antirickets vitamin. A deficiency in vitamin D, unfortunately very frequent in the Third World, provokes serious problems because of rickets (osteomalacia), causing a softening of the bones and stunted growth. It also plays a role in dry skin problems and psoriasis.

Vitamin D is present in egg yolk, fish, and liver. Cereals, vegetables, and fruit don't contain any. The sun's ultraviolet rays help to synthesize it in the skin. Hence, people living in sunny climes receive sufficient sunshine to avoid any vitamin D deficiency. Children need around 400 IU a day for their growth. This corresponds roughly to a teaspoon of cod liver oil. However, children who are often out in the sun need less. Too much vitamin D can result in excess levels of calcium in the blood.

Vitamin E

This is pre-eminently *the* antioxidant vitamin. It traps free radicals. It is destroyed by frying and by excessive exposure to light. It prolongs the life of red blood cells and improves iron retention, thereby helping to oxygenate the body. It apparently assists cellular nourishment and has an antiaging effect on mucous membranes. Its antioxidant properties protect the respiratory axis. Its action is synergistic with vitamin C, beta carotene, and vitamin A. Smokers need to take much higher doses of vitamin E than is the norm for the vitamin to have an antioxidant effect. Vitamin E is found predominantly in peanut oil, soya oil, olive oil, and, especially, wheat germ oil. The minimum daily requirement for a satisfactory impact is 200 mg. Sometimes, 400 mg a day is prescribed to help increase good cholesterol and decrease bad cholesterol.

The vitamin B group

Vitamin B1 acts on carbohydrates and increases cellular energy reserves. Yeast has the highest concentration of vitamin B1, which is also present in whole grains and dry legumes.

Lack of vitamin of B1 causes serious health problems. It provokes beriberi, but also neurologic problems such as polyneuritis (a nerve dysfunction caused by a deficient myelin sheath, causing wobbly legs, for instance). Beriberi is common in Asia and the East, due to the consumption of white polished rice. In its milder forms, vitamin B1 deficiency causes tiredness, irritability, and lassitude.

Vitamin B2 is synergistic with vitamin B1. Its action is also energetic. It can be found in dairy products, meat, eggs, green vegetables, and yeast. Its deficiency is rare.

Vitamin B3 or *PP*, also called nicotinic acid or niacin, intervenes in the synthesis of growth hormones. Working synergistically with vitamin C, it tones the respiratory tree. Found in most foods, it helps to strengthen vessel walls. Its deficiency can provoke pellagra, causing itchy dermatitis with redness, insomnia, and confusion. Cases of pellagra are rare in the Western world. Vitamin B3 is present in numerous foods: liver, lean meats, dry legumes, and beer.

Vitamin B4, or adenine, is an energetic vitamin.

Vitamin B5 helps with scarring, molecules used by neurons, and the synthesis of lipids and certain hormones. It is essential for hair and nails, but also for the ciliated cells of the respiratory tree. It facilitates the elimination of mucus. It is present in many foods.

Vitamin B6, or pyridoxine, provides energy to your cells, is antistress, and stimulates the brain. It intervenes essentially in nervous conduction and libido levels. It's found in yeast, dry legumes, and liver.

Vitamin B8, or biotin, helps to metabolize protids, glucids, lipids, and amino acids. Essential for growth, it acts synergistically with vitamin B5 and zinc to prevent hair loss. It's present in numerous foods.

Vitamin B9 deficiency causes anemia, tiredness, and intestinal disorders.

Vitamin B12 deficiency can bring on memory problems, tiredness, and anemia. Its presence is essentially limited to animal foods such as liver, poultry, fish, eggs, and dairy products. It is stocked by the liver. Four milligrams suffice to cover your requirements for several years.

Vitamin F, known as linoleic acid, regroups the essential fatty acids and diminishes the risk of arteriosclerosis. It is found in honey, almonds, and oils such as evening primrose oil. It plays a role in protecting the heart.

Vitamin K is essential for blood coagulation. It's found in broccoli in the ratio of 100 mg per 100 g.

The force of vitamins

Vitamins operate on three physiological levels. They have an enzymatic impact acting as a coenzyme; they have a direct action on the cell membrane or on its mitochondria; and they act on hormonal functions. A minimal daily dose is absolutely essential. This minimum depends on a person's age, level of physical activity, and intellectual activity. After this detailed if simplified description, I must stress the importance for voice professionals of vitamins A, C, D, E, B5, and B6, given the demands placed on them to be constantly dynamic, as well as mentally, physically, and vocally alert.

Minerals

Minerals are essential for your voice and organism. Iron, magnesium, and calcium are the most important minerals, along with phosphorus, sodium, zinc, and manganese.

Iron and Popeye the sailor

Iron is an essential element contained in hemoglobin (the pigment in red blood cells), in myoglobin (the muscles' protein), and in cytochromes (intracellular hemoproteins that play an important role in cellular respiration and the capture of oxygen). Iron contributes to the transport of oxygen in the body. Your organism contains only 3 to 4 g of iron. Yet this small amount is vital to you. Your daily requirement is 20 to 30 mg, given that not all the iron you ingest is absorbed. You only need 5 mg a day to nourish your body intrinsically. Nevertheless, your need for iron increases: when you exercise yourself or when you're very tired. Why?

Physical exertion increases muscle mass. Muscle injuries (such as a hematoma on a vocal cord) require proteins in order to mend. Hyperprotein diets require greater amounts of iron. In athletes, iron levels must be sufficient to allow respiratory and muscular efforts at a competitive level and to lay off the tiredness induced by anoxia or hypoxia (depleted oxygen levels in muscle tissue). Professional singers and actors bring into play 400 muscles. This makes them as much an athlete as the professional athlete.

In women, menstruation can bring about a significant loss of hemoglobin, and cyclical iron supplementation is recommended. The breast-feeding mother also needs more iron. You lose 1 mg of iron every day in sweat, urine, fallen hairs, and dead cells. This mineral is present in many foods—meat, fish, eggs, dry legumes. But the legend of Popeye the sailor isn't quite correct: spinach contains very little iron, whereas lentils have the highest concentration. Your intestines capture iron, but beware of meals that include a cup of tea or a glass of wine; their high tannin concentration blocks the absorption of iron by the intestines. Iron deficiency provokes considerable tiredness, anemia, impaired concentration, and paleness. Its prevalence increases with age.

Magnesium

In 1944, Mr. Kuch, a cattle breeder, finds his calves are dying. He supposes this is due to poor hygiene in the barn. He builds a new barn and paints it. The calves lick the walls and no longer die. Kuch finds out that the paint on the walls contains magnesium carbonate. Research into this mineral, essential to our organism, stems from his observation.

Your body contains around 25 g of magnesium, around eight times more than its iron levels. It is located primarily in your cells: 50% in the skeleton, 25% in striated muscles, and a little under 25% in the heart, liver, kidneys, and digestive tubes. Only 200 mg are located in hormonal tissue or in plasma. Magnesium is essential to us. Its absorption is facilitated by vitamin D and a protein-rich diet. Alcohol and saturated fats reduce its absorption. It plays a fundamental role in the formation of ATP and in the protection of our DNA. Magnesium intervenes in more than 300 neuromuscular and hormonal enzymatic reactions. On a daily basis, adults require at least 75 mg, the elderly require 420 mg, and infants 50 mg.

Pregnant women and breast-feeding women require 480 mg of magnesium per day. In 1998, a study in Europe of 5,500 people revealed that 75% of them were deficient in magnesium. This hypomagnesemia aggravates PMS with its migraine and pains. Sports help its absorption and galvanize its influence. Among other things, magnesium enables the use of glycogen, the body's natural energy reserves. Glycogen is also required for physical endurance activities. Thus, after a sustained effort lasting two to three hours, Ohla demonstrated a drop in plasmatic magnesium. Preventive treatment, two to three weeks before the effort, allows this problem to be circumvented and optimizes performance. A regular intake of magnesium is necessary for muscular and respiratory balance. However, in excess it can provoke intestinal disorders, and its deficiency causes tiredness and irritability and, notably, cramps. This tetany is evidence of a hyperreactivity of the neuromuscular joint.

Magnesium is found in numerous natural foods: cocoa powder, black chocolate, nuts such as cashews, almonds, or hazelnuts, soya, and wheat germ. Fish and oysters contain moderate amounts of it. Its presence is maximal in algae, 2.5 g for 100 g, versus 200 to 400 mg in chocolate. Vittel, Hepar, and Badoit mineral water have a high concentration of magnesium.

Calcium

Calcium is important in many ways, not only in bone tissue and hormonal secretions, but also in the proper functioning of neurons. Calcium is the prime constituent of bones and teeth. Moreover, it is essential for the efficient action of the heart, blood clotting, neuromuscular excitability, for short response times between the moment when the brain emits an order and the moment a muscle responds. To function optimally, it needs to be in equilibrium with phosphorus: the phosphocalcic proportion should be between 0.5 and 2. Calcium represents 1.5% of body weight, and 98% of it is in bones.

The daily requirement is between 600 mg and 1,000 mg. It is absorbed by the upper part of the small intestine. Its absorption requires a degree of acidity. Moreover, its absorption is regulated by hormones such as parathormones, the sex hormones, and vitamin D. Conversely, cortisone can prevent calcium from binding to bone. Calcium is a functional and dynamic element that varies according to level of activity. Consider a simple example: sweat. Physical exertion lasting over two hours can cause the body to lose 30% of its calcium, as demonstrated so well by Consolazio nearly forty years ago. Calcium is essential for all athletes, and notably for voice professionals, who sweat considerably.

Calcium is particularly active during the growth phase experienced between the ages of sixteen and twenty-five. It enables your bones to grow and speeds up nervous conduction. Its action is often synergistic with vitamin D. Our diet is full of it. The water we drink and cheese are our principal source of calcium. Note that cow's milk contains 1,200 mg per liter, whereas maternal milk contains only 300 mg. Its deficiency provokes rickets in children; in adults, it brings on tiredness as well as cramps, and, later, a demineralization of the skeleton (osteoporosis). Physical activity slows osteoporosis considerably. It is interesting that, today, most seventy-year-old women who participate in a sports activity regularly are able to keep osteoporosis at bay with prescribed calcium supplements and hormone therapy.

Phosphorus

Around 700 g of phosphorus are present in your body, of which 600 g are in the skeleton and 100 g in various protein, lipid, DNA, or RNA molecules. Our need of around 1 g per day increases rapidly with effort. It is absorbed by the lower part of the small intestine. It acts upon energetic molecules such as ATP and its derivatives. Present in the skeleton and in the nervous system, it is essential for cellular exchanges and for pH balance. The ratio of calcium to phosphorus must remain within a certain range. This means that if your body absorbs more calcium, the absorption of phosphorus must be lower, and vice versa.

Potassium

In the same way that calcium interacts with phosphorus, potassium interacts with sodium. Its roles are multiple. But its primary role is to assist in balancing intra- and extracellular fluids and proper cellular function. You require less than 50 mg of potassium a day.

Sodium

Sodium is essential for living beings. It stabilizes and regulates cellular exchanges. It modulates fluid reserves. It plays many roles, not only in cellular exchanges, but also in myofibril excitation and contraction. You need about 10 g of sodium a day. Six minutes after its ingestion, it's been absorbed. It reduces sweating and facilitates water retention. That's the dark side of the coin: water retention. If your diet is too salty, you increase your hydric mass and circulating fluids and increase the risk of arterial hypertension.

Iodine

Your body contains between 20 and 50 mg of iodine, primarily in the thyroid gland. This mineral is essential for the synthesis of thyroid hormones. It makes a major contribution to children's physical and mental growth. Iodine is absorbed into the intestine and is subsequently trapped by the thyroid gland. Any excess iodine is eliminated in the urine. An iodine deficiency causes the thyroid gland to grow into a goiter, which immediately affects your voice and singing. A goiter interferes on two levels. First, due to the compression exerted by the gland itself on the larynx, and second, through the reduced distribution of oxygen to the cordal muscles. The thyroid arteries, of which one branch is the laryngeal artery, nourish the vocal cords. When the thyroid gland expands, it requires an increasing amount of blood, to the detriment of the laryngeal artery that nourishes the vocal cords, and that now receives less blood. We call this "blood theft." Through its impact on the thyroid gland, an iodine deficit diminishes your mental capacities and your physical endurance. It is most prevalent in ocean fish, algae, and plants cultivated by the sea. Supplementation is rarely necessary.

Other minerals

Fluorine preserves your teeth and skeleton. It's well known for its protective action against dental caries. It's found mainly in water and fish. During childhood and after the age of fifty, 1 mg of fluorine a day helps to protect dentition and vocal health. Copper is an element involved in the synthesis of hemoglobin. Sulfur acts on respiration of tissue It increases your defenses against infectious aggressions. Zinc is fundamental for your organism and essential to many enzymatic reactions. It's present in fish, seafood, meat, and eggs. The daily requirement is about 15 mg. As for trace elements, research is currently attempting to determine their contribution.

Antioxidants and free radicals: preventing cellular aging

Why slow down oxidation?

Antioxidants and certain vitamins slow down the oxidation and aging processes of the body. Cut a slice of apple, leave it out, and in a few minutes, the contact with the air turns it brown. Take the same slice of apple, rub it with lemon juice, several hours will now pass before it turns brown. Thus, vitamin C has slowed the oxidation process, and in your organism this property promotes better resistance and improves performance.

What do antioxidants act on?

Antioxidants are medicines that act on free radicals, which have deleterious effects. They have a dramatic effect on the cell wall, which loses its permeability and is therefore unable to import needed nutrients and export unwanted toxins. This accelerated aging process proves fatal to the cell. To avoid this, antioxidants trap the unstable unpaired electron that triggers this chain reaction.

How do free radicals come about?

In the mitochondrion, a pair of electrons from the oxygen molecule can break away after an important energy exchange. This breakaway creates a celibate (unpaired and unstable) electron; if the electron isn't neutralized, it will provoke a denaturizing reaction on the cell membrane.

Free radicals are molecules produced by your organism when your body is attacked. This can be caused by pollution, excessive sun exposure, a brutal change of temperature or of humidity levels, tobacco, alcohol, or "affective pollution." This causes exaggerated aging of the tissues and unusual tiredness. These radicals free the celibate electron, which becomes toxic. This simple electron destabilizes the body's structures. Conjunctive tissue is the tissue most vulnerable to it. You owe the suppleness of your skin and of your mucous membranes to this tissue. It is composed of collagen, elastin, and hyaluronic acid, as well as proteoglycans that protect the tonicity of your tissues and ensure the elasticity and the youth of your vocal cords.

The battle for energy and endurance

This is where antioxidant vitamins and vitamins that fight free radicals come into play. If some suitable therapy doesn't block the celibate electron, the cell will lose its permeability, die, and induce premature aging. Thus, eliminating free radicals is essential for the survival of cells and the trace elements that help to neutralize them.

During the Olympic Games in Australia, 12 athletes were studied in endurance fields (marathon running and cross-country skiing). For nearly a month, six of them received a daily dose of 1,000 IU of vitamin E and 1 g of vitamin C. The other six athletes received a placebo. The study was a double-blind; nobody knew who was taking what. From blood tests carried out, an enzyme sample showed that the ingestion of a vitamin caused a 25% drop in oxidation. Moreover, endurance improved. These results show not only the undeniable benefit of taking antioxidant vitamins, but also that of associating muscular training with cardiovascular training for enhanced performance.

Cod liver oil and Omega-3, an interesting molecule of the 21st century

Cod liver oil ensures better physical resistance and improves mental concentration. Thanks to Claude Gudin, we now know why. Cod is a coldwater fish and it stores polyunsaturated fatty acids with very long chains. These lipids are beneficial to our organism. Cod feed on tiny fish that feed on microalgae. Microalgae form these long chains of fatty acids (with more than 15 carbon atoms), so these fatty acids are produced by marine plants.

Terrestrial plants also produce fatty acids, but in short chains (fewer than 15 atoms of carbon) that are less beneficial to our health. Animal fatty acids aren't recommended because they store saturated acids and, therefore, oxidize.

Cod liver oil has polyunsaturated fatty acids, which have a vital influence on our nervous system and our mental concentration. Our grandparents' generation gave their children a daily dose for a month every six months. Grandma knew what she was talking about! But now in the 21st century, cod liver oil has been "tamed" via Omega-3.

Omega-3 is the name given to a family of polyunsaturated fatty acids. Omega-3 is close to alpha-linolenic acid, or ALA. Like vitamins, it is essential to our life force. Omega-3 has 18 carbon atoms (plus 3 double bonds, e.g., 18, 3).

However, from the point of view of human nutrition, the long-chain Omega-3 fatty acids (eicosa pentenoic acid or EPA [20:5] and docosa hexaenoic acid or DHA [22:6]) are more suitable, as these are in the form required by our body. In theory, we should be able to synthesize EPA and DHA from dietary ALA, but in practice, this process is inefficient. Therefore, Omega-3 should be obtained directly from your diet. Oil-rich fish such as sardines and ocean salmon, and supplements such as fish oil and cod liver oil, are the richest and most readily available sources.

In 1996, the American Heart Association released its Science Advisory, "Fish Consumption, Fish Oil, Lipids and Coronary Heart Disease." Since then, important new findings have reported on the benefits of Omega-3 fatty acids on cardiovascular disease

But what is the link with the voice? A. J. Richardson has identified a link with dyslexia: brain scans of dyslexic adults via magnetic resonance spectroscopy have shown abnormalities of membrane phospholipid turnover linked to fatty acid deficiencies. Dyslexic adults show significantly more signs of this than nondyslexics. The severity of reading and writing difficulties in children with dyslexia has been associated with a lack of fatty acids.

Omega-3 fatty acids play an important role as structural membrane lipids, particularly in nerve tissue and the retina, and are precursors to eicosanoids—highly reactive substances such as prostaglandins and leukotrienes that act locally to influence a wide range of functions in cells and tissues.

Here are some examples of the consequences of an increase in free radicals: cramps, stress, insomnia, rheumatic pains, microvaricose veins, maybe aggressive premenstrual syndrome. The biological identification of the presence of free radicals in the organism remains very difficult in the present state of our knowledge. Only indirect clinical symptoms allow us to infer their deleterious effects. Prescribing a vitamin complex, notably vitamins E, A, B, and C, with Omega-3 fatty acids benefits people and helps to avoid this type of chain reaction and the precocious death of our cells.

Of interest is the fact that every minute of your life, nearly 10 million cells reproduce themselves in your organism. In other words, by the time you have read this page, you'll have around 25 million new cells in your body. It is never too late to take your health in hand!

Sugars, lipids, and proteins: energy for the voice

Sugars: first source of energy

Glucids (sugars) constitute an energy substrate that enables you to be effective over a shorter burst of physical activity. They play a role in replacing glycogen, your muscle fuel. For example, variety show singers, whose performance on stage is a real achievement physically, require anywhere between 5 to 10 g of glucids per kilo of weight. Paradoxically, they need glucids both before and after their physical effort, in order to avoid muscle collapse: the "tear at rest," the elongation of a vocal cord after the show. If professional voice users are obliged to raise their voices to speak after a concert or conference, they end up pulling on the already fragile vocal muscle, which is unable to withstand this renewed challenge and snaps.

It's a good idea to take an energy drink after a show or after an important vocal effort. This liquid nutrition is particularly recommended if you've lost a lot of sweat during the performance. Glucids are composed of carbon, hydrogen, and oxygen (their ratio is 6:12:6). When they are consumed, they release carbonic gas and water. Glycogen is formed from glucids, it's an instant energy resource.

Lipids: second source of energy

Lipids constitute an energy reserve used for a longer lasting effort, for example, if you're on stage every day or night for several weeks in a row. Like glucids, lipids are composed of carbon, hydrogen, and oxygen. Lipids include all the edible fats in our diet. In our organism, they break down into two categories. The first is tied to body build. It's part of a person's silhouette. The second forms an energy reserve that will be solicited for protracted efforts.

The fats that you ingest fall into two distinct groups: saturated fatty acids of animal origin or animal fats, and polyunsaturated/ unsaturated fatty acids derived from vegetables, plants, and certain fish. The distinction is an important one. Saturated fats promote atheroma, the plaque that can block your vessels and especially your coronaries, whereas polyunsaturated fatty acids have a protective influence on these very same vessels. The best known in the latter category are nut-based fatty acids and Omega-3 fatty acids. Weight for weight absorbed, lipids contribute twice as many calories as glucids and proteins, in other words, 9 kcal per gram, compared with 4 kcal per gram for glucids and proteins. Thus, when you eat, you would need to reduce the volume of lipids by half to get a comparable calorie intake. Your intake is smaller, but your physical capacity remains the same. Variety performers who perform every night, who dance and sweat and expend a lot of energy, need their daily dose of lipids and glucids to stay in good shape.

Proteins: the fundamental scaffold of your muscles

Proteins do not constitute a significant energy substrate, but they allow you to preserve your body's muscle and protein structure. Their contribution of amino acids determines your build and silhouette. Humans can't synthesize many amino acids, the fundamental building blocks of protein; you have to get them from your food. We don't have sufficient enzymes to build all these amino acids, the atoms of protein. When you swallow proteins, they're digested by the stomach and by pancreatic secretions before being absorbed by the intestine.

Proteins are present in many foods: eggs, milk, rice, certain grains, dry legumes (beans, dry peas, nuts), and of course, meat and fish. The daily requirement depends on your age: 2.5 g per kg per day for an infant, as opposed to 1g per kg per day for adults. These needs are increased by physical exertion, stress, vocal performances, and also by an infection or a psychological trauma. Proteins help maintain and develop muscle mass and enhance its adaptability to specific activities.

Moreover, proteins help to repair quickly and effectively microlesions in muscle fibers, such as result from overstraining the voice, as often happens in the head voice, which can only be avoided with proper training and diet.

Like sugars and lipids, proteins contain carbon, oxygen, and hydrogen, but also sulfur and nitrogen. The nitrogen atom specific to proteins plays a major role in rapid scar healing and in developing the appropriate musculature. Proteins play a predominant role in adolescent growth, in the development of the adult's body, and in hormonal balance. But above all, they ensure a regular turnover of your cells and, thus, the complete renewal every two to three months of most of your cells, excepting neurons. Their role is structural, not energetic. They can sometimes be called on for essential needs. They are essential for any protracted physical activity.

The cycle of energy

Animal proteins consumed by Man come from plants. Animals are grass and plant eaters; grass and plants are formed through photosynthesis, thanks to the sun. We are not far off our origins.

Salt and water

Hydration, and what we call our electrolytes, are vital for health.

Water: 85% of your body

Nearly 85% of our body is made up of water. All physical effort is dehydrating, as is any important vocal effort. But, and this is important, you are not always aware of this because you don't necessarily feel thirsty. Thirst isn't a reliable criterion of potential loss of water and electrolytes. Dryness of the larynx, maybe difficulties in taking a deep breath, the disappearance of certain vibratory frequencies in the high notes, the loss of *vibrato*, a toneless voice, these are the major symptoms of dehydration.

Muscle contraction provokes cellular oxidation. Of this chemical energy, 75% is transformed into heat and only 25% is transformed into mechanical energy. The heat generated by your muscles is brought close to the surface by the blood vessels, allowing you to sweat. You may sweat profusely and dehydrate too much, in which case you may have cramps. Also, in this case, the hydric loss is of course greater and the main electrolyte lost is sodium. That's why adding one or two teaspoons of salt to a liter of water can help preserve our precious liquids and avoid fast dehydration. Often, it's advisable to add an energy source to water, and I recommend this to all voice professionals. You should hydrate yourself at least every twenty minutes with a glass of water, taking care to wet your lips.

If a vocal exercise lasts longer than an hour, at least one liter of water is required to balance the organism, but this should never be drunk in one go. It should be drunk at regular intervals throughout the performance.

As we sing and speak only during exhalation, this controlled and often solicited breathing out is going to eliminate even more water. Try talking while you run, you'll soon be exhausted!

In the same vein, any food intake before an effort should be small to avoid gastric activity and a long digestive process that is greedy for energy. Thus, your body's muscles and your brain require vitamins, minerals, water, sugars, lipids and proteins in suitable proportions, as well as Omega-3 fatty acids: it is an "à la carte" menu.

The regular intake of water is crucial

The only universal rule for giving your best performance seems to be the regular intake of antioxidants; proper hydration before, during, and after a performance; training of the appropriate muscles, in combination with memorizing the vocal movements. Trace elements and homeopathy could be of interest, although no randomized study of their impact has been undertaken. Oscillococcinum and copper trace elements can help fight a viral laryngitis. To palliate voice strain, tiredness or laryngeal inflammation without infection, many singers and lecturers resort to arnica 7CH, and Bolchoi drops. These bring significant relief after four to six hours. They should be supplemented systematically with nasal baths using sea water.

Caruso was particularly attentive to his vocal health. This was no doubt the secret of his longevity. He rinsed his nose with a mixture of glycerids and sodium bicarbonate, which he also used to gargle with. He combined this with nasal instillations of boiled tepid water mixed with menthol and Vaseline.

Other well-known singers, actors, or comedians confess to downing a glass of Bordeaux wine before coming on stage, but none of them would risk drinking a glass of champagne or white wine, which dry out the vocal cords dramatically and considerably aggravate gastric reflux. Some lyrical singers and longstanding comedians are in the habit of wearing a neck scarf after a performance, or if their voice is tired, they place a hot compress on their neck every night.

Not only do voice professionals, no matter what their line of work, require a balanced dietary and physical activity program, they also require exceptional psychological and mental dexterity to resist the physical and affective vicissitudes of their way of life.

Hippocrates used to say: "Your diet is your first medicine." If you want to have and preserve a good voice, you need to follow this dogma rigorously, as well as have a good understanding of your muscular machinery.

The Voice brings 400 muscles into play

You must never stretch too much on the elastic cord

How do your vocal cord muscles behave? Muscle contraction is possible because of the structure of the fibers that compose muscles. These fibers slide thanks to myofilaments (named actin and myosin). These lengthen and shorten at will, a mechanical force is produced. During a vocal effort, the cordal muscles stretch to produce high notes and shorten to produce low notes. This action of the muscles is possible because of ATP.

The chemical energy of ATP is transformed into the mechanical and thermal energy of the muscular contraction (during this reaction, ATP transforms into ADP). Given that there's a finite amount of ATP in a muscle, ATP has to regenerate itself quickly to enable the muscle contraction to persist. Glucids are consumed.

1. The first step is always anaerobic: if the contraction lasts over a minute, the internal reserve is insufficient. The anaerobic action is exhausted. Thus, a muscular effort that lasts several minutes requires an aerobic action to make oxygen available, thereby ensuring the regeneration of ATP. This is what allows you to continue singing or talking for several hours at the same energy level.

2. The second step is aerobic. When your aerobic facilitator is in the presence of cellular oxygen, it draws energy from your intracellular chemical plant by oxidizing glucose and lipids, of which the cornerstone is the mitochondrion: this is your cellular respiratory chain. Proteins are rarely solicited.

When you oversolicit a muscle that doesn't have sufficient energy reserves and isn't suitably hydrated, its muscle fibers no longer slide as well and the muscle pulls. Emitting a high note or a low note requires the cordal muscles to contract. This exercise when practiced over and over hundreds of times can cause a traumatism. Microhematoma or hemorrhaging can occur. This normalizes in a few days, but there can be sequels. These sequels include a loss of suppleness in the myofibrils' sliding capabilities where scarring has formed. In other cases, when the cordal muscle is overstretched, for example in the very high notes, or when yelling, the amplitude of the fibrils' slide is excessive in relation to the length of the vocal muscle. The muscle is pulled and remains slack. It becomes atonic and bowed. This produces what is commonly known as a "breathy voice," with an oval-shaped glottis.

Understanding the mechanics of raising or lowering the voice helps voice professionals appreciate the importance of a proper warm-up of the vocalis muscle before performing, though of course each person's limits are different.

The phases of the muscular activity during voice production

During a vocal performance, you call on the energy provided by ATP in your muscles to control your muscles and to control your breathing. This energy comes thanks to three facilitators from three supply sources. They are a function of exercise and the intensity and duration of the performance, which are influenced by the activity of the artist, lecturer, teacher, lawyer, or politician.

- The first facilitator is anaerobic and non-lactic. An intervention of a few seconds at the start is sufficient to prevent the production of lactic acid, which asphyxiates cells.

- The second facilitator is anaerobic and lactic. It comes into play after 40 seconds of physical activity. The muscle uses the glycogen at its disposal and produces lactic acid, which needs to be eliminated. This is the case when you hold a sung note for more than 30 seconds.

- The third facilitator is aerobic. It is brought into action after 2 to 4 minutes of physical effort. Henceforth, ATP will have to be resynthesized, which is made possible by your reserves of glycogen and lipids. This is the case during a plea in court, a lecture, a declamation, or a concert.

The voice's health day in and day out

Good use of the voice requires voice professionals to be extremely attentive and focused. In this world where stress rules the day, taking time to relax is fundamental.

Daily physical exercise

The simplest exercise is to walk in an upright stance that positions the body correctly; hold your head up, relax the shoulders, stride out firmly, and breathe deeply. This simple advice helps ensure optimal vocal performance. The regular practice, at least three times a week for an hour, of a sport that solicits breathing (swimming, abdominal exercises, cycling, jogging, tennis) should be adapted to each individual's capabilities. Swimming stimulates all the muscles of the body. It isn't subject to the laws of gravity. In this weightless environment that is water, the cervical, dorsal, and lumbar vertebrae relax. Swimming, especially the crawl and backstroke, lengthens muscles naturally. The breaststroke develops the pectorals and the upper thoracic cage and offers the advantage of imposing a breathing rhythm and the need to control the exhalation perfectly, as in singing.

A combination of swimming and martial arts balances the body nicely. In martial arts, abdominal breathing and "*chi*" (energy) are fundamental to the adept's concentration. Perfectly mastered movements, controlled breathing, and remarkable concentration are the ground rules of the martial arts. They enable the harmonious development of the thoracic and abdominal muscles. To work these muscles, simple rules must be followed.

Aerobic classes with a good coach will also benefit, but not all sports are good for voice professionals. Some basic precautions must be taken in certain sports: jogging makes you breathe through the mouth, which dries the vocal cords after 100 meters. Therefore, you should not talk while jogging if you want to avoid a reactive laryngitis. It's best to leave equipped with a bottle of water and take regular sips every five minutes while jogging. This applies also to cycling. Wind dries the throat and nose.

Some sports activities are best avoided altogether: those that call on the sphincter muscles of the larynx to support a violent abdominal thrust, as in weightlifting. Weightlifting hypertrophies the ventricular bands and can damage the vocal cords.

Some practical advice

The muscular abdominal belt is the site of the voice professional's most powerful muscles of exhalation. It is, therefore, a good idea to keep these well muscled. You should consecrate twenty minutes of your daily physical activities to your "abs."

- Lying on the floor, feet blocked under some furniture and knees bent, do three series of twenty sit-ups.

- For the next exercise, lift your legs straight up at a 90° angle to the ground: lift the thorax off the ground to touch your feet in three batches of twenty sit-ups.

- The third exercise consists in pedaling with your legs in the air while lying on your back; an alternative is to keep the legs up in the air and bring the elbow to the opposite knee, again in three series of twenty sit-ups.

- To finish, lie flat on your back with your arms stretched out behind your head holding onto the foot of your bed (for example). Taking care to keep the small of your back flat on the ground to avoid lumbar strain, bring both legs up perpendicularly in two series of twenty leg raises.

- My advice is to adopt the following breathing pattern: two breathing out counts for every breathing in count, which should coincide with relaxing the abdominal muscles.

While swimming, the pattern for the crawl is three exhalation counts for every inhalation, whereas the breaststroke requires one exhalation count for every inhalation count. All sports bring balance to the voice professional. We've mentioned only activities that seem most appropriate. But obviously, whether it's fencing, tennis, football, brisk walking, or golf, any of these activities will help improve the body's resistance and mental concentration and eliminate toxins, all of which are indispensable to the balance of our organism.

Sleep: the cornerstone of the vocal athlete and of memory

Respect your sleeping hours

You must respect your sleeping cycle. This is vital. We each have an internal biological clock, our very own chronobiology, and must sleep according to its rhythm.

Deep sleep is the regenerating phase of sleep. Your pulse and breathing are regular, the muscles are relaxed. Note that protein synthesis and the hormonal secretions of the hypothalamus increase at dawn. This deep sleep represents, on average, 80% of your total sleep.

Paradoxic sleep, therefore, only accounts for 20%. It appears in the second half of the night. This is when you dream, move jerkily, have a faster pulse. The short, clustered waves of the electroencephalogram tell us that the brain is very active in this phase, whereas during deep sleep, the brainwaves are long and further apart. Paradoxic sleep is very important for our well-being, and especially for the maturation of the child's brain. In adults, it improves memorization of data acquired the previous day. Deep sleep is a universal feature in all animals, whereas paradoxic sleep is unique to birds and mammals. Paradoxic sleep and deep sleep alternate during the night. They alternate three to four times over a period of five to nine hours, depending on the individual.

Sleeping badly harms the voice

If you sleep little or not at all over a number of days, tiredness accumulates, your memory is affected, your vocal capacities weaken. This is the start of a vicious circle. Fatigue causes you to strain your voice; in order to be convincing and because you're not in full possession of your means, you force on the high notes, yell, and strain the laryngeal muscles. This is a first step toward nodules or an oval glottis (distended vocal cords that can no longer make proper contact). These muscular problems of the voice are exacerbated by problems on the mental plane affecting the voice professional's memory.

Mental fatigue and "the voice of the tiger" is gone

Cerebral tiredness also affects morale. Delivery speed slows down. The performer, lawyer, or journalist can't find his words as quickly. This problem isn't permanent, but it's demoralizing. It's caused by overexertion, being in poor physical shape, having a poorly balanced diet. It can be completely reversed within a few days; all it takes is rest, regenerating sleep, and proper nutrition.

My patients often complain of these problems. They can't get to sleep worrying about the morrow. They misuse their voices. A vicious circle is triggered. In these cases, sleeping pills may be required for a short period. This is where physical activity and a healthy way of life take on another dimension. Apart from oxygenating your muscles and brain, physical activity enables something else that's essential: the elimination of toxins from the organism during sports and the return to balanced sleep cycles.

Protect yourself from emotional aggression

We produce our own toxins

Stress cannot be quantified, but it generates certain toxins, which trigger manifestations that vary from person to person. "My stomach hurts": gastric pain is one type of manifestation; "I can't breathe": asthmatic type coughing is another; "My voice is broken": laryngitis is yet another.

Eliminating toxins

During physical activity, the metabolic rate of your organism increases significantly. Toxic substances are eliminated. More importantly, the hypothalamus secretes an excitatory hormone. Called endorphin, this hormone is well known to marathon runners. It galvanizes performance, whether on an immune, intellectual, physical, or vocal plane. Finally, to put it differently, if your organism has been polluted by "other people's pollution," or indeed by your own pollution, it will regenerate completely if you restore your physical and mental equilibrium.

We have the right to be tired

If in this 21st century Man has to pay particular attention to his physical health, it is because as mammals we were never conceived to live an entire day without physical activity. Indeed, only in the last century, people had to walk from one place to another, worked in the fields, and had to go about providing for their fare. Their organism burnt its reserves of glucose and fats and eliminated toxins quickly, notably through sweating. Their organism had to work hard and was healthy for it.

Fatigue is a signal sent by your organism to tell you that rest is required. This regenerating rest should be associated with immediate rehydration and appropriate nutrition. Indeed, you are allowed to get tired and you owe it to yourself to restore balance in your body if you don't want your voice to suffer. For this reason, it's not a good idea to automatically resort to medical treatment when your voice is tired, if the problem stems from overexertion.

Training and preserving the voice: permanent watchfulness is called for

It is best not to stray too far from your ideal weight

Two kilos is the most you should allow yourself to go over your ideal weight if you want to preserve your vocal timbre. In any case, your diet should include a reserve of protein to maintain effective muscle mass. If you analyze your eating habits, you'll no doubt find that, as a voice professional, you need to rebalance or supplement your diet. There's no escaping it; a balanced diet is a must. But what does it entail for the singer, the teacher, or the lecturer?

Dietary hygiene

- *During performance periods*—Before a lecture, don't ingest any dairy products, as they thicken mucous matter, and don't be tempted by a copious lunch that will slow you down, provoke gastric reflux, and make you feel tired because of the energy you expend digesting it. Go for slow burning sugars, such as pasta, rice, but also dry legumes; make sure you eat enough protein, as proteins are needed to correct or heal micro injuries of the myofibrils that make up the cordal muscles. Animal protein—meat or fish—is still the most effective protein. We've seen the importance of vitamins A, B, C, and E as antioxidants, and of Omega-3 fatty acids. Supplementing with minerals—iron, magnesium, calcium—improves performance. But, and this is important, this balanced diet must become a way of life if it is to improve your vocal performance significantly over the long run, added to which you must train your voice with moderation every day.

    Normally, you should eat three meals a day. However, if you are performing on stage for an hour and a half and sweat profusely, you're well advised to eat a meal consisting of slow burning sugars and fruit two hours before your vocal performance; then half an hour before the performance, ingest fast-burning sugars such as honey.

- *During the "interlude"*—When you're not performing, dairy products are essential (but should be avoided during your performing season as they can create thick mucus in your throat and disturb your voice). For example, at breakfast, milk, yogurt, cereals, and natural fruit juices can restore energy lost during the night. If you feel a little hungry around 11 AM, don't hesitate to have a snack (such as a fruit or an energy bar).

    You may sometimes indulge in a copious dinner, but be sure not to have it too close to your bedtime. Lunch should be light: fish or grilled meat, green vegetables, pasta, potatoes, fibers, and fruit. If you suffer from gastric reflux, avoid coffee and alcohol.

- *When you're in a rush*—If you're in a hurry and don't have time for lunch, you can make do with a healthy sandwich combining fish, meat, or egg with salad. By varying meals and keeping them light, you can often remain in remarkable physical shape, especially if you supplement, depending on your age, with trace elements, Omega-3 (1 to 2 g per day of EPA with DHA), minerals, and vitamins.

  If you feel momentarily "bushed," your voice will betray it. You should then eat some energy bars and fast-burning sugars, as well as drink a lot (water mixed with vitamins and minerals).

Sing, but warm-up first: agonist and antagonist muscles

The muscles of the whole body contribute to developing efficient breathing. Warming up the vocal cords avoids any risk of cordal strain. You must train regularly and both the cervical and the laryngeal muscles must be warmed up. You should never try to sing powerfully straight off in the high notes. The warm-up should be progressive, over a dozen minutes, starting with closed-mouth vocalizations, followed by vowel practice. Next, you should stretch your muscles by yawning and by flexing and extending the cervical muscles. This should be interrupted by rest periods of ten to twenty seconds. However, remain concentrated throughout. Vocal exercises are very useful. They ensure that vocal movements are memorized; they rehearse the movements of the vocal cords on certain frequencies and on how to adapt the resonators. Keep the exercises varied in order to avoid boredom.

In sports, as we saw previously, there are two ways of exercising: passively (for example, legs raised off the ground, immobile) and actively (for example, pedaling). The same applies in singing.

1. *Humming:* The passive workout of your pharyngeal muscular and respiratory muscles is done by voicing with your mouth closed, "mmmm," on different frequencies. It's impossible to strain your voice or dehydrate your vocal cords this way.

2. *Articulate active moves:* You then move on to the active work-out, bringing the muscles into play to emit vowels, to support singing, speaking, and prosody. Pass from the lower tones to the higher tones, then in reverse from the high tones to the low tones.

3. *Bring agonist or antagonist muscles into play* by practicing glottal plosives or a series of "ke-ke-ke-ke-ke." The abdominal and thoracic muscles control the power of the voice, in other words, of the exhalation. They allow excellent stability and protect the vocal organ. All the abdominal muscles are brought into play. Don't hope for that sculptured look with "abs" that look like a chocolate bar, especially if you have a little padding of fat between these muscles and the skin.

What is important is to feel your muscles working. At first, a sports coach can help you to develop your muscles harmoniously, just as the singing teacher will teach you how to place your voice, how to project and control it, and also how to yell.

The recovery period: eliminating lactic acid

Training your muscles enables you to progress, quickly at first, then increasingly more slowly, at the same time as you have singing lessons. Singing lessons teach you to break new boundaries at each class to continuously improve your tessitura and develop better vocal resistance.

1. The recovery phase after a performance is very important. The lactic acid buildup caused by the physical exertion, and the toxins produced by the emotional strain of the performance need to be eliminated: relax the pharyngolaryngeal and abdominal muscles, breathe deeply, and enjoy a moment of calm for a few minutes.

2. This recovery phase is often neglected. Yet it is this phase that will guarantee the quality of the next performance. A few minutes of voicing practice with the mouth closed after a performance can help to relax and loosen the laryngeal muscles. It's the same as stretching after sports.

3. If you feel any pain, or have strained your laryngeal muscle and perhaps caused a hematoma during or after a phonation effort, it's essential to rest your voice immediately and seek appropriate treatment.

4. In some relatively rare cases, there are pseudocramps: certain frequencies are painful, sustaining a note becomes impossible. If this happens, stop rehearsals or the show immediately, and seek medical advice. Dehydration can cause laryngeal pseudocramps. The dehydrated muscle is no longer supple and can't recover. It loses its elasticity, and without this elasticity, the singer is helpless. Drink often.

5. As for muscle strain (you are all familiar with it for having experienced it, whatever your sport), the voice professional experiences it as a toneless voice that's slightly painful. It's due quite simply to a deficient elimination of lactic acid (remember the aerobic facilitator) that can provoke microlesions of the muscles if the voice is forced. Singers, actors, or lecturers should modulate their voice and drink energy beverages.

Finally, if you want to avoid a very dry environment, it is advisable to have a humidifier in your office, dressing room, or conference hall. Prevention of strain is the objective of a good physical workout, avoiding memory lapses is the result of daily mental exercise.

Voice and chronobiology

We humans are sensitive beings and we each react differently according to time and place, according to the time of day: this is known as "chronobiology." Some voice professionals prefer to sing, teach, or play toward the end of the day. An obvious reason for this is our daily hormonal cycle, notably as regards cortisone and melatonin.

- Cortisone peaks twice in our organism: at dawn and in the late afternoon, around 5:00 PM. At dawn, our thyroid hormones also come into action. This is when our vocal tonus is at its best. Cortisone's early-morning peak is one reason why sleeping in is counterproductive, as cortisone peaks again around 5:00 to 5:30 PM and increases muscle tone;

you can perfectly well indulge in a beneficial after-lunch siesta before a concert and be in good form for the performance.

- Melatonin regulates our waking and sleeping cycles. Voice professionals who travel a lot and cross different time zones can adjust the daily cycle of their hormonal secretions by taking melatonin in pill form. Melatonin is a hormone secreted by the pineal gland at the base and in the center of our brain. It is itself regulated by the alternation of light and darkness. During the day, our hydric impregnation also changes. In the morning, we are more pumped up with fluid than in the evening. Our voice is half a tone lower in the morning than in the evening.

How to prevent a vocal injury

Twenty-four-year-old Mr. H. Y., just starting out on his career as a professional singer, consults me to learn how to manage his voice and avoid vocal injury! He wants to know how to protect his larynx.

Before I examine his vocal cords, paradoxically, I begin by checking out his stance. His posture will give me the key to how he projects his voice. The way Mr. H. Y. stands, breathes, braces himself on his two legs, is a first indication of the power behind his voice. Whether a variety show singer or an opera singer, a theatre actor, or a film actor, a teacher, or a lawyer, the same rules apply. His work instrument is his larynx. Singing in front of a microphone is different from giving voice without any artificial acoustic aid. The sensitivity of the microphone correctly transmits not only the vocal register, but also the timbre, the pianissimo, or the forte. The existence today of exceptional acoustic equipment means that there's no need to strain the voice. The quality of a recording depends not only on the singer's mastery over his or her voice, but also on the amplification given by the recording equipment. This amplification is a double-edged sword. It brings out what is beautiful and exacerbates what is mediocre. The intensity or power of the voice becomes an element that's always relative—to other sounds, other musical instruments, other voices.

The problem is different for actors and singers who perform without a microphone. In this case, both the spoken voice with its prosody, and the singing voice, impose the need for rigorous vocal technique.

H. Y. asks me: "Is there such a thing as a vocal gift?" A combination of parameters, both objective and subjective, can indeed allow one to contemplate the possible existence of a vocal gift, and, more precisely, whether the stimulation of harmonics in early childhood will allow one to be gifted or not. Music instruction and vocal instruction are both necessary if such a gift is to develop and endure.

Having a gift is wonderful, but a career is built on hard work and passion. Being gifted may be necessary, but hard work and vocal exercises are vital to the longevity of the voice professional's career.

Singers are slaves of the register that mother nature endowed them with. Tenors or bassi profundi, lyrical sopranos or altos all have different laryngeal configurations. There is no point in going against nature. Nature enables the creation of harmony; we just try to improve on it. Thus, the artist's temperament in the true sense of the word is a determining factor in his career. His conviction and his passion will serve his vocal art. His motivation will provide the source of his creativity.

Taking good care of the voice is a must; the vocal Stradivarius will give of its best only if the artist protects it.

Chapter 16

The voice is on

"Tous les hommes sont des comédiens,
sauf quelques acteurs."
("All men are comedians, except some actors.")

Sacha Guitry

The words that escape from our mouth
no longer belong to us

According to the Greeks, Man is a living being gifted with speech. Speech and reason, science and the soul are essential manifestations of the verbal expression that defines Man. Without a spiritual dimension, the voice professional becomes mechanical, a robot. The melody of our soul is also the secret symphony of the cosmos.

Homo vocalis has to go through many stages to get from the infant's cry to the controlled voice projected on stage, in a lecture hall, or in a court of justice. Each child redefines his own evolution of sound, of cries, of language, of the voice. We start out as infants, we suckle. We are helpless. We cry, but we have no voice. Then we become a child. *Infant* denotes a being that can't talk, a being that vocalizes, groans, grunts, and babbles. The spoken word is the final outcome of this primary evolution that creates our thinking faculty, a faculty that then uses words to create its own verbal expression. Our verbal expression is a message to others, but also to our self. Speakers and listeners follow a code, a grammar and a syntax, words and silences, rhythm and prosody.

The word remains our prisoner as long as it hasn't been pronounced. As soon as it escapes us, we become *its* prisoner.

The left brain is all about mastering language, text, and vocal articulation. This mastery requires a contribution from our emotions, from our imagination, from harmonics: that's the right brain's territory. The balance between our right and left hemispheres is influenced by our mother tongue.

Our voice can change. Individuals who are autistic, in a coma, or who lose their voice after a psychological trauma (psychogenic aphonia) can no longer communicate orally. Their communication with their inner self becomes hidden. For some years now, vocal expression has seized people's imagination. Karaoke is a way of expressing oneself through song that's both liberating and colorful. Some consider it as therapy, as appeasement, as an escape from their stressful life; others do it purely for fun, as a way of letting off steam. When the voice switches off, it is often in reaction to intellectual pollution, to an affective shock, or to an attack on our psyche.

Yet being quiet, remaining silent, retreating into muteness is also a way of saying something, is it not? According to Talleyrand, one of Napoleon's ministers, "men were endowed with language so that they could hide their thoughts." Yet even though some of us can't talk because we have too much to say, the voice remains a fantastic medium for release, as demonstrated by Sigmund Freud. Psychoanalysis caricatures "the voice is on." It reveals the hidden face of the right brain that our rational brain does such a good job of protecting. If I make you speak, I teach you to listen to yourself, I show you how liberating your own vocal expression can be.

Language associates phonemes, expresses our personality. Although speech is different from song, its musicality, intonation, intensity vary in accordance with the emotion expressed. Speech reveals our homeland, the province we come from, the village we were born in. Any Frenchman is familiar with a regional accent from Paris, Marseilles, Lille, or Saint-Malo.

The melody of the voice that has taken a given stage varies in frequency, intensity, rhythm, and duration under the influence of language.

Rhythm and acoustic intonation, notably in songbirds, are also a language of sorts. They condition Man's interpretation, for example: "la, la, la!" and "la, la, la?" signify something quite different. Being understood hangs not only on the meaning of the words spoken, but also on prosody (the melody of our vocal expression) (see Plate 25). Our voice is sexual: angelic in the child, feminine or virile after puberty. The voice in a given framework, your vocal expression in the language you speak, will range over nearly two octaves in Russian, one and a half octaves in English, and barely one octave in French.

We build our voice in our inner cathedral

The voice finds its impulse in the lungs' outward flow, which is the voice's creative energy. The trachea carries puffs of air toward the vocal cords, the organs that give our voice its timbre. They transform the flow of air puffs into a vibrating force. This virgin wave will receive its show apparel in the resonators between the pharynx and the nasal fossae, between the tongue and the lips. The voice's melody is born. It can be modulated and analyzed by the brain. Is it now the human voice? It is not far from it. The vocal edifice is in place, chaos will give it life.

Our voice demands the presence of noise, this aperiodic sound that is irregular and unpredictable. It's composed of our exhalation that bumps into and over the landscape of our internal space between the vocal cords and the lips. It's the organized chaos of the canvas of our vocal timbre, which metamorphoses itself into speech. Its noise is the landscape in which the scenes and characters of our voice are going to take place. This same noise clarifies or dampens our vocal expression. Too salient, it distorts; too pure, or not sufficiently present, it makes us sound like robots. For a voice to be beautiful, there must be neither too much nor too little noise accompanying it. Chaotic acoustic harmony is pleasing to the ear.

Every vocal artist, every singer or actor, lecturer or lawyer has a specific resonance that he develops and exploits, but to be harmonious, the voice must also have its share of dissonance. Man's resonators are all delicately curved and rounded, as if their intent were not to injure the voice. The musical instrument that most resembles the human voice remains the violin. The violin's shape is almost sensual, somehow disquieting. Man Ray, an exceptional photographer, immortalized it with his "Violon d'Ingres," in which the back of the woman represents the instrument. The tessitura of a violin approaches that of the female voice. *Vibrato*, *legato*, or *piccato*, the violinist's action is the same as the singer's. The alchemy of the vocal tessitura is born of our internal mechanics.

Our ear is the orchestra leader of our spoken voice. It regulates the voice's power, frequency, musicality. It calls on the left brain to deliver the right intensity and pitch of vocal expression. It calls on the right brain to contribute sincerity, harmonics, passion, shouting, dialogue, and fervor. What power, and yet how fragile when ill prepared.

The technique of the spoken word

Before you use your laryngeal instrument, you have to prepare it, place it correctly, harmonize it; you practice a few rotations to position the cervical vertebrae, you verify your posture and support. You do all this in a few dozen seconds, much as when you check things out quickly before driving off or attaching your seat belt. Then you are ready, free to sing or speak.

For voice professionals, learning to place the spoken word is as important as learning to sing is for the professional singer. Speaking comes naturally when talking among friends, but much less naturally when you have to speak in a conference room, in a court room, or in a classroom six hours a day. The spoken voice requires of us a specific posture of the neck, torso, and stomach, as well as an upright stance. To blossom forth, the spoken voice requires lack of tension, freedom of expression, physical and respiratory suppleness.

Voice therapists make an important contribution here. They should be the teacher's or the lawyer's first port of call, because voice therapy is as important for them as their theoretical knowledge. To become a sports coach, you have to learn not only how to teach (pedagogically), but also the movements and workings of the body on the gymnastics apparatus, on the mat. or while running.

In my opinion, the same applies to voice professionals. They must learn the movements and workings of the larynx if they want to train the larynx without risk of injury to the voice. The "vocalist" who is tense and rigid, who holds himself with shoulders raised, head jutting forward, and spine rounded, will not captivate his audience for long. His voice tires, loses timbre and harmonics, becomes hoarse. Singers or actors who are stiff as a broomstick will not get very far either. Their voice is at the service of their words and their intelligibility to the audience. The beginner is going to shout from the throat to be heard at the back of the room.

But the voice is a fluid that passes through the phonatory tract like water in a riverbed. It flows. It doesn't force its way through, it follows the natural lay of the land. Mechanical equilibrium is important, but no more so than the equilibrium of the body or the mind.

Mastering one's voice comes with experience and technique. This technique must be simple, it must allow the "vocalist" to use his vocal instrument without constraints: as he wishes, when he wishes, but always conscious of his limits. He adapts his technique to his voice should his voice start to tire. To do that, he needs to know his text. Technique is never but a means to play a role. The credibility of the interpretation comes from the strength, equilibrium, and apparent ease of the artist. Laryngeal muscular tension and body tensions should never exist. Tension can only disserve. Sometimes a deep breath is the way forward.

The voice dances with the body, vibrates with it, it only metamorphoses our breath into voice. Gerard Philipe and Michel Simon in the movie *La beauté du diable* (The beauty of the devil) show their mastery of every vocal technique, with oh such different results.

The drama teacher who respects his pupils' timbre and melody is able to give them the proper knowledge of their instrument while preserving its individual identity. The teacher must adapt himself to each pupil, correcting faults without necessarily eradicating them completely, always respectful of personality.

- The key here is not to correct a fault with another fault.

For example, suppose your hip has rotated downward and to the left: a heel-piece placed under the left foot is a preferable solution to compensating by keeping the right knee permanently bent. Careful observation of the posture of voice professionals as they breathe provides a good indication of the stability of their upright posture between the inhalation and the exhalation. The rules have been the same for centuries, only fashions change: from Arletty to Simone Signoret, from Delphine Seyrig to Isabelle Adjani, from Marilyn Monroe to Lauren Bacall, the voice varies in clarity, in tone, in breathiness. What has remained a constant is the public's need to understand the "vocalist."

The scream slashes the silence

The actor or singer, lawyer, or lecturer projects his voice. If he wants to whisper, his whisper must be heard at the back of the theater, courtroom, or lecture room. When he shouts, he must be able to shout without injuring his voice. His technique guarantees the preservation of his instrument.

You can't hear yourself the way others hear you. Here's the proof: block your left ear and recite a sentence out loud. Block the right ear and recite the same sentence again. It will sound different to you. The feedback won't be the same. Stereophony enables you to regulate your vocal expression. This underscores the importance of the receiver, of the listener, but where the expression is emitted is also important.

The voice comes forth from the mouth, delivered into an external world that is aerial and vibratory. Noise exists in this external world outside the boundaries of our body. For example, in a concert hall, there's a noise we're all familiar with, known as "background noise." It's around 12 dB, the hall's "breathing, bouncing off the walls." Rehearsing in front of an empty hall is very different. The lawyer pleads in a full courtroom: the power and harmonics of his voice are perceived differently by the spectators and by him. Actors and comedians know how to use both, their voices and their bodies, their vibratory presence and their physical presence. They draw their energy from their audience. To exist, artists must have an audience. There can be no acting without a spectator.

The memory blank

A musical melody is never forgotten, it doesn't go blank on one. It comes from our right brain. Our spoken voice reflects who we are with our weaknesses and strengths, our oversights and our reference marks. It has forged the education of our thinking and the imprint of our culture.

Memory is essential to our staged voice. Drama schools normally only teach vocal technique; I often think it regrettable that they don't make it obligatory to also learn techniques for learning text by rote. Our memory needs to be titillated, trained, and perfected. Indeed, there's a play called *La baie de Naples* (Naples' bay) that actors often test each other on to train their memory.

Different techniques can be used to memorize a text: you can learn the first sentence, then the second by repeating the first, then learn the third by repeating the first and the second, and so on. This gives some logical continuity to the memorization of a text. Often people think that repeating the same text for hours on end helps to internalize a part. In fact, this isn't so. It has been proven that concentration can only be excellent over a moderate time span, which for a given text is forty-five minutes.

If you work for three hours on the same text, you'll know it less well and interpret it less well than if you had studied three different texts each for forty-five minutes twice a day. Prosody is also a learning prop, especially if learning verses. The caricatural aspect of prosody was exploited by an amusing sketch that delighted several generations with its multiplication table: "two times two four, la-la-la-la."

But to remember a text, you have to want to learn it. Motivation is the key driver of our memory. Yet we can all be victims of a memory "blank." An intriguing expression, as if we had a hole in our brain. Memory blanks are more likely if you learn a text in several chunks: twenty minutes today, an hour tomorrow. This way, you don't have time to put in place the proper memory circuits efficiently. On the contrary, going at it over and over again, disciplining yourself and challenging your memory are essential. Then the memorized text will come back to you quite naturally; all you will have to do is interpret it.

But memory blanks and memory capacity call on very specific areas of the brain and specific brain circuits: I can recall where my glasses are almost instinctively, but I have to remind myself that I have a meeting scheduled for a certain time. In the latter instance, memory is brought into play on two levels: to memorize the time and to memorize what I must do at this time. Thus, there are several mnesic menus. It is true that some people use the sound of their own voice to help them memorize text. Others use the text itself as a visual prop to help them memorize a poem: "the word 'sun' is the first word on the left of page 7 . . . " Memory is something that has to be continually practiced. If it's more alert in adults than in the elderly, isn't this because we stimulate it less after the age of seventy?

Several levels of memory

The very sophisticated world of Cerebropolis

It's interesting to note that repeating a text—and this is especially true for actors—activates numerous areas of the brain (the right cerebellum, the insula, the frontal lobe) during the initial memorizing of the text. Thereafter, rehearsing the text stimulates only the anterior insula. Our neurons are economical in their efforts. After all, the words are the same.

What goes on in our brain? How are these different memories organized? Which complex circuits, out of the billions of connections already formed, is the brain going to seek out to feed the singing voice, the stage voice, the memory of a song heard twenty years ago that fills us with nostalgia?

We know that every day after our birth, we lose millions of neurons, but remember we have around 100 billion. So we're still capable of learning a play like *Le bourgeois gentilhomme*, by Molière, at eighty. Man reigns supreme in this respect. The feedback of our hearing is the key for our memory. Without memory, we're deprived of language. Without memory, the comedian or actor, the lawyer or teacher are deprived of their work tool. Our voice requires permanent memory training. The number of neurons we have is only one aspect. What is incredible is the number of connections that each neuron can develop. Computers are a long way off from being able to mimic this environment. Moreover, computers will never know what it is to feel pleasure! This affective component cannot be measured, but it's fundamental for artists. The more you stimulate your memory, solicit it, implicate it, the more it will generate new neuronal connections, facilitating the integration of a text, a song, or an itinerary: creation begets creation.

As time goes by, we ask our brain to store and preserve an increasing volume of memories.

- These memories may be recent, it's what is known as our anterograde or short-term memory. Located in the middle of the brain, it lodges in the hippocampus. This is where memories are stored initially before they go to the cortex (the surface of the brain) to be stored in our long-term memory. There they are engraved, leaving an indelible mark that enables us to retrieve them decades later. The most serious disease involving our short-term memory is Alzheimer's, a disease caused by cerebral lesions in this area. It produces anterograde amnesia: recent events can't be recalled.

- Our long-term memory is in the cortex. When a stroke affects this area of the brain, aside from engendering motor problems, it causes retrograde amnesia (events in the distant past can't be recalled).

We have five different memory recall systems

Thus, our memory isn't restricted to one part of the brain. It calls upon complex systems located in three areas of the brain: the cerebellum that harmonizes our memories, the limbic brain that controls our emotions, and the neocortex that enables the mechanical integration of this memory, whether verbal, physical, or visual. The neurons are the cables that connect up these regions.

1. *Our short-term memory* (in the hippocampus): I have a coffee, five minutes later I can remember this. Our short-term memory can house between five and seven items of information.

2. *Our skills memory* (in the cerebellum and central gray matter): responsible for what we do in automatic mode: driving a car, riding a bicycle, swimming. These automatisms survive even in amnesia. They are rarely forgotten or interfered with. This type of memory is also called into play when we memorize text. It is highly dependent on the brain being stimulated (the parietal cortex and the fusiform gyrus).

3. *Our factual memory* (in the prefrontal cortex) rules our behavior and enables us to do several things at once. It doesn't exceed a few minutes or hours. Whereas our short-term memory enables us to recall something without conscious effort, our factual memory does require conscious effort. We go after the information, we decide to recall it. For example: I look for a telephone number. I take the telephone book, I recall the name I want to look up. Then I memorize the phone number. I return to my phone, I compose the number. A few minutes

later, if I have not decided to memorize it, the number will be forgotten. This cascade can be interrupted by an external event that distracts me, then I have to start the process all over again. This memory can be called on for the initial memorization of text. In Broca's area, the phonemes that are memorized are repeated mentally. This is an auditory memory, stocked by articulated language. Speakers use it a lot. If the storage is very short-term, the information is held in the supramarginal gyrus.

4. *Our episodic memory* (in the hippocampus and frontal region) is our long-term memory. It enables us to remember our childhood, events tied to our family, to people around us, many years ago. I can remember my first bicycle; it was red, with four wheels.

5. *Our semantic memory* is particular. It's housed primarily in the cortex of the left brain (mainly in the frontal cortex and the posterior neocortex of the left hemisphere). Like our factual memory, it's an explicit memory. Using various mnemonic techniques, I can recall the different muscular insertions of the vocal cords: this is my semantic memory at work. A conscious effort is required to retrieve these memories that go back a long way, things we learned, things that were imposed on us, the movements involved in singing or speaking. It's one of the cornerstones of our emotional makeup.

As incredible as this may seem, when we are missing a word that's "on the tip of our tongue," it's registered in a precise part of our anatomy: the perceptual trigger of the word is in the right lingual gyrus. The occurrence of memory blanks, though not always avoidable, can be reduced by learning text in a more concentrated fashion instead of spreading it over the day or several days. When you have a word on the tip of your tongue, it's often because of a momentary blockage caused by another word that is screening the one you want from your active recall.

This tip-of-the-tongue word is often a word that doesn't mean much to you. It has no connotations; it doesn't evoke anything for you. It's asemantic. The memory circuit, that it belongs to, is too well hidden. But just let it go and your automatic memory, via another circuit, will retrieve the word for you from the depths of your brain a few minutes later. The pleasure derived from singing, from speaking, from acting, the pleasure derived from having a vocation rather than a mere job, greatly enhances the mnesic capacity of our brain.

Our memory isn't a computer system, it's full of emotional subtlety

These different memories interconnect, relay each other, complete each other. Different neuronal circuits and their interconnections make this magic possible. But as in the case of the singing voice, the stage voice, the voice that interprets Shakespeare or Molière, or argues a plea in court based on key points of the case that have been memorized, synaptic connections aren't like computer connections.

We're not dealing with a binary system: yes-no. It isn't a "black or white" system. These synapses are the transmission links between two neurons. The information is ferried by the neuron thanks to an electrical signal. Chemical substances allow the information to pass from neuron A to neuron B. The amount of this substance is determined by the amount of information that has to pass. There's an emotional component involved. The quality and quantity of information will vary according to the volume of chemical substances delivered during the transmission. Is this not one of the unique aspects of our emotional world? Is this not why Man is perpetually creative and never has strictly identical gestures, unlike a robot?

Thus it is that the now famous quote from Shakespeare "To be or not to be . . . " can be repeated thousands of time by the same actor, but never in quite the same way. He no longer has to be conscious of his technique, his recall of the text isn't conscious. He lives his text. The art of the artist lies not in recall, but in interpretation. His memory is his cerebral instrument, his larynx, his sonorous and acoustic instrument, his voice, the reflection of his emotions.

The capacity of our memory doesn't alter with age, or very little. Actors have no problem learning new text.

The following anecdote corroborates the existence of this capacity in all of us. Subjects aged between sixty-three and ninety-one were brought together once a week for a one-hour German lesson. After three months, they passed tests that are normally passed after three years of German study. Their cerebral connections had built all the necessary circuits for this rapid memorization. Yet time scales vary. In the time dimension, a year is a tenth of a ten-year-old boy's life, whereas it's but a fiftieth of the life of a fifty-year-old. Time goes faster at this age. Even emotion is affected by the theory of relativity.

Memory's friends are sometimes our foes

I have often been approached, be it by teachers, singers, or actors and asked to prescribe miracle medicines to boost a failing memory. Some medicines can help, but the only effective therapy in the long-term is practicing memorization. Practice is essential. The alchemy of the expression and memory imposes the need for a healthy lifestyle, a diet rich in fruit and antioxidants, regular sport, and especially, regenerating sleep. Indeed, our orchestra leader, the brain, eliminates its own toxins and resources itself while we sleep.

What was I to say to the comedian who reported back to me: "Doctor, since you asked me to give up smoking, I can't work, I can't remember my lines." It was imperative that he give up smoking as his voice was raucous from a lesion on a vocal cord. After the lesion was removed by microsurgery, all was well. He had gone back to work nine weeks later with a perfect timbre, but his interpretation was mediocre because his memory was giving him trouble. What was going on? He had put behind him the stress of the operation. From an anatomic point of view he was cured, but he was dependent on tobacco and was perturbed. It seems that nicotine intoxication had helped him to memorize his lines. Indeed, we know that the tar content in tobacco can produce malignant lesions and that its nicotine content can produce vascular lesions, but it's also true that the same nicotine is a stimulant that influences the hypothalamus and the hypophysis. It increases hormonal secretions affecting vigilance. I referred him to a cardiologist, who prescribed a nicotine patch. Decreasing concentrations of nicotine delivered by a patch over a period of three months allowed him to "kick the habit."

Some people's capacity for memorization is outstanding. Not everyone is an athlete with the potential to compete at the

Olympic Games. But through practice, each of us can attain satisfactory results without being a champion. The same applies in the memory field. Some voice professionals have outstanding abilities as regards their memory skills, others' memory skills are not as good, but they're still excellent artists. This inequality in memory skills is notable in young chess players. Practice is critical, but aptitude and talent are irreplaceable. When the memory has been strongly solicited, rest intervals are required to give the organism time to regenerate its internal energy.

Stress on the memory side

Stress influences our emotions, but also our memory recalls. We know that the feeling of being "under pressure" causes the secretion of three types of hormones: endorphins, cortisone (corticosteroid hormones), and epinephrine (a member of the catecholamine group, which also includes norepinephrine and dopamine).

Excess epinephrine increases the heart rate, but especially memory blockages, the dreaded memory blank, the stage fright. Our synaptic connection doesn't allow us to retrieve the required word or sentence during a performance. Some voice professionals who are regular victims of this panic may resort to beta-blockers.

The cortisone we secrete is a stimulant and an energizer. Endorphins, secreted under certain types of stress and also during sports activities, are a real drug. They accelerate our memory activity and capacity. They galvanize our interpretation. They dispel all shyness and overcome stuttering, as was the case with that wonderful actor Roger Blin.

Voice and controlled silence

Inner silence is the edge between emptiness and vibration, between yin and yang. It feeds off our harmonics and vice versa. Although the intonation or musicality of our voice doesn't change, whether we're on stage at the Comédie Française or in front of a film or television camera, the way we use our voice does. The real voice professional transmits his message not only through his words, but also through the silences between his words. As Lacan said: "A shout is an appeal, but first and foremost it calls forth silence."

When a lawyer improvises a plea to defend his client, he must bring his client's case into his memory to select key arguments from it. He will use his eloquence to back them up, this being a key element in his repertory of skills. His timbre will convince, the words he has memorized being merely a vehicle for passing on information. But he also uses silences, with all that they imply, as a form of dialogue. During counsel's address, during a lecture, in Hamlet's soliloquy, the silences between words impart rhythm and emotion, impose silence on others and for others. Indeed, silence allows whoever is listening to develop their own inner silence, to become a mere receptacle, and, thus, free their mind of all interference from their own memories. They are then open to register fully the new information they've just heard.

Roger Blin stuttered badly off the stage, but never in *Hamlet*. Louis Jouvet had his stuttering under complete control. Born on the 24th of December, 1887 in Brittany, this first-class pharmacist stuttered as a child. He had complete control over his stuttering when he acted his part in Molière, Pagnol, or Jules Romain works—I recall his exquisite interpretation of Dr. Knock—"Does it tickle or does it itch?" Later, he was able to master his stuttering in his everyday life as well. "I said strange . . . very . . . sstrange." This prosody, so typical of his vocal print, was a key part of his charm and personality. He had tamed his vocal expression, the text became a vehicle for his emotion.

The artist's skill and the power of the stage voice, are expressed in the artist's capacity to interpret text with silences and to play with silence and harmony.

In a court of law: The voice is an offensive and defensive weapon

You enter the courtroom. The accused is isolated in his box. The trial begins. All communication here is oral. The voice is a weapon used both for attack and for defense. It can betray the innocent person with an unpleasant voice, just as it can make innocent the guilty person with a seductive voice.

The bailiff announces the president and his two magistrates with a loud:

"The Court."

As required by this impressive protocol, everyone rises. The president in his red robe is accompanied by his two deputies. The defense advocate and the prosecutor are present. The jurors are drawn at random from electoral rolls and take their seat if neither the defense counsel nor the prosecutor object.

The trial starts. The president asks the accused to stand and to reveal his identity, profession, birth date, and address before the facts are stated. This is the most crucial moment in the trial. The jurors get to know the accused through his voice.

"The voice" reverberates in the court room, introducing emotion.

The accused has come to life, he has just introduced himself. He exists. Another voice is now heard: the court clerk reads out the accusation. Anything not covered by the clerk will be revealed by the witnesses.

The witnesses each take their turn on the witness stand. No document exists, other than perhaps photos. All is reduced to voice, intonation, and rhythm, punctuated by silence and noise. As Andre Gide noted in 1912 in his *Souvenir de cour d'assises* (Memories of an Assize Court) "the jurors are glued to their seats by the vocal power of the pleading."

It is now the prosecutor's turn to rise in his red robe. He imposes respect. His voice becomes his attack weapon. The president, defense counsel, the accused, and the jury listen in complete silence. The voice now plays its part conveying information and emotion. The prosecutor's voice is his weapon. He knows how to use it. His verb is seductive, authoritative, perforce accusing. But if his pleading goes on for too long, his voice may tire. If he does not place his voice correctly, it will weaken. He will then lose some of his persuasiveness. To convince, he must maintain the right timbre. He needs to conclude strongly, vigorously, and with conviction to announce his conclusions with the eloquence of the orator. No one has interrupted his requisition; he demands an exemplary sentence in a loud voice in awed silence.

The defense advocate now rises in his black robe. The contest of eloquence now begins. The requisition has caused such a shock that everyone is impatient to hear the first words of the defense advocate, or should I say, the striking timbre of his voice. Will he be convincing? Will he be listened to? For the time being, he is not arguing his case. He first has to hook his audience in. Surprisingly, it's the silence following his first words that will confirm if his voice has struck the right note, if it was powerful enough, neither too loud nor too soft. If too loud, it interferes with the intelligibility of his text and he loses his audience. If too soft, his listeners are no longer captivated and drift into their own thoughts.

Pleading is all about words, rhythm, and silence. The emotional component is as important as the argument. He makes his final argument. The president asks the accused if he has anything to add. His voice and his timbre are the last vibratory elements that the jury will hear before the verdict.

The jurors deliberate, having heard *the voices*. Personal conviction is the final decisive phase each of them must bring to term. Objective and subjective arguments are all amalgamated deep inside them. The timbres, first of the president's voice, then of the accused, then of the witnesses and of the advocates, will play a major role in their final decision.

Their personal conviction comes from talking to themselves. It is their inner voice, able to make abstraction of the others, nevertheless influenced by the affective charge of the harmonics of the voices heard in court, where the oral character of the proceedings reigns supreme.

The advocate's voice is his weapon, his passion is his arrow, his conviction is his target. When he addresses his audience, indeed he calls upon reason, but more so on emotion, which is highly intensified by the formality of an Assize Court. Advocates are past masters of the affective vibration of their address, they are supreme orators.

In this ritual of justice, the vocal dimension is enhanced by the setting of the tribunal. The president, the magistrates, and the prosecutor are on a higher level than the other members of the court, who have to look up at them. Defense counsel, the jurors, and the accused look up at them. The voices on both parts are amplified in this universe in which the sentence distresses or delights, in which the human voice is the vehicle for the decision process, in which the group judges the individual.

The power of the politician's voice

The target of a political address is the crowd at a political gathering and each of us watching the television screen. Television is a remarkable amplifier of emotion. It reaches millions of people, as opposed to only a few thousand in a hall. It allows sincerity to shine through and is fatal to the sham. A look, the movement of an eyebrow, the posture of the shoulders, the gesture of a hand, a facial expression, these are all dead giveaways as the words pour forth. Seduction won't do the job, the politician must deliver a verbal message that is coherent and must demonstrate inner harmony. His exhalations during his speech carry his message. They impose a rhythm and a technique that the politician must be thoroughly at ease with. If he has mastered the technique of declamation, he is able to forget his voice and think only of his message, of his powers of persuasion, of the "off-the-cuff" improvisations that characterize the genius of these splendid orators. And yet, how often does one hear, after a political speech, the comment that the politician moved well, spoke well, or that his tie was a good choice? The content of his address seems secondary. Is the problem that oral communication is thought to lack sincerity, or could it be that our society is so submerged by voices that we no longer pay attention to them?

We are submerged by a multitude of voices. Paradoxically, in this world of oral communication, physical appearance has become paramount; we live in a world of pretense. We listen to silences. But, all too often, the journalist reading the eight o'clock news has thirty seconds to make his pitch. No more silences between words, no room left for comprehension. The viewers are shown what amounts to political video clips, instead of receiving political information. The same phenomenon happens in radio broadcasting. The broadcaster behind his microphone receives signals to ensure he is as brief as possible. It's impossible for him to sound natural. From listening serenely, we've been hustled into receiving a frenetic message of what is considered newsworthy. Superficiality has stolen the march on sincerity. Appearance can be misleading, not so vocal utterances. We need to restore our inner harmony, have the courage of our convictions, and communicate them to others in order to be heard and to give our voice back its voice. Only then will adolescents be able to identify themselves with the heroes of oral communication. Asphyxia by the media is threatening our acoustic wave band. Too much information is making us "deaf" to all of it.

When the voice becomes ambient noise

Does the voice still exist? We hear voices in meetings, on the street, in restaurants, but don't listen to them anymore; worse still, we have become indifferent to these ambient noises. In another register, when a child does his homework, he listens to music on his Walkman, with the television on, providing a backdrop of noise and images. He doesn't hear anything. He isn't communicating, these voices are just a backdrop, he doesn't register any verbal or harmonic messages. He is part of the "zapping" generation. Insulation and loneliness are exacerbated.

Is this vocal pollution becoming destructive? Maybe not, but it does generate indifference to dialogue. Paradoxically, in the 21st century, in spite of the telephone and three hundred television channels, our individual vocal space is shrinking. Yet the collective vocal space is overdimensioned. Is silence dead? If we could relearn to hear the footsteps of a child in the street, or the rustling of the wind on the streets, we would be a step ahead in the re-education of our affective perception of vibrations. The verbal onslaught we are subjected to isolates us from our inner self. Talking with someone nourishes our thoughts, but listening to all this one-way communication atrophies our interpersonal skills and experience. Beethoven's deafness didn't stop him from listening to music in his head. Some people hear, but never listen.

In a restaurant, a couple dine. These days, it is not unusual to see couples who don't say a word, except to order or to answer their mobile phone in plain sight on the table. Elsewhere, they settle down in front of the giant screen, relieved not to have to converse. The voice as a means of communication is turning into mime. Words are swallowed, barely pronounced. Yet conversation is an essential learning ground to construct our thinking and provide some logic for our future. Theatrical plays, true popular entertainment, prompted discussion. Their popular comeback in theatres and cultural centers is a great initiative for re-educating the voice and communicating with others, and one that gives you the freedom not to "zap" anyone.

Our body, instrument of the voice

Unhappy equilibrium between the void and harmony

The voice is an instrument, an entity that is immaterial yet always present. The magical alliance between body and soul is its alchemy. The voice is intrinsic to Man through its affective charge, and extrinsic to Man in that it results from the mechanical metamorphosis of our outward airflow into vibrations. There are as many different voices as there are grains of sand in the ocean. Six billion *Homo vocalis* each have their own voice, their own vibrations. Vocal technique tames these vibrations to harmonize them within our deepest self. Our voice is a weapon. It attacks, seduces, destabilizes, awes. It is both offensive and defensive. It also brings us ecstasy in prayer or in incantation, hope or sacrifice in certain rituals like voodoo.

Vibrations are an unstable equilibrium between silence and noise. Thus, the voice carries messages between you and me and to myself. Thanks to the voice, Man finds solace in the memory of his mother's melodies, urges himself on in competition, argues with himself to reach a decision. These days, certain voices try to imitate instruments, but for millennia, instruments have tried to imitate the voice.

The actor's voice: from the individual to the group

This voice seduces us. In our society, the artist is the square peg in a round hole. He perturbs and yet he enthralls. His emotions are heightened, be it in the depths of sadness or in the ecstasy of joy, torn between life and suicide: never far from the edge. His voice is his emotion. Respect it. When you boo an actor, you hurt his inner self and insult his passion. When he interprets an artistic work, his vocal mechanics no longer exist for him, they are as natural to him as walking on stage. His artistic sincerity stems from the harmony between his affect and the way he has dressed up for the part he has to play. The actor brings to life the words that Corneille, Victor Hugo, or Samuel Becket put on paper. He makes their words vibrate, resuscitates characters that have been dormant for years. Respect for the author's creation, its vocal rhythm, its romance is inscribed in a setting carefully drawn by the author. The highlights, the way the character is brought alive, are contributed by the actor, just as Henri Alcan provided a touch of magic through his *chiaroscuros* in Jean Cocteau's film *La belle et la bête*. The actor's voice is the vibratory wave that transfers his emotion to his audience. The sham is quickly unmasked and often punished by the return of the breaking wave that frequently injures the ego of the artist who hasn't been authentic in his interpretation. Conversely, the artist must not go too far and hijack the author's creation. He would not be forgiven if he were to falsify it.

The voice seduces

Italy, country of the bel canto, has music coursing in its language. When an Italian speaks, the vowels sing. The opera merely pays homage to the voice. The artist goes on a voyage of self-discovery with every performance. An original creation takes form. It is authentic, it is sincere, it enthralls us. Western song is built on a solfeggio that is familiar to our ears. The Hindu language and Hindu music explore different harmonics. In India, improvisation reigns supreme. The frequencies heard there may offend our ears. Their consonance and dissonance disturb us. They use a quarter and an eighth tone intervals, which we are not familiar with. In Europe, I'm familiar with the established scale, I'm in a safe zone; it's Western and it's rational.

In Asia, I'm plunged into a chaos of harmonics, into an emotional abyss. Yet Asia's language and her music, have their own words, their own vibratos, their own rhythms and ornaments. As I listened to these harmonics, I understood the importance of those odd harmonics that perturb me, but are indispensable to the landscape of our spoken language. The major scale is a supple waveform in which consonance rules; in the minor scale dissonance prevails. The major scale is given its true value by the minor scale.

In difference lies the very richness of our culture. This mixing has enriched the melody of our voice, spoken and sung. Sadness vibrates in the minor third, joy in the major third. The feeling that emerges is the secret of music's emotional vibration. It shuns boredom, the cult of uniformity, the monochord voice. This seductive voice caresses and reassures. Melancholy sprinkled with major pitches, against a background in the minor scale, charms. A slight veil accentuates the dissonance. This discordant combination, punctuated by silences in a deep register, gives what we consider today to be a voice full of charm. Happily, it can't be synthesized.

The voice owes it to itself to seduce. It is sexual, it is the Cupid of our soul. Cyrano projects his voice and Roxanne succumbs, irreversibly touched by it in the deepest folds of her vibratory being. Our voice can be esthetic or charming. It casts a spell. It carries emotion and fantasy, it inscribes itself in the landscape of our internal vibration.

Chapter 17

The singing voice

"A mysterious force drives me toward an unknown goal.
As long as I haven't reached it, I remain in vulnerable.
The day I shall be of no use to it, a puff is all
it will take to knock me down."

Napoleon

From Malibran to La Callas, they had the splendor of life
in their voice and they always had that mysterious force.

Emotion and reason pass through the singing world

To sing is to turn silence into melody

Singing draws on two distinct aspects of Man's nature: emotion and reason. The singer stimulates both. When he sings, he is the song. But to sing is not enough. He must also seduce the ear, interpret every concert as if it were a new creation, express passion, emotion and the intimations of the opus. If he is to achieve these difficult results, if he is to carry the listener along in this sung harmony, give him the wherewithal to dream and make him vibrate in his heart of hearts, the artist must be gifted not only with that indefinable something that we call the affective inspiration of creation, but also with the required vocal technique.

The otorhinolaryngologist (ORL) or the phoniatric specialist is the violin maker who fine-tunes the laryngeal instrument. The vocal "Stradivarius" is in there, unique to each artist. The singing teacher guides as necessary the varied movements of the virtual bow that caresses the words.

What is a great voice?

Lyrical art is alchemy between voice and orchestra. It imposes concessions on both sides and a perpetual openness to the ever-changing interplay between the musical instrument, the voice, and the audience. But because of its constraints, opera has prescribed different vocal registers, or tessitura. Going back over nearly four centuries, what do we understand by a great voice, a diva, an outstanding tenor?

Singers have to deal with their own problems of expression, but they must take the credit for taking into account not just the opus, but also the personality of the conductor. Indeed, it is he that conducts the harmony of the instruments, from the violin to the piano, from the brass to the double-bass, as well as the precision of the singer's musical instrument. Opera fans enjoy the opera as much for the spectacle as for the music. Operas dazzle, seduce, fascinate.

A great voice is the voice you listen to impervious to the technique behind it; it is the voice that makes you vibrate through its range, its power, its timbre, but also through its subtleties and silences. Spectators eagerly await the performance of the tenor or the soprano. They lie in wait of the singer's exploits; a counter *C* is impossible without mastery of the appropriate technique.

Thus, the classification of voices in opera was adopted merely for the convenience of simplification, to establish reference points. A given tessitura doesn't suggest the limits of a voice, merely, which, this voice is at ease in this register.

In his given tessitura, a singer can sing effortlessly for several hours. This doesn't mean that he can't sing higher or lower, all it means is that the *passagio* comes naturally to the tenor, whereas the basso profundo will find it a little tricky. Certain bass voices are able to sing as high as a tenor, but it is not natural for them. It tires their voice. In the same way, a butterfly swimmer is perfectly capable of swimming a two-hundred-meter race in breaststroke, but will get better results in his own specialty. There are exceptions. Being able to do it doesn't mean one should. It is in singing school, be it of the lyrical or popular category, that technique fine-tunes the voice. Each vocal group harmonizes with the others and weaves a musical symbiosis with the orchestra. A voice defines itself through its register, its power, and its timbre. It strikes a chord in the spectator, plays with the scale. It is at times clear, at times dark, at times strong, at times soft. The vocal register enables us to classify singers.

The vocal register

The feminine register

The female voice has been classified into five categories:

- The soprano voice should be singled out. Considered the highest voice, the term also applies to boys with a voice in the range C3 to C5 (258-1034 Hz). The vocal cords of a soprano are normally around 16 to 18 mm long. The highest voice among sopranos is the soprano coloratura. We come across it in the *Lakmé* melody of the opera by Delibes, on which Mady Mesplé left an indelible stamp in 1953. She excels in her vocalises, in her trills and ornaments.

- The lyrical soprano, also called mezzo-soprano, is a more powerful voice. Its goal is not to reach the very high notes. The timbre is rich, with a special mordent. The volume is ample. The repertory is also rich, a good example here being Katia Ricciarelli, an Italian soprano who was superb as Mimi in *Bohemia*, or as Marguerite in *Faust*.

- The dramatic soprano is a well-known timbre in Wagnerian operas, but also in Italian operas—for example, Violetta's part in *La Traviata*. The medium or mezzo-soprano is very rich and powerful, with vigorous high notes. The timbre is darkly colored, always velvety, with richly hued harmonics.

- The alto is a deeper voice, between A2 and A4 (217–870 Hz). The vocal cords in this case are between 16 and 20 mm long. It is a voice full of charm and nicely set off by Wagnerian operas or bel canto parts.

- Finally, the contralto, the deepest female register, is a vocal tessitura that often has recourse to the chest voice, something that cannot be said of sopranos. The contralto is found in Rossini operas. The register ranges from G2 to G4 (193–775 Hz). The length of the vocal cords is between 18 and 22 mm.

The male register

The male voice has four registers:

- The tenor ranges from C2 to C4 (128–520 Hz), with a vocal cord length of 20 to 22 mm. The voice is high-pitched and powerful, the timbre warm and seductive. The purists make a further distinction: the dramatic tenor, whose weight and vigor match the rich subtlety of the timbre's tessitura. Parts for tenors are legion, from Mozart to Wagner, from Rossini to Verdi. The maestros of this register, be they opera tenors, lyrical tenors,or dramatic tenors, are among others Enrico Caruso, Luciano Pavarotti, or Roberto Alagna.

- The countertenor (known as *haut contre*— high counter— in French) uses a head voice with specific resonances that enable him to have an extremely high-pitched voice, notably in operas by Gluck or Lulli. It is in a category of its own. A wonderful interpreter of Baroque music, sometimes likened to the tessitura of the castrati, although the countertenor and the castrato have nothing in common, his vocal cords resemble an anatomic sketch. He has the larynx of a child, but the muscles are those of an athlete. The vocal cords are long (25 mm) and very fine (between 3 and 4 mm). The their variation in length between the high-pitched voice and the low-pitched voice is impressive: around 27 mm in the high pitches compared with 10 mm in the low pitches.

- The baritone, ranging from A1 to G3 (100–390 Hz), has vocal cords that are 22 to 24 mm long. The baritone excels as Don Juan in Mozart's opera, Figaro in *The Barber of Seville* by Rossini, or Germont in *La Traviata*. A distinction is made for the Verdi baritone, as exemplified by Ruggiero Raimondi's voice in *Don Giovanni* or *Don Carlo*.

- The bass ranges from C1 to E3 (65–325 Hz, and for the purist, the basso profundo, stable at 60 Hz) with a length of vocal cord of 22 to 26 mm. The voice is voluminous, enveloping the spectator. The timbre is powerful and firm. It makes a striking impression from the start. It is Sarastro's voice in *The Enchanted Flute*.

The power or intensity of the voice

The grand opera voice such as Roberto Alagna's strikes your eardrum with a power of 120 dB. The standard opera voice has an intensity of 110 dB. The intensity of the comic opera voice is 100 dB. The operetta voice raises 90 dB. The cabaret voice or amateur singer has a intensity of 80 dB. The normal spoken voice raises less than 70 dB. We shall see later that the voice's intensity is also influenced by the acoustics of the hall.

The timbre of the voice

The classification of timbre is highly subjective. One can differentiate timbre on the basis of color, dark, clear, or even white. In terms of volume, timbre can be said to be rich or poor. The mordent of the timbre refers to voices that are silky and fluid versus those that are rough and rasping. Finally, the width of the voice refers to voices that are fragile or consistent, heavy or light.

From Malibran to science

Manuel García, the father of laryngology in 1854

Laryngology, the science of the larynx, was born in 1854, thanks to Manuel García. He was admired for his talent, but also for his fascination for the vocal instrument. This singing teacher is the brother of "la Malibran," an outstanding soprano, and of Pauline Viardot, a lyrical dramatist. When Manuel's father performs in Rossini's *The Barber of Seville* in New York on November 29th of 1825, Manuel García is none other than Figaro. His sister, "la Malibran," in those days known as Maria Félicia, sings Rosina's part. The opera is a big success. On the 23rd of March, 1826, Maria Félicia marries the banker Eugène Malibran and becomes "la Malibran."

La Malibran tolls the knell for the castrato

Born in 1808, Maria Malibran abandons the stage in 1836, at the age of twenty-eight. Manuel Garciá senior, her father, had given her first music and singing lessons. She was said to be able to sing while crying.

In fact, she pushed herself constantly to perfect her vocal organ. In her crusade of the lyrical song, she manages to dominate her vocal technique. She is a mezzo. Her register has an astounding range from G2 to counter E5. She speaks foreign languages fluently thanks to her father, who often traveled with her.

She can sing her repertory in English, French, Italian, or German. In January 1828, at the Paris Opera house, she's acclaimed for her interpretation of a Rossini repertory that she had worked on with her father in New York. Her fans don't comment on her technique, they are subjugated by her performance. In the 1830s, she divides her work between Paris, London, and Brussels. In Naples, she sings for the first time Bellini's *I Capuletti ed i Montecchi*. Then, following in the footsteps of the castrato Farinelli, she performs at la Fenice in Venice on the 2nd of April, 1835, in *The Barber of Seville*. Her performance creates such a sensation that a theatre near the Rialto is named Malibran after her. Other sopranos, such as Giuditta Pasta, the top romantic diva, try to emulate her, but pale in comparison.

In the early autumn of 1836, Malibran goes horseback riding in the countryside. She is a few weeks pregnant. That morning, fate calls. The horse bolts and she falls off. Her foot is caught in the stirrup. She is dragged for several hundred meters. She loses consciousness for a few minutes, then comes to her senses. But the show must go on. She is due to perform in Brussels and in Aix-la-Chapelle in the next few days. Nothing could be more important. She honors these engagements. Back in Manchester in September, she loses consciousness at the end of the concert. She dies on September 23rd at the age of twenty-eight.

A soprano of extraordinary charisma, she had dethroned castrati. Other divas succeeded her, but none could rival her, including Jenny Lind, nicknamed the Swedish nightingale, or Henriette
Sontag. Only Maria Callas, the diva of our times, was able to pick up
the gauntlet. Malibran, adulated by her admirers, leaves a big void
behind her. She was called "La Diva" because she had a divine
voice. Alfred de Musset writes: "She exerts on us from a distance
her charm, her empire, her fascination." Lamartine dedicates the
following quatrain to her:

> Beauty, genius, love was her middle name
> Inscribed in her gaze, in her heart, in her voice,
> Her soul was represented in heaven in triplicate
> Weep, Earth! and you Heavens, welcome her three times.

To strain the voice is to lose it

Pauline Viardot loses her voice

Manuel García's second sister, Pauline Viardot, was at the start of
her career when her sister's came to an end. Henri Malherbe, a
critic of her era, often comes to converse with her to remain close
to Malibran's spirit. Pauline Viardot, a pupil of Liszt, has a pleasant
voice and is a talented pianist. A contralto, her register is also
uncommon: from the low C of the tenor (C2) to F5.

Born on the 18th of July, 1821, Pauline García, later Pauline Viardot, like her sister sings in several languages and travels extensively.
Théophile Gautier, on October 14th, 1839, wrote on her account:
"She is a first class star. She possesses one of the finest instruments
around." A friend of Chopin, she is very fond of him. In 1853, she
performs in Moscow, then in Saint Petersburg. She meets Turgeniev
there and has a romance with him, returning to Paris in 1856.

A terrible fate awaits Pauline Viardot's voice.

- Her voice is going to suffer the whims of the music maes-
  tros. Berlioz leads Beethoven's *Fidelio* and Gluck's *Alceste*.
  However, the vocal register is too high-pitched for Pauline
  Viardot.

- She asks Berlioz to transpose it. He refuses. Although her tessitura is ill-suited to singing in *Alceste*, she decides to do her best, determined to interpret the part.

- She strains her laryngeal instrument. She goes beyond her vocal capacities, exceeds the limits of her laryngeal tolerance, of her suppleness, of her muscles. This takes its toll very quickly. When the curtain falls, the audience acclaims her. No one suspects that anything is wrong. But she knows that something has just gone wrong, her voice hurts. The opera is a success, but it will spell the end for Pauline Viardot. Her voice has just broken. Her singing career is at an end.

Henceforth, her broken voice forces her to retire from the stage. In 1863, she leaves Paris and takes up residence in Baden-Baden. Later, she writes oratorios and musical comedies with her friends Jules Massenet and Gabriel Fauré. She founds a singing school that will make a great contribution to the singing voice. She dies in 1910.

The artist's sincerity is his weak point

Technique should enable singers and other voice professionals to avoid accidents such as Pauline Viardot's. A vocal injury can be irreversible, but prevention is the guarantee of a long career. The artist's capital is his voice. The singer sings with his whole body. He vibrates from the tip of his toes to his hair roots. His larynx, both cord and wind instrument, is only a transformer, converting aerial energy into vibratory energy.

As any athlete, from the start, the artist trains in harmony all the structures that contribute to his vocal performance. But in doing so, more than in anything else he does, the singer, actor, or comedian should never test the limits of his or her voice. The generosity and sincerity of these artists is both their strength and their vulnerability. They want to offer us all their emotion. Yet they must learn to be selfish and keep in reserve 30% of their capacities, otherwise wear and tear, physical and emotional frailty, will inescapably induce a vocal accident.

To sing is to harmonize science and emotion

Singing transforms the body into a musical instrument

Without technique, you can't get a violin to sing. The fingers of the left hand take up their position on the strings. The right hand guides the bow and slides it across the strings to create the vibration that will charm us with its melody. It is under the spell of the artist's affect. The virtuoso can practice fifteen different notes per second, correctly position his index finger to the nearest millimeter, memorize all the body's movements during an apprenticeship that is often long and difficult. Thereafter, he will focus solely on interpretation. The coordination between the right hand and the left hand is orchestrated by his brain. The same circuits are at the singer's disposal for manipulating his internal musical instrument: the vocal tract.

Learning to sing means teaching your body to become a musical instrument that communicates, resonates, controls itself. The harmony of your vocal expression, of the melody, of gestures is but the outcome of the tough school of the singing voice. It calls upon reason and affect. The right brain is emotion. It perceives harmonics, shapes, the environment. The left brain decodes rational information, the solfeggio, enables the memorization of words and of mechanical movements of the larynx. The two are intimately connected. Moreover, the cerebellum is solicited to balance the harmonics.

Training the voice means preserving the voice

The cerebellum plays a primordial role in your sense of balance on Earth. It is dependent on Earth's gravity and enables us to know where up and down are, whether we are leaning to the left or to the right. A few weeks spent in weightlessness traveling in space and your sense of balance changes. The cerebral circuits of an astronaut's cerebellum diminish and regress. As the cerebellum's balance function hasn't been stimulated by Earth's gravity in space, the related cerebral circuits haven't been stimulated. Back on Earth, the astronaut can't walk straight, he staggers about, he has lost his sense of balance. He has to readapt and stimulate his nervous circuits again.

Similarly, if a singer stops practicing his art for a few weeks, he loses some of his technique. Conversely, the more he sings, the more neuronal connections are going to be formed in their thousands, creating complex crossroads that contribute to building and improving his voice. This apprenticeship begins in childhood and continues throughout life. Stimulating our brain on a daily basis keeps the singing process alive, and so much more. But that is another story.

Man, in contrast to artificial intelligence, derives pleasure from his artistic creation. The singer needs the precision of a sculptor to sing in tune, the coordination of an acrobat to adapt his vocal instrument, the balance of a dancer to judge the projection of his voice, and, last but not least, he needs a musical ear to modulate his acoustic emission.

The singer's nodule and poor technique

A poorly adapted technique can lead to nodules on the vocal cords. Some remarkable singing teachers, including Mady Mesplé and Yva Barthelémy whom I have known since 1982, helped me gain a better understanding of the art of singing. The technique of a highly experienced teacher can rebalance the voice of certain sopranos and erase the scar left by nodules brought on by ill-adapted and poorly understood techniques. A well-placed voice is a sign that the singing teacher has adapted himself to his student, not that the student has adapted himself to the teacher.

This precious gift of yours, your voice, must be managed. This cannot be left to the singing teacher or to the voice therapist. Given that your larynx is always there for you, always available, it is up to you to spare it, to avoid soliciting it inadequately, for example, singing *a capella* for friends, in a noisy setting, after a concert or a conference. You must also avoid laughing out loud without restraint, ostentatiously and loudly, as this sometimes traumatizes the vocal cords. But this is not always possible, when a teacher comes home, she should endeavor not to raise her voice with her own children.

The position of the body

The uprightness of our bipedal body has contributed over millions of years to the emission of our voice. Thus, whether you are singing, lecturing, or pleading, you must harmonize your technique, your physical movements, and your mind in order to optimize your vocal impact.

The pupil learns different techniques, but must first assimilate the fact that the voice is a transfer of energy—from air into vibration. Technique and a good memory for music and words are important assets for the apprentice singer and comedian.

Being an artist is not a job, it's a vocation. An artist isn't a "9 to 5" artist. Artists are born artists and remain artists all their lived. For the voice professional, the way forward begins with being attentive to others, being sincere. Talent is the development of a gift peculiar to each person. This hard work, this dedication to always do better, to sometimes suffer, to be often surprised, are indispensable ingredients of the life of a voice professional. The school of lyrical singing, drama, comedy, teaching, law is the school of life. The spontaneous voice, the action-reaction voice can be soft, hard, unequal, or shaky. When you are about to declaim, to teach, to sing, you must be in control of your voice. It becomes the vehicle for the text. It gets rid of parasites that could provoke a badly placed emphasis, an irregular intensity, or a hesitation (unless the latter is intentional). Coaching a pupil to become a voice professional, be it a future teacher, lawyer, or artist, means teaching him to adopt the correct dorsal-lumbar and cervical postures, and the right physical attitude for vocalizing. He must sing in front of the mirror, correct himself, visualize his own musical instrument, of which the main component is his larynx, but also his physical appearance, his stance, and his body language.

A small standing exercise

The clue is simple: it's the position of the feet.

- First example. You're standing with your legs glued together, leaning slightly forward, heels off the ground, as if to better convince the spectator. The chin juts forward; it's hard for you to keep your balance, difficult in these conditions for your declamation to be loud and convincing. The position is unstable. To sing a melody, be it a lyrical or popular melody, you need to be rooted to the ground. The same is true for public speaking.

- Second example. You stand with your legs slightly apart, but with toes raised: the weight of the body is in the heels. This is also destabilizing.

- Third example. The singer is rooted solidly to the ground. "He's comfortable in his jogging shoes." The arches of the feet are solidly grounded. The legs are not glued together. Neither are they aligned. It all looks easy. The declamation is even and powerful. The aria is strong and projects easily to the back of the opera house. All it takes is a well-braced position and a pair of suitably comfortable shoes, and the rest of the body will feel the center of gravity of the voice in the pelvic girdle and project it to wherever it sees fit.

The center of gravity of the voice

This stability is maximal in the ventriloquist. Indeed, on a special scale that enables one to weigh each leg separately, one observes that if the ventriloquist holds his puppet in his right hand, it unbalances the body and the scale registers a few more kilos on the right leg. The practice of this art induces a pathology that the ventriloquist has to rectify regularly. The normal procedure entails a visit to a chiropractor, who rebalances the center of gravity of the voice, which shows that a center of gravity of the voice does exist. This stability can also be sought out in motion. One has to learn how to move on stage. The body's center of gravity is located just below the navel. It is well known in the martial arts.

The pupil's stability, his control of his movements, of his facial muscles, of his eyebrows and eyelids (he must observe himself in the mirror), the mastery of his breathing, the rhythm of his voice, respecting appropriate silences, these are the cornerstones of his apprenticeship.

The wall, the mirror, and the singer

The novice singer often practices at home at his piano. If his piano is up against the wall, he will be disappointed in what he hears, because the resonance of the room isn't the same as at his singing teacher's; indeed, he is practicing his singing close to a wall. It's pointless for him to strain his voice trying to achieve the same retro-control, since the ingredients have changed. He may create vocal cord pathology, such as nodules or soreness, by pushing his voice. A simple suggestion can set this right: all he has to do, though it is easier said than done, is move the piano.

The child's singing voice

Learning from the first intake of air

Artistic expression depends on the education and on the apprenticeship of the singing voice in Man's offspring. The development of a musical ear since infancy shapes the singing voice. The baby develops vocal acuteness for singing by listening to his mother humming on the edge of the bath and by being plunged into a musical world. Mothers are our original singing teachers. Little by little, the infant constructs his mechanical pharyngolaryngeal function; he stimulates the various cerebral areas tied to musical art.

From what age can a child join a choir?

We know that the fundamental frequency of the spoken voice is the baseline of our harmonics, and that this is around 180 Hz in men, 220 Hz in women, and 300 to 450 Hz in children. The soprano's singing voice varies from 260 to 1300 Hz, the tenor's is between 120 and 520 Hz, that of a bass is between 65 and 325 Hz. A child sings practically always in the vocal register of his head voice. He is physiologically incapable of emitting the lower pitches of the register in a chest voice, which is one octave below the head voice. Thus, women and children have basically the same register. Puberty is vocal revolution time.

The novice choir singer needs to undergo an apprenticeship. He needs some basic knowledge of solfeggio, which means he must be more or less able to read. He can join a choir from the age of seven. Some stand out within a few months and are oriented toward a career as a soloist. When a child first discovers his singing voice, it is surprising to hear him say: "Is that me making all that noise?" The soloist in a choir is an individual in the service of the group. He is a full member of the group. He resonates with the group. He gives the *A* note. His vocal orchestra backs him up. A soloist is chosen on the basis of his voice, but more so on the basis of his personality, a strong personality, often keen to imitate the singing teacher because he identifies himself with him.

The very young soprano discovers his vocal register. Toward the age of eight or nine, he discovers his full child's voice, his timbre. He shows a new side to his personality, a mixture of self-confidence and sensitivity. In my opinion, this sensitivity remains one of the key aspects of the child's singing voice. Affect is an indispensable ingredient in the soloist's career.

The tessitura of the child's voice

A child can be a soprano or an alto. The child alto is one octave higher than a tenor's voice, though with less harmonics. It is closer to the woman's singing voice, which is one octave higher than men's. Thus, the child alto and the adult tenor can sing in the same register one octave apart. This lends a special beauty to certain requiems that harmonize children's choirs with adult voices, sopranos and altos with tenors and countertenors. The charm of a musical palette that mixes high and low pitches seduces us and gives us some insight into the power and beauty of castrati voices, whose range covered the child's soprano register and the adult's tenor and bass registers.

Francis Bardot, children's choir leader at the Opéra de Paris until 1999, gave concerts with his choir throughout the world; he informed me that children (predominantly boys) in his choir, but also in other choirs, be they French or Anglo-Saxon, Italian, or German, change tessitura after puberty.

We came to an extraordinary conclusion:

The child sopranos become bass singers, not tenors, and the child altos become tenors, not bass singers. Thanks to this choir leader, I was able to do some fascinating research. I followed these children over a period of twenty years, I saw their voices evolve from childhood to adulthood, from the age of seven to around twenty-five or thirty. At puberty, these young adolescent singers change register and are confronted with the metamorphosis of a breaking voice. True, as always when dealing with humans, the above observation is a guideline rather than a rule, it isn't a certainty. But in over 95% of cases, we observed this evolution among the boys as they became adult.

Enrico Caruso was an alto singer in church choirs during his childhood before becoming one of the greatest tenors of the early 20th century. Chaliapine was a soprano before puberty. His voice became one of the most beautiful deep voices on record. Some say he was a bass, others consider him a baritone, but his register was amazing.

Why doesn't the child soprano become a tenor?

This brings us to ask ourselves: why does a child soprano not become a tenor? Why does the alto not become a bass or a deep bass? Frequently, the child soprano is relatively tall and slim. His fine vocal cords produce high-pitched harmonics in his resonance chamber. This contrasts with the alto child, who tends to be stronger and rounder. His vocal cords are also thicker. This gives him a deeper timbre. When his voice breaks, the tall slim boy becomes even slimmer and taller. His pharyngolaryngeal resonator becomes correspondingly more spacious. He is now endowed, as we have seen, with the larynx of a bass singer. Whereas the larynx of the alto child still reflects the roundness of his physique, one might say, thus normally he preserves his powerful larynx, with shorter vocal cords than the bass singer, and more to the point, a more concise resonance chamber that is shorter and stronger. He gravitates naturally to a tenor's voice.

You'll notice that we've said little about young girls. Indeed, things are much simpler in their case. When their voice breaks, the singing voice remains in the same register.

Until puberty, children use the same singing techniques, whether boys or girls. They almost always use the head voice.

The mature larynx places the voice correctly

The vocal technique of the opera singer demands a body that is almost fully developed, mature and structured, and an attitude of mind that is serious, determined, and thorough. This is why it's advisable for youngsters to embark on advanced studies from the age of eighteen in the case of boys and seventeen in the case of girls. Many voice professionals, such as comedians or actors, have a register that spans about two octaves. With practice, the singer and, indeed, the schoolteacher who teaches singing, rapidly develop a register that covers three octaves.

In women, the vocal cords are about 18 mm long, with a diameter of 4 mm; in men, they are 20 to 23-mm long and 5-mm wide. Regarding the female tessitura, although some predisposing factors do exist, the tessitura is difficult to predict on the basis of anatomic criteria. I've seen coloratura sopranos become superb lyrical sopranos after ten years of career. On the other hand, I have rarely seen altos turn into sopranos. The coloratura soprano often has smaller vocal cords than an alto, and her larynx is on the whole also more compact.

In men, it is easier to get a fair idea of tessitura by observing the larynx. We've demonstrated this. However, there would be absolutely no point in trying to be an "anatomical fortune-teller." The singer's anatomy gives some pointers, but can never be a firm predictor of his tessitura. In the end, vocal technique and experience will count for more than the muscle structures we may observe.

Singing techniques: an "à la carte" menu

Vocalizing and breathing techniques, or how to control one's singing in five exercises

Vocal techniques are based, among other things, on a vocal onset or attack, in which the stroke of the glottis is perfectly controlled in relation to the desired volume. The ability to deliver an *i* or an *a* with an even volume and on the same frequency for 15 seconds is evidence of the degree of control that is a prerequisite for vocal emission. Having thus sustained the vowel, free of parasites and in the timbre that was intended, the singer then repeats the exercise in *vibrato forte*, and again in *pianissimo*. This is done for *a, e, i, o, ou*, first taking each note singly, then practicing the whole scale.

To vocalise

Manuel García's remarkable description of the vocalization exercise for singers, written nearly a century and a half ago, has been used by numerous singing teachers. The five main exercises are summarized here:

- The first type is the sustained or *portato* vocalise: like the bow that glides smoothly across the violin string, the exhaled air slides over the vibrating vocal cords smoothly and continuously, without a break.

- The second type is the *legato* vocalise, in which the singer passes seamlessly from one note to another without any interruption, as if our vocal instrument were a slide-trombone producing a smooth flow of tonalities. This exercise demonstrates the agility of the larynx, and especially the singer's respiratory control. It is advisable to begin the exercise properly hydrated, as it makes important demands on the lubrication of the vocal cords and their elasticity.

- The third type is the marked or individualized vocalise: each note is distinct, emphasized, without being detached from the others. The airflow is intensified, which intensifies the sound, then it is diminished. Here the abdominal muscles play a key role. The control exerted during the exhalation phase that accompanies certain martial arts movements, or the breathing exercises in *tai-chi*, are of precious help in understanding the essence of this vocal and respiratory exercise.

- The fourth type is the chopped or *staccato* vocalise: the notes are produced using a hard glottal attack to separate them from each other. This technique enables the singer to deliver a series of brief, isolated, and repeated sounds. The exercise also tests the singer's mastery over volume and projection as well as speed of delivery. This is done in quadruple time: the note rises from *pianissimo* to *forte*, then it returns to *pianissimo*, then it's emitted solely in *pianissimo* before rising again to *forte*. These exercises are done on a single note then on the whole scale.

- The fifth exercise is the sustained *vibrato*. The technique consists in sustaining a *vibrato* for ten seconds in medium and in *piano* on every note of the scale. This exercise develops proper control of the support provided by the abdominal muscles.

From medieval song to rock and roll

The passagio: head voice and chest voice

The distinction between the head voice and the chest voice has been made for centuries. In 1602, there were three types of song: church chanting, chamber music songs, and theatrical airs. At this time, Giulio Caccini makes the point that "one should be careful not to disperse the meaning of this word." The importance of the passagio was recognized in 1562 by Giovanni Camillo Maffei, a singing teacher in Naples. He set the ground rules at that time: complete aperture of the mouth, low position of the larynx, control over the breathing, the diaphragm, and the abdominal belt. The same technique is still used today. But the maestros who best exploited the *passagio* are the castrati, whose physiological conformation allowed their voice to range over at least three octaves.

The distinction between chest voice and head voice was well known even before the beginnings of opera. It was toward the end of the 16th century and early in the 17th century that the voice of a soloist accompanied by a choir first made its appearance in opera. The melody was still important, but understanding the text became crucial. The soloist became the star, overshadowing Madrigal polyphony, in which several voices perform together. In those days—and according to some, this still applies today—improvisation often enabled each singer to contribute a personal touch to the performance. Each singer took the liberty of adding his own ornaments thanks to his mastery of vocal technique.

Ornaments are a suite of notes that are added to the main melody without altering the main melodic line. Usually, the singer practices these ornaments in *legato*, passing seamlessly from deep notes to high notes and from high notes to deep notes. A trill is the rapid alternation of two adjacent musical tones.

The male chest voice

The chest voice is richly hued. Its register covers around three octaves, starting from the deep *ut* or *C* of the cello. Singers specify that they have the impression of vibrating all over, but more so in their thorax and resonators. This chest voice can range from C1 in the lowest bass to E3 in the high notes. It is a technique that requires excellent respiratory control. The outward air stream is powerful. The voice muscles, be it the neck muscles or the laryngeal muscles, are contracted. The abdominal belt is tonic. This mechanical approach ensures that the register comes from the chest, but limits the singer, who can't go higher than E3. To reach the higher pitches, he has to pass to the head voice.

The male head voice

The head voice gives him a register of F2 to G3. In counter alto, the voice can range as high as C5. Chest voice, head voice: between the two some have created a transition space for a mixed register. More natural, softer, the mixed voice is never pushed and never strains. It ranges between C2 and C4.

The female chest voice

In women, although this is rarer, the chest voice that is used for normal conversation can be used in song to go down to D2 and up to F3. It is used for 2 to 3 notes normally. Women don't need to develop a head voice, they have it naturally. This probably explains why sometimes hearing some well-known singer speak can be a disappointment, as some singers have an unpleasant chest voice despite having a superb voice when they sing.

The mixed voice

On the whole, variety singers have a middle register or mixed voice. It is a slightly veiled, somewhat sensual voice; the singer isn't looking for perfection in the high pitches. This mixed voice is nothing new, the troubadours also sang this way. Already at the beginning of the 17th century, Adriano Banchiari proffers the advice to sing with moderation, even in the high notes, to ensure the perfect intelligibility of the words. In effect, he was advocating the mixed voice.

Vibrato yes, *tremolo*, absolutely not

The vibrato

But what is a *vibrato*? Used by the lyrical singer or the variety singer, the *vibrato* lends rhythm to the voice, which seems to pulsate 5 to 7 times per second. This contrasts with the wobbly voice, or *tremolo*, which pulsates around 3 to 5 times per second in both the spoken voice and the singing voice. Sometimes the elderly speak with a *tremolo*. The *tremolo* should never be used in singing, it is a sign of poor technique and lack of experience, whereas the *vibrato* is a vibratory amplifier. The *vibrato* enables the singer to increase not just the clarity and carrying power of the melody, but also its emotion. It adds to the richness of the harmonics. It also allows frequencies to be amplified, but by no more than a semitone. Indeed, our ears can only detect the *vibrato* amplitude if its amplitude exceeds a quarter tone. But if the amplitude exceeds three quarters of a tone, the voice trembles.

In the same way as the violinist's finger pinches the violin string and gives it a periodic movement that is also 5 to 7 times per second while the bow glides on one of the violin's four strings, the vocal *vibrato* is under the direct command of our brain. It sets up a wave of vibrations 7 times per second in perfect harmony, coordinating not only the exhalation of the vocal instrument, like the bow, but also the periodic movement of the pharyngolaryngeal apparatus. The *vibrato* accentuates the strength of the harmonics created in the larynx. It considerably augments vocal intensity. It enables the singer to be heard from the back of the concert hall. It is clearly perceived by the ear as a succession of regular waves that accompany the melody.

Observing the vocal cathedral

If you observe the larynx during the *vibrato* and look at the voice with the help of the videostroboscope and its 2,000 images per second, the sight of the vocal cathedral is breathtaking. At first, while the voice is flat, the emission of an A3 causes the vocal cords to vibrate at 440 vibrations per second. The *vibrato* then gets underway. Its perfectly controlled, regular rhythm vibrates 7 times per second throughout the entire vocal edifice with the vocal cords in its heart, and this enables the very same frequency that is produced by the vocal cords to be a semitone below or a semitone above the 440 Hz, every seventh of a second.

Singing and clear diction: not always easy

The intelligibility of the voice

Aside from register, acoustic intensity is another key aspect of the singing voice. The voice carries *a capella* and must carry across the orchestra pit. The carrying power of the voice depends of course on the singer's technique, on his resonators, on his harmonics and formants, but equally on his build. His vocal power must in no way compromise the intelligibility of the melody's verbal content. The vowel remains the kingpin of the singing voice. It is what makes the popularity of Italian opera. The singer's diction, elocution, and rhythm not only help spectators to hear what is sung, they also help them to hear what the music has to say. This whole—carrying power, harmonics, vocal warmth—creates the timbre characteristic of each singer and gives the singing voice its beauty and dream quality.

As an aside here: it is much more difficult for singers to be easily understood in the high register than in the medium or low register. This is why nasal phonemes are rarely used in the higher register, and the bel canto is practically the only exception to this rule. The artist must have excellent diction and articulate precisely if he is to be understood. This may seem evident to theater actors and lyrical singers, but sadly it appears to be a lot less evident to a number of variety singers, who, quite frankly, should take elocution lessons before pretending to be voice professionals. Their artistic sincerity isn't in question.

Sound engineers: not always present

For the past fifty years, progress in acoustic techniques has never ceased. Sound engineers achieve miracles. Thanks to them and to their instruments, artists' voices are set off with all the qualities and defects that make their charm. The microphone enables us to hear a voice 100 meters away.

No need to have a chest like Caruso or Maria Callas, who sang *a capella*. Yet if a star can be created in a few months, these interpreters of the vocal arts will often take singing lessons to consolidate their career. Not many young singers have the right technical baggage. They throw themselves into the adventure of our modern musical comedies without any concern for the discipline that the singing voice requires. Even if singing comes naturally when celebrating with friends, if you make it your career, you have to learn your trade properly.

The gift is turned into an art

Singing professionally undeniably requires a predisposition. It also requires regular work and a healthy way of life. The gift is turned into an art. The voice of the variety singer or lyrical singer depends on its height, timbre, intensity, from the pianissimo to the fortissimo. It must respect the music, its tempo, its rhythm. It must bear the singer's stamp in its harmonics, execution, and clarity of delivery. The vowels transport the melody, the consonants give it rhythm, the silences shape its landscape.

The learning curve: from school to Broadway

The rules must be learned

The lyrical singer isn't going to risk interpreting an aria or a solo part from *La Traviata*, *Carmen*, or *The Enchanted Flute* without a long and arduous apprenticeship. Lyrical artists and musicians who perform on the stage of an opera house bring to account several years of apprenticeship in prestigious music schools. Many have the calling, few make the grade. The novice singer, about to embark on years of study and the solitary apprenticeship of singing, must be persevering.

At every concert, the opera singer or the singer of musical comedies does a marathon performance on stage, sweating under his stage costume. He is surrounded by other artists whom he interacts with. Actor and musical tragedian, he acts not just with his voice, but with his whole being. But in contrast to singers in musical comedies on Broadway, in London or in Paris, who perform six days out of seven, to preserve their voice lyrical artists only sing three times a week.

To preserve the musical voice instrument

For over four centuries, lyrical singers have imposed the rules of their apprenticeship and vocal rhythm. It would be wise to apply the same rules to the artists who perform in today's musical comedies, at the very least, rigorous knowledge of vocal technique to avoid voice strain and the appearance of cordal nodules, and the observance of vocal rest at least twice a week. If you consider that these musical comedies are on normally for six months, often putting on two performances a day, you have some idea of the achievement of these modern day lyrical artists.

More often than not, variety singers or comedy singers sing with a microphone, but occasionally they might perform at a concert *a capella*, and demonstrate a remarkable display of technique. In France or in North America, we are lucky to have many professional singers with a perfect mastery of singing technique.

Some novice singers in quest of early glory are willing to take short cuts, a dangerous practice. Good technique is a must. It's unthinkable for a professional singer to have poor technique, or no technique! It can be learned after the first "hit" if it hasn't been learned before. It's the guarantee of a long career, rather than a few months of glory, as is too often the case today, sadly.

Singers have become a marketing product. This is not art, but it is a choice! The arena is the television set, the gladiators are the singers, the spectators are the jury members who give the final sentence. The execution is cruel. The winner becomes a legend. I am impressed with these gladiators of modern times!

The singing voice on stage

Singing lessons throughout one's career

During the making of my first movie, *The Vocal Print*, in 1985, a basso profundo from the Paris Opera House, Mario, explained to me:

> "When you're starting out your career, singing is easy, natural, but its mechanics are unfamiliar. The singer doesn't see his vocal instrument. His voice is there with him, near him, inside him. He can't touch it. It carries the melody, the lyrics, it carries emotion of course, but so much technique, so many hours, so much hard work are required to master it, and especially, to preserve it!"

What more could I add?

The singer of texts, the lyrical poet, forms yet another category. Often on his own on stage, guitar in hand, the melody is a prop for his poetry. It amplifies it.

All singers should continue singing lessons throughout their career to avoid getting into bad habits. Who knows why, these are the ones that stick! When tired, the singer compensates by slouching—back bent forward, head low, breathing shallow. The tendency then is to push on the larynx, which amounts to correcting a fault with another fault. I often recommend a series of four to six voice therapy lessons per year to get back to the basics of the physical and postural dynamics of the spoken voice or the singing voice.

The singer belongs to his public

The pop singer performs on stage with an orchestra in a loud acoustic environment. The sound engineer mixes the instruments and the singer's voice and creates harmony on stage for the music. A variety concert is the equivalent of a 110 meter horse race with fences. The singer "jumps" from one song to the next. On stage, the singer sweats, dehydrates, and gives himself to his public. It is a vocal effort, a muscular effort, but also an incredible mental performance. The symbiosis between singer and public is impressive. He is challenged to transcend himself. It's a challenge he must face night after night. His career imposes a healthy way of life.

The denominator that all these singers have in common is this harmony between them and their public, this transcendence of the individual who becomes the emotion of the group. Height and intensity are parameters of the song the singer can repeat, timbre is not. The first two are Cartesian, the third is an artistic parameter.

To sing is to adorn words with music and silences. Respect of silences in order to involve the public, to be compelling, to make the audience hang on every word, is an essential ingredient for voice professionals.

The same words and melody recreate a new "singing art"

The singer speaks two languages: music and lyrics. The note is a letter, the syllable a beat, the sentence a melody. He's capable of seven to twelve tonalities per second. In effect, he builds a project in his mind that has a given rhythm. Memorizing the muscular coordination delivers the vocalization, but if that were all there was to it, he would just be parroting.

A master painting is unique. It is an artistic creation. Take the same painting, reproduce it thousands of times, and all you have is printed paper, industrial decoration. In the same way, a bad singer is an industrial decorator of songs. The singer who is a real artist is an interpreter; he transforms every song into an intangible masterpiece of human vibration that brings pleasure. Like any painting by Salvador Dali, Rembrandt, or Fragonard, the singer's voice is unique, but the similarity ends here, because his voice disappears in space and time.

The musical environment

In our quest for the sublime in song, in our passion for voices that seduce us, we must not forget the conditions that these lyrical singers must satisfy. First, there's the larynx. Then there's their interpretation, which the public is sole judge of. The interpretation is influenced by the singer's surroundings, which change all the time.

A singer needs a public: the public is in a hall; this hall has specific acoustic characteristics. The following figures give some idea of the constraints that artists perform under. The carrying power of the voice is influenced by the size of the room or hall. Without a microphone, in an opera house of 30,000 m², a volume of 120 dB is the equivalent of the noise of a plane taking off 25 meters away from you. In a standard opera house of 16,000 m², 120 dB is the equivalent of a plane taking off 4 to 5 m away. In comic opera, 110 dB is the equivalent of a distance of 2 meters. In a small show room, 80 dB are sufficient for the singer to be heard. You'll recall that ordinary conversation raises 60 dB and the ticking of a mechanical watch 30 dB. These figures give us a better idea of the power generated by these opera singers performing without microphone and how important it is for them to adapt their voice to the hall.

To interpret is to forget about technique: emotion has no scale, only hues

Memorizing the movements of the "singing mechanic"

In singing, technique and apprenticeship are the fundamentals of any singer's career. We know that the voice is characterized by its pitch, intensity, and timbre. We know that the audiophonatory loop allows retro-control of the voice. We also know that the basics of singing technique associate respiratory control with control of subglottic pressure and proper alignment to allow the outward airflow to reach the vocal cords and the pharynx. The trachea, the larynx, the pharynx must be in a trajectory which to be efficient should have maximal verticality. Finally, the singer's diction, the way he places his tongue and lips, determine the final conformation of the sung phonemes. Each vocal register requires a different technique, be it the chest voice, the head voice, or the falsetto voice. The singer has to take into account his natural register. He can't change everything.

Artists, be they adults or children, learn the mechanics of singing. For example, it is known that, in order to memorize the movement of a backhand or a forehand in tennis, the movement has to be practiced at least eight times. Moreover, the brain takes about 4 seconds to integrate this information in its memory bank. By analogy, teaching a student a vocal technique requires him to memorize the muscle movements enabling him to produce precisely the intended tonality, with the desired volume, the desired hues, and the required intense vibrations in the proper parts of his body. This proprioceptor memory filed in the left brain is brought alive during the artist's performance by the emotional world of the right brain and the limbic brain.

The artistic approach

The clinical, physical, and medical approach can never supersede the artistic approach. The gap is filled by the singing teacher and the drama teacher, who insist not only on voice projection into the face mask, not only on the artist's posture and elocution, but also on the artist's interpretive skills.

Cyprien Katsaris plays a Chopin waltz. This outstanding pianist imposes his imprint and makes us share his emotion. He makes us forget about technique or the piano, he transcends us. Each interpreter leaves his personal mark. The body of the artist, assisted by muscle tension and the jointed agility of his fingers, strokes the keyboard or pounds it. Hands, elbows, arms, shoulders, and chest all play the piano. This way of playing is overseen by a conductor, in this case the auditory perception of the pianist. It takes into account not only what the pianist feels, what he hears on stage, but also what the public hears. His public is his emotional amplifier. It boosts his performance, enabling instantaneously a richer interpretation of the music. "I play a lot better, I make the piano sing far more effectively; I share my emotions through my mechanical interaction and derive extreme satisfaction from this, both physically and emotionally: it's like an auditory orgasm." Thus did Cyprien Katsaris explain to me the artist's symbiosis with his instrument and with the music he interprets.

Emotion has no scale, only emotional hues: sorrow, melancholy, anger, laughter, joy, enthusiasm, serenity, ecstasy. The same goes for the singer or actor. His musical instrument is inside him. The way he strokes his acoustic jewel depends on his frame of mind. It is true that life's circumstances can perturb his interpretation. If there is harmony between his life and his feelings of sadness or joy, the work he interprets becomes a unique artistic work and not just a technical feat that makes us say "What great technique!" which is a far cry from "What a stunning interpretation!" In the first case, we admire the trapeze artist, in the second, we share his emotion.

A regular "hitch" on the same note: technique isn't always to blame

A mechanical problem

Janette, a Belgian singer in her forties, has had trouble sustaining a particular note in the medium register for nearly a year. It is always the same note. Her singing teacher thinks the problem has to do with her passagio, often a culprit. But although Janette applies herself assiduously, the break in her voice persists. She becomes obsessed with the faulty note. She decides to consult me because of it. Otherwise her singing voice is satisfactory.

Using my videostroboscope, I am able to view her vocal cords vibrating in the medium register. The guilty party is soon discovered. The vibration is blocked by a microcyst on the right vocal cord. It gives the impression of a surfboard on a breaker, interrupting the fluidity of the vibration. This causes the voice to break and disrupts the smooth transition from low pitches to high pitches. As the problem is causing her psychological stress in her singing and she's already had a year of voice therapy, we decide to operate. Laser microsurgery enables her voice to recover. Here, technique wasn't at fault. Only the cyst, the size of half a grain of rice, was to blame.

Faking the passagio*: it's possible*

But habitually, vocal technique is to blame. Then the break takes the singer by surprise. It does not happen consistently, but it happens in the *passagio*. The voice isn't correctly placed. One comes across it in certain tenors whose chest voice is above E, but also Also in certain sopranos in the head voice, an octave above the tenor's voice. In this case, the sustained vocalise is being neglected. To avoid this type of problem, singers must keep the pharynx and larynx contracted, at the same time controlling the smoothness of the exhalation. Professionals are well aware of this. Some have confided to me that, if necessary, they manage to fake this by staying with the note on a sustained vowel, instead of pronouncing the end of the word. Indeed, if they were to finish the word, they would have to articulate a consonant, and that would destabilize the vibration of the vocal cords. The vowel, support of the singing voice, is able to create the impression of an even timbre, of continuous sound from one tonality to another.

Singers, yes, but not always by chance

The greatest singers of our era, Maria Callas or Luciano Pavarotti, Mario Del Monaco, or Renée Fleming, Jessy Norman, or Céline Dion, have something in common: their childhood was steeped in music. In the 1980s, Jerome Hines' remarkable research among one hundred lyrical singers established that more than 90% had been steeped in the world of music from the age of three.

Knowing how to rest before a performance

Placido Domingo, born in Spain, begins his career as an opera singer in Mexico in 1959. His parents manage a theater. Music is his first language. He considers Caruso his spiritual master. So much so that he knows the first recordings of this tenor by heart and builds his technique by listening to Caruso's vocal register. As any great artist, the night before a concert he speaks very little and grants few interviews. He takes care to have a good night's sleep. On the day of the concert, he has a light lunch. He often takes a siesta and then goes to the concert hall. He warms up his voice for half an hour before going on stage. These rules that safeguard the health of the voice are observed by practically all voice professionals.

Limit your singing to 70% of your capacities

Roberto Alagna, a remarkable tenor who received the Pavarotti prize in Philadelphia, was brought up with popular music from his early childhood. His father and uncle, both of Italian origin, were also singers. The vocal qualities of his father, who is a tenor, intimidate him. He only begins to sing around the age of fifteen. Not lyrical songs, but modern "pop" songs of his generation. He lives his passion to the hilt daily. He regularly sings in cabarets, and indeed continues to do so until the age of twenty-four. One night, someone is impressed with his voice. He is told that he has the voice of a tenor. He has just made the grade! His voice, therefore, has a place in the lyrical landscape. He reaches a decision: he wants to become an opera singer. His international career is about to begin. Levon Sayan, his coach, sees to the programming of his concerts to spare his laryngeal instrument. Indeed, it is important to fix limits for oneself in this artistic profession in which emotion has no brakes. The tenor's voice is superb, his vocal cords reveal an impressive laryngeal instrument. But he never oversteps the musical boundaries he has set himself.

After attending a performance of Puccini's *La Bohème*, in which two perfect voices harmonize together—that of Roberto Alagna in the role of Rodolpho and Angela Gheorghiu (his wife) in the role of Mimi—I noticed that neither the tenor nor the soprano seemed tired after their performance.

The interpretation of Rodolpho revealed a sunny, natural voice with a clear timbre. Mimi's charm and sensuality lent a touch of magic to the opera. The conductor pointed and manipulated his stick to better show off these exceptional singers to their best advantage. It was they who imposed the rhythm, not the score. This tenor explained to me that he uses only 70% of his capacities when singing, "that way, if I'm stressed or bothered, if I have a little acid reflux, I have a security margin that allows me to still deliver a good performance, despite my stage fright. My nerves penalize me, but only a few seconds, then they galvanize me. I'm very careful about what I eat before a performance."

The professionalism of these two singers is ensured by their remarkable vocal technique, which they train daily to be able to forget about it while they perform. The timbre and interpretation of this tenor have enhanced the popularity of opera. His lifestyle, the professionalism of his concerts, and his calendar of engagements demonstrate the rigor that is required in his line of work. On stage, he transports one into the world of bel canto.

Preserving one's voice at any age

Charles Aznavour preserved his voice intact after his duos with Pierre Roche in 1942 and later with Edith Piaf. His laryngeal instrument did not alter over the years. This athlete of the singing voice kept the same timbre and warmth in his voice. Performing for an hour and a half was no problem for him. This gifted artist could only have become a singer, given the emotional environment of his childhood: a baritone father, a comedian mother. The musical world that bathed his ears led him quite naturally to perform on stage at the age of nine. He is a wonderful example of the fact that a well-trained voice can survive a career of more than fifty years practically unchanged. This agility has to be backed up by a good memory and cerebral dexterity, both indispensable to the artist's long-term survival. An aging voice was something he never knew. The artistic rigor, professionalism, and concern for his health with which he guided his career were astonishing. He knew how to spare his resources by organizing quiet moments in which he could rest his voice and recover his strength. But don't imagine that he did nothing then: between each series of concerts, the artist was perpetually creative.

Head voice and chest voice: a long learning process

Luciano Pavarotti's story, as described by Jerome Hines, tells us the mystery of this voice. L. Pavarotti, a superb tenor born in Italy, in Modena, is steeped in music from a tender age. At the age of eight, he joins a church choir. He begins to sing with the Metropolitan Opera of New York in 1968, in the role of Rodolpho in *La Bohème*.

When he lives in New York, south of Central Park, and sets off for the concert hall, he covers himself up like a mummy if it is cold. Covering not only your neck but also your torso and head is one of the best protections against laryngitis. For he can't bear to cancel a performance: he considers this as a defeat. At nineteen, he begins his professional studies as an opera singer, in Modena, Italy. Arrigo Pola, a tenor of that era, helps him to get started and teaches him the basics of lyrical opera for nearly two and a half years.

His teacher's approach is unusual.

- The first six months are consecrated to vocalises and cor-rect posture. He works on the position of the tongue, which is low in the chest voice and like a dome in the head voice, while the membrane between the larynx and the cricoid is contracted. The transition from chest voice to head voice is difficult. The consecrated term for this is *passagio*. He works on that and nothing else. Thus, he wants his student Luciano to understand how he should open his mouth, how he should place his jaw, how his face and larynx should feel, as well as the rest of his body, and finally, how he should memorize every vowel in relation to every note and to a given degree of loudness. These vocalises allow him to assimilate one of the biggest hurdles a singer faces: the *passagio*.

- The next two years are devoted to learning the classical bases and to improving his understanding of the first six months. Indeed, understanding is not sufficient, he must now assimilate the *passagio*. Luciano Pavarotti recognizes that it took him nearly six years to master it. During the initial six months, his efforts discourage him. His voice doesn't carry the way he intends. Sometimes, his face becomes congested with effort, he practically passes out from lack of air. No matter how hard he tries, what comes out is not to his liking.

- The difficulty lies in allowing the airflow through quite naturally, like water flowing in a riverbed. After several months, he understands and is able to feel that mastering the technique requires not only positioning the tongue correctly, but also the following paradox: the thoracic, laryngeal, and pharyngeal muscles must be relaxed, as when one yawns, and the muscles are contracted only during the *passagio*, to support the transition from the chest voice to the head voice. How is this done? It requires perfect control of one's body: the larynx moves up higher in the throat, contracts just enough to allow powerful notes in the higher register, but not so much that the larynx feels tight. At the beginning, certain notes are chopped. Regular practice, perseverance in improving technique without ever injuring the larynx, and experience allow him to finally master the natural (the word is well-chosen) *passagio*.

Luciano Pavarotti, the tenor, becomes a singing teacher. He too gives technical lessons, and it is now his turn to demonstrate to his students this practice at which he's now a past master. His mastery over it enables him to describe it perfectly. He makes the point that during the *passagio*, he leaves less space for the ascending airflow in his vocal tract. But as soon as this tricky moment is over, he re-establishes the normal amount of space in his resonators and larynx. This pseudo-compression, "*passagio* with tightening," as the artist specifies, is specific to him. Nevertheless, other tenors also use this technique, in combination with projecting the voice into the face mask, a technique commonly used by lyrical artists. Notably by Roberto Alagna, who specifies the importance of acquiring solid basics before launching into difficult operas such as *La Bohème* or *Tosca*. The tenor braces himself, using the abdominal muscles during the whole sung phrase as it transits from the chest voice to the head voice. It is the center of gravity of his voice, just below or level with the navel. This abdominal muscular belt, this center of vocal energy, is essential to a singer's balance, to the stability and correctness of his voice, to the vocal expression of the comedian.

This center of gravity of the voice is itself a guarantee against vocal strain and facilitates the artist's control over his vocal power, frequency, and timbre.

The artist and his ritual

Pavarotti has his technical ritual: doing scales, controlling his abdominal breathing, ensuring he can anchor himself to the ground to bring his vocal power up from the ground. If he has to perform, he makes sure he gets a good night's sleep the day before, he rests his voice, speaking little, using it sparingly for over thirty-six hours. He gets up around lunch time to be in the best possible shape for the concert that night. As soon as he gets up, he vocalizes for three to four minutes, takes a light breakfast, then vocalizes for a couple of hours. After that, he remains mute, doesn't sing. When he arrives at the concert hall half an hour before the concert, he again solicits his laryngeal instrument, but for no more than five minutes, practicing scales with his mouth closed, then with his mouth open. He ends this warm-up singing with a full voice for two to three minutes.

Every artist may have personal habits just before a concert, but a vocal warm-up followed by a few minutes of concentration and isolation just before meeting the audience are essential for any artist. For the emotional load that these thousands of spectators direct at the artist as soon as he comes on stage demands an unusual degree of self-control.

The singer's device

Singing in tune

Singing in tune is important for the melody, but respect for rhythm and silences is also important. Memory plays a crucial role. It will appeal to the cerebral projections of audition, language, music, and also affect.

The singer's memory can fail him. This is where experience is critical. He will automatically substitute one word for another, because the memory lapse will affect a word, never the music. Once we've memorized what we have to reproduce singing, once we've internalized this luminous energy, we become its transmitter. This alchemy brings into play mechanical, cerebral, and emotional systems. During a vocal emission, if you sing frequently and you're not a real professional, you improvise a few notes here, a few notes there. You touch up the paintwork of the music you've just seen and heard. You dress it up your way. You give it the flavor of your own imagination. The feedback of your voice enables you to know deep down whether you are right on, in the true sense of the word, in relation to height and rhythm, but also interpretation. However, the other one, the one listening to you, informs you that you are not in tune. This means that your feedback isn't working properly. It isn't well adjusted. If you block one ear while you sing, you can often correct your voice and fine-tune it. Also, it is easier to sing in tune in a tessitura that suits your natural register.

The singing instrument

The vocal emission, we have seen, flows through the cathedral of our instrument. The flow of air skirts the different asperities it encounters along the way: a stalagmite such as the epiglottis, a stalactite such as the uvula. Aerodynamic turbulence is inevitable. In this edifice, the unfurling sound meets the tongue, a prime factor in word formation. Intensity depends on amplitude and, therefore, on the vibration of the cordal mucous membranes during the exhalation. The singer can bring its volume up to 80 dB. Its height, which depends on the length of the vocal cord, can go up to A3 without problem.

The singer has one major obligation: he must control his exhalation. No parasitic muscular contraction must interfere with this respiratory phase. Throwing your chest out abnormally is not a good technique. It raises the clavicles, and hence the shoulders; it unbalances the muscles that insert onto the clavicles. These muscles are important for placing the voice at the right height. This speaks much about the importance of abdominal breathing, or more precisely, thoracoabdominal breathing. To support the loud emission of a fairly long phoneme, the breathing must be abdominopelvic. To produce variable intensities and fast changes of tone, such as *staccatos* with *pianissimo* and *fortissimo*, the role of the intercostal, abdominal and subnavel muscles is essential. The verticality of the spine lends excellent stability to the voice.

The good teacher isn't always the obvious one

Finding the right teacher

The singing teacher ensures that the pupil learns techniques that are suitable for him. Certainly, you need to find the right teacher, someone who doesn't tire you and that you appreciate, because changing singing teacher every year is only going to set your apprenticeship back.

To give you a similar example, if you play tennis and learn the backhand, some coaches will tell you to hold the racket with one hand, while others tell you to hold it with two hands. Who is right? Whom should you heed? Every coach will cite a tennis champion who uses his technique, but these coaches all forget that each person is unique and that the technique must be adapted to the player's body, and not vice versa.

Changing teachers mixes techniques, perturbs your individual sense of singing. The student loses self-confidence. "I'm no good." Not at all! Choosing the right singing teacher is a question of seeing whether there is harmony between teacher and pupil, whether there is an emotional bond, so vital in this tough school of the arts. The first teacher may not be the right one for you, never mind, persevere until you find the one who can best bring out the artist in you.

The good singer is not always a good teacher

The fact that you are a fine singer doesn't mean you can be a fine singing teacher. Often the maestros, the very best, have tried to impose their way of doing things, and that's not right. Each singer has his own personality, his own alchemy between his vocal tool and the art of singing. After thirty to forty-five minutes of a singing lesson, the student should feel good. He should never, but absolutely never, finish the lesson feeling tired, hoarse, or frustrated. He should be enthusiastic. His voice should be clear. "What a pity it's already over!": that is what the pupil should say at the end of the lesson. A dose of admiration associating technique and emotion is essential to ensure the pupil wishes to attain the standard the teacher is asking of him. There should be no constraints, other than the wish to excel. If your right hand is contracted, if you move your toes, your voice can't be clear because the whole body is not free to vibrate.

The voice is a horizontal keyboard that moves us

Singing liberates the body. When you sing, the idea isn't to try to push your limits at every moment. You should conceptualize your voice in the horizontal plane, not in the vertical plane. You shouldn't think "I'm going to raise my voice up to counter C"; rather, you should think of your voice as a flat keyboard and think "I'm going to sing along the keyboard to counter C." The challenge here isn't to reach a certain note to impress the audience, but to move the audience, to make the audience vibrate on the day.

On the day of the Olympics, on opening night, the audience is in the hall, the critics are there also, this is the time to give 70%, maybe even more, of your vocal power, of your technique, of your self. Experience closes the gap between apprenticeship and performance. Talent feeds today's performance and tomorrow's artistic career.

The singer must dominate his voice, but his voice should never dominate him or intoxicate him. Like Narcissus, he would risk disappearing into his own mirror. He must not become the object of his own success.

Ivry Gitlis once said something surprising. A fan comes to see him: "Master, your violin is exceptional, what beauty, what music!" To which he answers "Stick your ear to the violin." Naturally, the fan heard nothing. The violin was only the instrument for Ivry's emotion, for his technique. The same goes for the larynx; it exists only because of what moves us.

The tool must be protected

Hydration

This was discussed previously in the chapter on "The health of the voice." I just want to call your attention here to the importance of the vocal tract's rather special lubrication. This essential role is performed by the salivary glands. They moisten the lips, the mouth, the pharynx. Stage fright often dries the mouth and throat, but very quickly, in a matter of seconds, saliva flows again, the adrenaline surge has passed. This is why artists are often advised to suck on honey drops or lemon-flavored gum. Lemon excites the taste buds. It is also a good idea to drink a few sips of water at room temperature, or better still, some hot tea made with honey, lemon, and salted butter.

It's either chili con carne *or singing*

The influence of the abdominal and pelvic belt is well known. A few years ago, I'm called out to attend an artist with a weak voice. He awaits me anxiously while the orchestra continues to play to keep the audience entertained. He looks livid and pale; he's in a clammy cold sweat. He hasn't forced his voice when the orchestra tuned up (the artist tunes his voice to the acoustics a few hours before the concert). His vocal cords are fine, his neck is relaxed. But he doesn't feel well. Further questioning reveals that he ate, or rather gulped down, *chili con carne*. It's now perfectly obvious: he has a bad case of indigestion. The digestive toxins and the flatulence brought on by them are preventing him from controlling his voice properly. I give him an antispasmodic injection. An hour later, he feels better. To the public's delight, the concert resumes after a delay of over an hour. This all shows how rigorous singers need to be about their diet just before a vocal performance.

Allergic to the stage

Allergy to the dusty environment of the stage can affect the nose, larynx, trachea, and bronchi. Artists risk finding their vocal tract penalized. Nowadays, problems are increasingly caused by the air conditioning and by pollution. This is why, if singers know they are vulnerable, they should take their precautions and follow a preventive treatment. Some theaters are notorious for their dusty environment.

Plastic surgery of the neck may affect the voice

Losing the high notes

Clara, a forty-year-old coloratura soprano, is working on a Mozart repertory for an upcoming concert at the Châtelet. "My voice has been weak for the past fifteen days," she tells me. Given that her spoken voice is excellent, that her vocal cords are superb, and that her transitions are nice and regular, it seems to me that only tiredness can be the culprit. But it seems this isn't her wont. A few minutes later, she explains her problem in more detail: "I can sing normally in *fortissimo* and *pianissimo*, the *vibrato* is difficult but possible, but I can't play with my voice. I've lost the very high notes and my high notes aren't particularly stable. I can't count on them." This professional singer of international renown is due to sing in an opera in three weeks. Like a detective, I try to line up the exhibits of this strange story.

Normal examination?

Indeed, her neck is normal when I palpate it, her breathing is normal, the verticality of her vertebrae is excellent, she has no apparent gynecologic problem. She doesn't suffer from any premenstrual vocal syndrome. Her vocal cords are normal, whitish, and pearly. They move quite normally. Even the partial loss of her high notes and of her *pianissimo* remains a mystery. I explore her larynx with high-speed cinematography. Still no clues. What's going on? Could the problem be psychological? Given the personality of this coloratura soprano, this seems highly unlikely.

Trying to understand what path this patient's voice took that led it into trouble. I ask her what went on before this episode. "Nothing that I recall."

Nothing that I recall . . . but!

There's a short silence for a few seconds. I remain perplexed. Then she adds, embarrassed: "Ah, yes! Two weeks ago, I had botulinum toxin injected into the wrinkles of my neck to get rid of them." I would never have guessed she'd had this injection, as six months ago her neck was hardly wrinkled at all. It hadn't appeared in the press either. It all becomes clear. The master clue has been unveiled. Botulinum toxin causes a slight paralysis of the muscles and thus diminishes wrinkles. The muscle concerned is the neck muscle just under the skin, level with the cricothyroid membrane of the larynx. This paralysis does not affect the spoken voice or the singing voice in the man-in-the-street, but it does affect the voice in its extremes. Indeed, the small prelaryngeal muscles at the level of the cricothyroid membrane are essential for adjusting a counter *C*, for controlling a *pianissimo* or modulating the register.

Thus, Clara is suffering from the temporary and unsuspected consequences of an injection of botulinum toxin. Certainly, the dosage is very minimal and the effect wears off in time, but what a worrying situation for this lyrical singer! To accelerate the elimination of the toxin, I recommend that she massage her neck morning and evening.

Stimulating lymphatic drainage and blood flow in the neck area accelerated the elimination of the negative side effects of the injection, and she was able to sing three weeks later thanks to her perfect mastery of technique.

The thyroid gland and a voice's career

The thyroid goiter

One can't discuss pathologies of the singer's voice without reference to the thyroid gland and the importance a goiter can have on one's career. The goiter is a large thyroid gland with a number of cysts and nodules inside it. This hypertrophy of the thyroid can constrict and create a diversion of the trachea. It may tighten the bottom of the larynx. The goiter gets in the way of the respiratory axis, and also of the organ of the voice. Singers are, therefore, often advised to have it removed.

This surgery isn't without risk. Indeed, if the recurrent nerve or the superior laryngeal nerve is touched, this can affect the voice. Respectively, the recurrent nerve commands the laryngeal mechanics that open and close the vocal cords, but also elongate and shorten them. The superior laryngeal nerve is in charge of the laryngeal mechanics controlling high pitches and the sensitivity of the larynx. In most cases, surgery on a goiter goes well. But one has to mention the possibility of permanent alteration to the voice. This postsurgery complication can arise due to an injury of the laryngeal nerves, or, and this is more frequent, due to the nonvascularization of laryngeal nerves that weren't sectioned (all the vessels proximal to the nerve are ligated to avoid bleeding). This lack of vascularization means the nerve is no longer properly oxygenated. This problem isn't predictable. Very often it's reversible. In these postsurgery problems, the voice is veiled, weak, or else one or both of the vocal cords can be paralyzed.

Another accident can occur: operating on the thyroid gland brings one close to the cricothyroid membrane. Retractile scarring of the latter can perturb the voice in the high notes. This is why surgery is only justified in two cases: if a potentially life-threatening cancer is suspected, or if the goiter risks jeopardizing the patient's career.

A diva is operated and sings using a new technique

Brigitte, a forty-year-old English mezzo-soprano who was operated on for a goiter two years previously, complains of needing to clear her throat. She consults me for this problem. She makes absolutely no reference to any voice problems: "I've been clearing my throat constantly for the past six months." I ask her: "After your thyroid operation, were you at all bothered?" "Not really," she explains, "six weeks after the surgery I was able to sing correctly and so I didn't see any need to have my vocal cords checked. It's true I battled a bit with my high notes in the beginning, and I had to change my vocal technique because I felt things were somehow different inside of me. I have the impression my vocal instrument has changed. That's to be expected, isn't it? I adapted my technique to find the same harmonics again, or close."

When I examine her, the scarring of the neck is remarkable, almost nothing is visible, the laryngeal cartilage under the skin is normal and slides on the subcutaneous muscle without any retractile scarring when she swallows. The left vocal cord is less mobile. It does not move much. There is a partial paralysis of the left vocal cord; only a few branches of the recurrent nerve have been damaged during the removal of the thyroid gland. The right vocal cord is perfectly mobile. Surprisingly, during phonation it remains tonic, in other words it contracts partially. There is no ankylosis of the cordal joint. A few days later, confirmation of a partial lesion of the recurrent nerve of the left vocal cord and of the good health of its superior laryngeal nerve is provided by a test: an electromyogram. Thus, in the high pitches the right vocal cord stretches and partially extends the left vocal cord sufficiently to allow satisfactory tonality, which is exceptional. Using a technique that she herself discovered, created, and adapted for herself, Brigitte manages to continue performing as an international diva.

However, listening to recordings of her voice pre- and post-surgery, one can detect a slight veiling of the voice, that, according to many critics, adds to its natural seductiveness. But I still hadn't elucidated the reason for her frequent need to clear her throat. After a more thorough examination, the diagnostic for this complaint which motivated her to consult me isn't the partial paralysis of the vocal cord, which hasn't perturbed her; on the contrary, it's quite simply pharyngitis caused by secondary gastric reflux, brought on by the great stress she is under due to her frequent travels.

Thus, Brigitte compensated remarkably for her handicap by adapting her technique. She found for herself, nearly two years ago, a new vocal print that according to some is more original. She has turned her handicap into a trump card that adds to her charm.

Story of a wounded voice: Maria Callas

From Manhattan to Athens

The great voices that have succeeded each other since the 17th century on the Italian, Anglo-Saxon, Germanic, or French stages have all left their mark. Aside from Malibran, Callas marked the 20th century. Maria Anna Sophia Kalogeropoulos, alias "La Callas," was born on December 2, 1923, in New York. Her Greek parents arrived in the United States in August of the same year. Her father, a chemist in Manhattan, changed his name to George Callas. Maria Callas begins piano lessons at the age of nine and adores singing. Already as a small child, she was frustrated by her sister, who was the favorite child. She had learned music and singing, well before Maria, leaving Maria no room for self-expression. In 1937, Maria returned to Greece with her sister and mother. This separation from her father is very hard on her.

The artist becomes "La Callas"

She enters the Music Conservatory of Athens. Her singing teacher, Maria Trivella, leads her to her first prize from the Conservatory. In 1940, she begins a brilliant career with the national theatre of Athens. She receives an ovation at La Scala in Milan on December 7, 1951 for *I vespri siciliani*. Later, Elizabeth Schwarzkopf will comment about her: "Why should I play Violetta (in *La Traviata*), when another artist, 'la Callas,' does it to perfection?" A turning point in her career makes her lose 30 kg. Indeed, her obesity was tiring her, she couldn't bear it any longer. She lacked agility on stage.

Maria Callas considers herself an athlete. She specifies: "I had to carry an extra 30 kilos on my back before my diet. My game was difficult, my voice was heavy and lacked agility." Her faculty for self-criticism was always one of this diva's strong points. From then on, she sticks to a rigorous diet. On October 28, 1956, she performs for the Metropolitan Opera of New York in Bellini's *Norma*. It's a triumph, with sixteen curtain calls.

A stage performance that ends in drama

On January 12, 1958, she sings *Norma* in front of the Italian President Giovanni Gronchi and his wife at the Rome Opera House. The night before, she had seen the New Year in style, staying up late at the Degli Sacchi Roman club. She isn't in great shape, and neither are her vocal cords. Even whispering is difficult. Thirty-six hours later, she's on stage, but not her voice. Her doctor and friends ask her to cancel, she won't hear of it. From the first few notes, her voice sounds laborious. At the end of the first act, she has to abandon. The press is scathing.

Tired, Maria Callas sings her last performance

On May 29, 1965, she plays *Norma* at the Opera Garnier in Paris with Fiorenza Cossotto in the role of Aldalgisa, who is pushing her notes to the maximum and imposes a much sustained rhythm on Maria Callas. The audience witnesses a veritable singing duel in the finale. Maria Callas faints on stage at the end of the first scene of Act II of *Norma*. She is almost comatose. Her arterial tension is weak. After the show, she is exhausted. She decides then and there to put a stop to her career.

Yet she keeps receiving offers. Aged forty-nine, on October 26, 1973, accompanied by the tenor Giuseppe Di Stefano, she presents a recital in Hamburg. After singing all around the world, she gives up, for good this time, on November 19, 1974, and dies on September 16, 1977. Two years later, her ashes are scattered in the Aegean Sea.

Her presence is Virtuosity

Callas often said that behind a trill, there's often an intention. She specifies that a pause can signify more than a note and, finally, that bel canto is not about singing a note below or a note above, but about attacking it head on. She's perfectly aware that the ear requires one-fifteenth of a second to register the voice, and that, therefore, it is best to ignore a second note that would follow the first note too quickly, rather than risk a faulty vocalise.

Callas generates electric vibrations all around her. When she doesn't sing, notably in *Norma*, among other operas (Norma was the opera role she played the most in her career, eighty-nine times in fact), she fixes her partner with such intensity that her gaze is a real presence. Her corporal expression on stage is spontaneous, but always intended. "Best not move your hand unless it is ruled by your emotions and your heart," she used to say. Sincerity was her motto. Any repartee must sound as if it is being sung for the first time. Naturally, each performance has its rules, but it's like a signature: always recognizable, always written by the same hand, and yet never the same. The singer must read between the notes and not just read the score. Passion for one's work, or more exactly for one's art, is what feeds creativity.

But Maria Callas exceeds her own limits, she loves a challenge. Bored by the long notes of the bel canto, she asks the orchestra leader to shorten them. Unlike many singers, she warms up her voice singing fairly heavy opera, such as *Il Trovatore*. Thus, does she fine-tune her breathing, her suppleness, her purity, and vocal color. Her voice can be dark, mordent, but always exceptionally virtuoso. The lyrical artist serves the composer, and not vice versa. It is essential to respect the creator of the lyrical work. The public is captivated by the sincere artist who sometimes uses a language that's difficult for the public to grasp. Opera school teaches one to feel every note, to differentiate a *legato* from a *portato*, to pronounce a word without distorting it, and, especially, not to betray the composer, something Maria Callas mastered well. This remarkable diva was pure emotion. Her fragility was that of all artists who give themselves to their public without holding back, and who live solely for transcending through vibration.

Imagination and vibration

The "body instrument"

The singer is an instrumental body. He shares in the magic of vibration and harmony, he transcends matter with sound. He gives the composer's notes their freedom. His voice is infinitely varied. He knows how to tame a note to make it his own. He creates his own internal vibration. He can become a slave of his voice. Balancing on the tightrope of vibration can be delicate.

This same vibration bears the seal of the singer, the actor, or comedian. It rocks his audience. It organizes his acoustic environment. The singer projects his voice, but remains viscerally caught between the *yin* and the *yang* of the breath of life. He communicates the affective vibration we all carry inside of us. This biological envelope of ours can't resist the seductive plea of his voice to please his fellow human being.

Each being has his own specific resonance: here nothing is linear, all is curved. In this context, two and two don't necessarily make four. Our voice, so fragile, can be astonishingly fiery, powerful, and energetic. It pitches the soul, renders our auditory space, metamorphoses vibration into emotion. It enlightens silence. The space that surrounds us shares in our inner silence. The authenticity of our verbal expression is in harmony with the sincerity of our being.

Dissonance and consonance

Yet in our daily lives, in urban settings, on the road, civilization attacks us with its noises. Our hearing has become a mere filter that battles to recognize the voice that speaks to us. This acoustic pollution often distorts, sometimes asphyxiates our perception of the vibratory world of music and of living beings. This acoustic violence in this present generation is extreme, both in terms of loudness and in terms of its intensity and register. Only one element remains immutable: the association between dissonance and consonance.

The power of this vibration of the senses finds expression thus: a major third fills you with joy, a minor third inspires nostalgia and melancholy. The one exists only by contrast with the other. This is where the minor third becomes dissonant in relation to the major third. This sensitivity is evident when Yehudi Menuhin plays the violin. Indeed, here notes are not imposed the way they are in piano. They are not preformed. He is free to disaccord a natural chord of the violin. He becomes a magician of all that is possible.

The opera uses the voice as a jewel case for its melodies. The singer proceeds at his own rhythm, his body is the suppleness that enables him to give his voice a semblance of lightness. All he is doing is setting free inner frequencies that settle in space. Nothing can give you a sense of this more spectacularly than being with gypsies whose song draws you into their universe.

The strength of the singer is that he creates his own vibratory tone between joy and sadness, between enthusiasm and despair. This "body-spirit" pair vibrates as one. Partition is served by technique, emotion is served by the voice. The balance between the inner self and its external space comes from the power of the vibration.

The voice is painted with emotion

Painting and sculpture have their props—space, canvas, bronze, marble. The singer works in time-space, in the chiaroscuro of the vibration of one's being. The setting, with its costumes, arrangement, and play of lights, condition the spectators. The synergy that the artist creates is his charisma. His own emotion is amplified by his public. It takes on a different dimension. The artist feeds off the affective charge of the public and returns it magnified a hundred times. It's no longer a voice you listen to, it's a melody, a melody that charms you, seduces you, transports you. This is characteristic of this intangible and ephemeral art that leaves its mark in our memory.

Part 3

The mystery of the voice

Chapter 18

The castrati

Are castrati not men assigned to serve the Muses?

A voice from the past

A voice is absent from today's vocal panorama: the voice of the castrati. These lyrical artists who appear in Italian opera from the 16th century left their mark on a whole era. At one time adulated by royalty, the public, and by the Church, their feminine voice, their power, timbre, and harmonics enthralled listeners for over three centuries. The opera raised the status of the castrati thanks—one could say—to the Catholic Church.

Indeed, women weren't allowed to sing in churches. Castrati singers made their first appearance in the Sistine Chapel in 1562. Their singing was heard there for the last time in 1903. Pope Leo XIII then formally forbade them entry. The last castrato to direct the Sistine Chapel Choir was Alessandro Moreschi, who left us a recording of his voice on a wax cylinder.

How did they come to sing in Church?

High pitch and sacred chanting

In the 15th century, a few castrati arrive from the Orient to make a name for themselves. They penetrate the liturgical world. They are associated with the high pitches of sacred chanting. At the end of the 15th century and in the early 16th century, they are practically indispensable in the Sistine Chapel. Why? Gregorian chanting has a very high register that demands a quality of elocution close to perfection. At first, these asexual voices bordering on the divine were rare. Falsetto voices were tried, but they were too expensive to hire. Bringing castrati over from Spain was also prohibitive. And so it came about that from 1592 to 1605, Pope Clement VIII encouraged castration. At first, castrati were sought out for sacred chanting, but they were rapidly also sought out for secular music.

Georgina's escape ushers in the era of the castrati

An incident accelerated the career of the castrati within the Church. In 1686, the Duke of Mantoue, invited by the Pope, attends high mass and that same evening a concert by the singer Georgina. Her bewitching, superb voice is accompanied by castrati voices. Before the Duke's departure, the Pope, Innocent XI, asks his guest what he most appreciated during his time in Rome. He was expecting the answer to be "The high mass." But without hesitation, the duke answers: "The voice of the singer, Georgina." Scandalized, the Pope decides without further ado to have any female singers refusing to leave Rome locked up in a convent and to forbid women to sing or act in the theater. He has Georgina summoned, but she manages to escape through a hidden corridor. This prohibition, initially applicable only in Rome, was later extended to the whole of Christendom by Pope Clement XI, who decreed: "No person of the feminine gender is allowed to learn music with the intention of using her musical knowledge to become a singer. Indeed, one knows that a beautiful woman singing on stage yet purporting to preserve her virtue can be likened to someone aspiring to jump into the Tiber river without wetting his feet." This prohibition went a lot further than Saint Paul's in his first epistle to the Corinthians (XIV, 33–35): "*Molieres taceat in ecclesia,*" in other words, "Women are forbidden to sing in churches." Ipso facto, chanting being an indispensable religious prop, the door was now wide open for castrati.

Farinelli: how is it that this castrato has such a powerful voice?

The voice of the castrato: not quite an asexual voice

With a reach of more than three octaves, the castrato voice exerted its fascination as early as the 16th century. Its characteristics are strictly the consequence of hormonal castration, not of emasculation. We now know that the voice is subjected to our sex hormones. The voice is influenced, of course, by our genetic heritage, but more so by androgens as regards men and by estrogens and progesterone as regards women. These hormones only appear after puberty; therefore, a child's voice will remain "feminine, angelic, asexual" if, and only if, a man is castrated before he reaches puberty. Indeed, if he's castrated after puberty, it will have no repercussion on the voice, which will stay the same, namely, masculine. This is because testosterone has a definitive influence on the organism's muscles and cartilages: so much so that any woman who takes male hormones will find her vocal timbre becoming irreversibly masculine.

Where does the power of the castrato voice come from?

The castrato's voice has never broken. He keeps his child's voice, but has the morphology of an adult. He keeps the child's high-pitched harmonics with a component and warmth of the adult's low-pitched harmonics.

Why, in spite of having no male hormones, does the castrato nevertheless develop such male vocal power, an intensity and a force of exhalation so completely out of step with the high notes he's capable of producing? In fact, though testosterone has no more influence on Farinelli, he still has a residual hormonal environment due to his XY sex chromosomes: an environment formed by several nonsexual hormones, namely, thyroid hormones, corticosteroids, and growth hormones.

The delicacy of the vocal cord muscles and the pharynx is due to the absence of any impact of testosterone. Growth hormones and thyroid hormones, the secretions of which are greater in XY than in XX, and are not produced by the testicles but by specific glands, play a part in the energy, power, and morphologic build of the castrato. These different characteristics produce a hybrid individual. His energy and appearance are those of a man. His long and delicate muscles are those of a woman. Sometimes he appears gynoid.

The association of a feminine timbre, none other than a child's timbre unadulterated by testosterone, with the masculine vocal power produced by the significant presence of hormones, notably growth hormones among others, is more readily perceived. Farinelli has a falsetto voice, or countertenor. Castration has preserved his soprano voice, with a vocal register that has grown from three to four octaves. He can sing a succession of trills and cascades with astonishing ease and passes from the lowest tones to the highest in one-fifteenth of a second. This agility of the vocal muscles is natural and readily executed.

Farinelli was able to sustain a note for nearly two minutes with apparent ease, whereas a professional singer is rarely able to hold a note for more than forty-five seconds. Thus, the power of his exhalation and his reserve of air, prior to the vocal attack, are impressive. The resonators are also subject to hormonal impregnation, which explains the spellbinding quality of his harmonics, that women, but also men, find so seductive. Women faint like groupies at the Olympia hall. The beauty of choir singing is derived partly from the combination of high-pitched harmonics with low-pitched harmonics that provide both a support and a background for the higher-pitched harmonics.

Castration: a surgical procedure performed by the barber

The castration of a castrato wasn't the total ablation practiced on eunuchs. The technique was well-oiled. The idea was to "annihilate" the testicles, to prevent any secretion of male hormones. According to Charles d'Ansillon, who published a treatise on eunuchs in 1707, the child was first drugged and left in a hot bath to partially anesthetize him. An incision was made just above the testicles. The spermatic cords, with their spermatic canal, arteries, and testicular veins, were tied. This ensured rapid necrosis of the testicles within ten to fifteen days. But the necrosis could be partial, which explains why certain castrati were able to have an erection and were proud of still being libidinous.

In those days, the surgery was performed by barbers. The intervention was only of interest if it was done before the age of twelve, when a child's voice begins to break. The decision to castrate a child was often a consequence of his poor social background. Indeed, castrati could hope for a career and decent remuneration. It was said that parents only decided to castrate their child with his approval and that of his singing teacher.

According to Pope Clement VIII, these children pledged their voice to the "Kingdom of God." He had prohibited them from marrying.

Carlo Broschi: the young Farinelli

Farinelli, whose real name was Carlo Broschi, was a career singer for seventeen years. Born on January 24, 1705 in Andria, near Bari, in Italy, he is probably the best known castrato of the 18th century. A modern singer, he surprises his public. His pure, perfect voice, soprano and alto, angelic according to some, penetrating and luminous, makes light of registers with disconcerting ease. His father, Salvatore Broschi, is a highly ranked civil servant in the service of the King. Young Carlo sings from early childhood. According to his older brother Ricardo who followed him throughout his career, he had a very beautiful voice. A horse-riding accident endangers the life of the future Farinelli. He has to be castrated in order to be saved; castration "is" his only chance of survival. Strange that castration should have been this child's only chance of survival. Was this an excuse? In those days, the surgical act of castration was officially prohibited unless motivated by medical reasons. However, it is hard to imagine that a nobleman would castrate his son secretly in order to protect his own financial future, which was what usually motivated this type of illicit practice.

How Carlo Broschi becomes Farinelli

So Carlo Broschi, son of a noble family, is castrated at the age of nine and becomes Farinelli. Absolutely brilliant, knowing how to take full advantage of both his voice and his charm, he travels throughout Europe giving concerts and recitals. His reputation is acquired in Italy. His teacher, Nicolo Porpora, was born in Naples in 1685. Son of a bookseller, one of many children, Porpora puts on his first opera, *Agrippina*, in 1708, at the age of twenty-two, in his hometown. The success is overwhelming. In his operas, confusion reigns. Men play female parts, women play men's parts. But there's also a third "sex," the castrato, who is able to play any part. Porpora discovers his prodigy when the child is eight. The child, Farinelli, a genius of lyrical art, is about to start his apprenticeship with Porpora, and remarkable though this apprenticeship was, it was also a real challenge to human nature.

He takes his young pupil to Rome, for the 1721 to 1722 season, to interpret his operas at the Aliberti Theater. Farinelli is a huge success. For his first performance, he is made to sing on the market square with a virtuoso trumpet player. It is clear to all and sundry that a duel has been staged between a wind instrument, the trumpet player, and a wind and cord instrument, the larynx. The public is expectant. The two artists are about to confront each other. According to the writings of the journalist Sachi, the melody begins with a note held in *fermata*. The trumpet begins the note softly, holds it from *pianissimo* into *fortissimo* for so long that the public's enthusiasm is at its highest pitch. Everyone presumes that Farinelli will never manage to sustain this crystalline note. But he sustains it for so long that it unleashes explosive applause and cries of admiration. Farinelli goes further. He sings the musical phrase again and adds brilliant trills to it that no one before him has ever attempted. The vocal virtuoso had just emerged.

The singing technique of the castrato

Farinelli owes his surprising agility and the range of his register to the breathing technique he learned with Porpora. A technique inspired by Giovanni Andrea Bontempi's book, *Historia musica*, published in 1695. It advocates a Spartan education of implacable rigor that calls for physical resistance, mental prowess, culture, and harmony. The rhythm it sets is impressive: over six hours of exercises a day.

In the morning, the castrato pupil sings difficult works for one hour, then practices his trills for an hour, followed by an hour of *passagio*, and an hour spent studying words and phonemes, after which there's a final session rehearsing with his teacher. The afternoon is consecrated to the study of music and literature, as well as vocal technique in its minutest detail. The last hour of singing of the day is spent in front of the mirror. The pupil must listen to himself, admire himself, look at himself. It's true that the mirror is a corrective instrument. Observing his reflection enables him to control his body: nothing must move. While he sings, his legs, abdomen, thorax, face, and mouth are set. The singer must be well grounded. The technique is at its zenith.

Of course, being a castrato and having an unusual laryngeal, thoracic, and auditory predisposition endows the castrato with an unusual pneumophonic (respiration and vocal cords) and audiophonatory (hearing and retro-control of the voice) loop. Farinelli is pure voice. His seduction is based solely on his voice—indeed, unlike Nicolina, another castrato of his epoch, he's awkward on stage. He isn't able to use his body as would an actor. In 1730, in Venice, Farinelli interprets the role of Darios in *Idase*, a work composed by his brother. The public's ovation is exceptional, as reported by articles at the time: "The first note, pianissimo . . . the others exploded in a succession of passagio that were so fast that the violinists could barely keep up." He knows how to charm the crowds and carries the lyric to its zenith. He is a vocal musical instrument. Engaged in Spain, he becomes the personal singer of Philip V, and also of his successor Ferdinand VI, in 1737. Legend has it that he sang for the King every night. Farinelli's influence over the King is practically that of a Prime Minister. He leaves Spain at the instigation of the queen mother, Elizabeth Farnese, whose son, Charles III, becomes King. Back in Italy, he founds his own singing school. He retires to his villa in Bologna and dies in 1782.

The physical appearance and libido of the castrato

The larynx is unusual

In 1865, Dr. Edouard Fournier, a laryngologist, gives us a remarkable description of the castrati's vocal cords, considering the means at his disposal back then. The laryngoscope has just been invented, but is difficult to handle. The castrato's larynx is smaller than a man's. The thyroid cartilage is softer, it can easily be depressed with the fingers. The Adam's apple is hardly visible and hasn't calcified. The neck is long and slim. The larynx inside is very narrow. The vocal cords are fine. The vocal cord, when compared to a ribbon, is wide at the back and thin at the front, which is unusual. This glottic configuration lends a remarkable natural predisposition for singing in a high register. But it requires the singer to clamp the two vocal cords together very tightly to enable them to vibrate and to avoid any air escaping and veiling the voice. These days, the explanation for this singular anatomy is simple. In a "normal" man, the calcification of the thyroid cartilage facilitates the insertion of the cordal muscle on the cartilage, thereby strengthening it and enabling it to have a strong and wide tendon, while the body of the muscle is more developed and more resistant.

How does the castrato's physical appearance change over the years?

How does the castrato's morphology adapt to the lack of male hormones? This is described in detail in research carried out in 1976 by Dr. Pelikan, a Russian doctor from Saint Petersburg. He identifies two morphologic types: tall and thin, like Farinelli, and strong and gynoid, like Nicolino, Senesino, or Bernacchi. The castrati were callow and their hair was dense and plentiful. They were taller than average, with unusually long arms and legs. Their thoracic cage was impressive. Their bearing was relaxed, limp, with little tonus. Recall an anecdote about Casanova, who in 1745 was strolling in the streets of Milan and took a seat at a cafe with his friend Gamma. He's impressed by an abbot sitting close by. His face is attractive. "Judging from his hips, I took him to be a girl in disguise," he comments. To which Gamma answers: "That's the Abbott Bepino Della Mama, a famous castrato. He can prove to you whether I'm right or not."

With the passing years, the castrato's voice becomes deeper and his morphologic traits thicken. Some stop singing to become actors around the age of thirty, others (such as Nicolino) sing into their fifties. Their morphology becomes a handicap for their singing. They acquire a belly and this makes them look gynoid.

Their striated muscles, deprived of the influence of male hormones, weaken and lose their tonus.

Yet on a sexual level, the castrato remains a man attracted to the opposite sex, although with a significantly diminished libido. There have been cases of castrati with diminished but persisting sexual powers. Their castration was incomplete from a mechanical point of view, therefore, a low level of testosterone continued to be secreted in quantities sufficient to maintain the libido at a minimal threshold, but below the threshold required to allow the development of the secondary sex organs and male muscles.

When, why, and how did castrati first make their appearance?

Well before the Egyptians, castration was practiced as a sacrifice to the gods and goddesses. Priests emasculated themselves in order to devote themselves "body and soul" to their gods and to sacrifice what is most precious to a man.

Nearly two thousand years BC, in Ancient Egypt, Nabucco emasculated all his prisoners to be surrounded solely by eunuchs. Evidence of the existence of castrati can be found in China in the twelfth century BC, as well as in India some time later, then in the rest of the Oriental world.

In Ancient Greece, priests, notably those of Diana of Ephesus, suffered the same fate. Hippocrates differentiates eunuchs from castrati even then:

> Eunuchs can't beget children because their seminal conduits have been obliterated; indeed, there are vessels that bring semen to the testicles, and other vessels that are smaller but very numerous, connect the testicles to the penis and determine its rigidity or flaccidity. These are all removed by the castration; which is why one can't breed after this operation. In castrati, torsion or compression has crushed or obstructed the seminal conduits; the testicles and vessels remain; they harden, become callous and can neither stretch nor slacken.

Castration is also practiced by the Romans. The ceremonies that accompany self-emasculation take place in March. They are often associated with the sacrifice of a six-year-old bull, as the cult of Cybelia and Atys, introduced to Rome in 204 bc, is commemorated in March. As mythology would have it, the Phrygian goddess Cybelia loves the shepherd Atys. He falls in love with Sagaritis, a nymph. Cybelia can't bear this and to punish Atys, she plunges him into madness. He emasculates himself, which proves fatal.

Eunuchs were expected to keep guard over women and girls and their voice was of no interest. Indeed, they were emasculated at any age, which was not the case with castrati.

In those days, there were three categories of castrati: *castrati*, who underwent a complete ablation of their external genitalia; *spadones*, in whom only the testicles were missing; and *tblibioe*, who underwent a simple compression of the testicles with alteration of the seminal canal.

The first castrations carried out on Christian soil took place in Rome in the 1st century AD, despite castration being forbidden and despite laws decreed by the emperors, notably Nero and Antonin the Pious, under whom castration was punishable by death.

The castrati's path from the 16th century to the early 20th century

The castrato was the popular and operatic singer of his time

- At church—On September 27, 1589, the Pope officially authorizes castrati to sing in his apartments in the Vatican Palace, in the Capella Pontificia, later renamed Capella Sixtina (the Sistine Chapel). The Sistine Chapel could seat a choir of twenty-four singers. In 1562, under Pope Pie IV, this edifice is host to the first two castrati, Francesco Torres and Francis Co Soto Lengua, two Spaniards. Henceforth, the music is adapted for these new singers. The castrati who later also take their place in this choir in Rome sing like sopranos, some like altos. Loretto Vittori, an Italian castrated before puberty, is engaged by the Vatican in 1622, at the age of twenty-two. Not only does he sing at mass in the Sistine Chapel, he's also a variety singer in the princely morning-rooms of the epoch. He performs with other castrati, such as Marc Antonio Pasqualini.

At the end of the 17th century and in the 18th century, there are around one hundred soprano and alto castrati in Rome, around thirty in Venice in the Basilica San Marco, another fifty or so in the Basilica San Petronio in Bologna: this in response to the demands of the Catholic Church. From the 18th century onward, the castrati desert the churches and basilicas for concert rooms, theaters, and opera houses. Over sixty opera houses were built in one year in Venice alone.

The sacred chanting of castrati first made its appearance at the start of the 16th century, prior even to the beginnings of opera. It's performed *a voce piena*, that is, with a full voice. It takes advantage of the resonance chamber of the chapel and harmonizes with the vibratory space of the choirs. This alchemy delivers an acoustic creation in which words are hardly articulated; only the melody, ornamented with vowels; allows vocal transcendence.

- At the theater—Castrati voices are at the height of their glory at the beginning of the 18th century. Indeed, little by little this hybrid and bewitching voice begins to dominate baroque operas. In 1720, Farinelli plays the part of Queen Berenice, then in 1725, of Queen Cleopatra. To counterbalance the male singing parts given to women, or more exactly, to castrati, men's parts are given to female singers dressed up as men, which shows how little importance was attached to the sex of the voice. The role of Anthony, in Hasse's *Anthony and Cleopatra*, is interpreted in 1725 by Vittoria Tessi, a contralto, giving the repartee to a Cleopatra played by Farinelli.

The relation between voices and parts is astonishing. The great lovers, the battle heroes, are played predominantly by castrati, not by male singers. Male voices jar on the public's ear. They find little favor, are considered too unpolished, too coarse, too deep, all in all too masculine. Men's parts are taken by transvestite women. The music is written for "precious" voices, light and crystalline. The public is entranced by high registers. The only deep voices that are accepted and appreciated are bass and deep bass, thought to incarnate the wisdom of the Ancient world.

The fascinating voice: from the castrato to the diva

What a strange voice

How strange is this castrato's voice! The castrato's pitch does not go as high as children's. His timbre is different from men's, different from women's, different from children's: it is a vocal hybrid. "Once you've heard it, there's no chance of you're confusing it with another," according to writings of that epoch. The castrato must have had exceptional technique.

Yet castrati become progressively scarcer on stage and are dethroned for the first time by the best female singer of her time, "la Malibran." Her singing in the high registers has a divine quality. And indeed, henceforth, great female soprano singers will be known as "divas."

For all that castrati were important lyrical artists in Italy, such wasn't the case in France. We recall here the great irony with which the minister Mazarin greeted castrati.

A fragile voice

But castrati can also lose their voice. Francesco Antonio Pistocchi, born in Parma in 1659, loses his voice, it seems, after practicing a vocal technique that wasn't suited to him. A soprano, he then has to adapt to a new way of singing to become a contralto. He contributes the notion of a natural singing style that respects the individual. He privileges the melody by imposing a clear elocution. He inspires the vocal techniques of Farinelli, but also of Vittoria Tessi, a contralto, and of other castrati. His merit lies in having passed on the message that singing is an inexhaustible source of harmonic variety, and in having taught different musical styles all based on the same vocal technique, much as a piano can be used to play a Nocturne by Chopin, or a Gershwin score.

The 18th century produces a host of reputed singing teachers, such as the remarkable castrato Giuseppe Aprile, teacher and interpreter, born in 1732 in Martina Franca, near Tarento. He was castrated when he was eleven. He gave his first performance in Naples in 1753. He founded his own school of singing in Naples.

The castrato is also an actor

This is especially true of Nicolino, whose real name was Nicola Grimaldi. In 1709, he performs in London. It will be said of him that he expresses his voice right to his fingertips and that a deaf person would be able to follow him, understand his text, and feel his singing. Like Farinelli, he is said to have exceptional breath and tessitura. But Nicolino has more than one bow to his arc. He is a great theatrical actor. He can create the illusion that he is singing while speaking. He recites to music. He teaches castrati the *passagio* technique and especially, how to place the voice for the head voice. He creates fast variations between *pianissimo* and *fortissimo*, between high pitches and low pitches, structuring the technique around breathing. Later generations will base their technique more on the chest voice, as taught by Farinelli. This technique enables singers to draw their vocal power from the chest and to support it with their abdominal and pelvic muscles. Virtuosi of this technique, aside from Farinelli, include Bernacchi and Carestini. Carestini kept a soprano voice until the age of twenty-eight, then, very quickly, his register dropped down to alto. From a reach of three octaves, he passed down to two octaves.

Castrati disappear from the scene

In the early 19th century, Giovanno Battista Velluti was one of the last known castrati. The curtain falls; Moreschi was the only castrato to have recorded his voice on a wax cylinder in 1904. The story of the recording is droll. The greatest tenor of that epoch, Caruso, was to be recorded by The Gramophone Company, later known as His Master's Voice. In 1902, technicians arrived in Milan to immortalize the tenor's voice. Encouraged by the success of the recording, the company decides to record Moreschi and the Choir of the Sistine Chapel in Rome. Four recordings were made on the 11th of April, 1904, with Moreschi as soprano castrato, Giulio Bianchini as baritone, and Dado as bass. The Choir was directed by Baron Kanzler. But this wax cylinder is of mediocre quality and, today, despite our technological know-how, we are unable to reproduce the sound satisfactorily.

Charm and seduction: the giddiness of the voice

The castrato made his public dizzy. He challenged the usually accepted margins between man and woman. He could control the *legato* to perfection, tying notes together seamlessly, in contrast to the *staccato* rhythm of the spoken voice. He was also able to play with the roundness of his voice, preserving unusual power for the *vibrato* that lasted for several dozens of seconds. Note that nowadays, professional singers demonstrate all these characteristics, be they lyrical singers or popular singers. Countertenor voices fascinate us, they make light of registers in ways that enchant us.

The fascination with Farinelli motivated the 1994 movie by G. Corbiau, a motion picture that was a great technical achievement. The castrato's voice was reproduced by combining, indeed, fusing, the voices of Derek Lee Ragin, "a male alto," one of the foremost countertenors of our day who did the high notes, and Ewa Mallas-Godlewska, a soprano, who sang the low notes. So the *passagio* between these two voices was perfect, with no possibility of guessing who is singing (the singing formants at these pitches made a perfect match). Thanks to the technique used, the film gives a good idea of the castrati's now lost voice. The impressive success of this movie is no fluke. In today's world, we need something extraordinary to make us vibrate: the vocal challenge that makes light of the limits of our vibratory world hypnotizes, fascinates, and makes us dream.

Chapter 19

Impersonators:
contortionists of the larynx

The impersonator is the caricaturist of the voice.

Is the impersonator a clone, the twin of the original?

The hereditary aspect of Man is inscribed in his genes, of which there are nearly 30,000. Heredity determines that you have your mother's brown eyes or your father's blond hair; this is your appearance, also called your "phenotype." More precisely, the color of your eyes will depend on two chromosomes, each of which has a color gene. Brown eyes are their external manifestation, but you may have a dominant brown gene on one chromosome and a recessive green gene on the other. As the green gene is recessive, only the color brown is imprinted on the iris. Thus, our phenotype is only a partial manifestation of our genetic cartography.

Monozygotic twins are veritable clones, identical at the genetic level and often identical in their external appearance. The 30,000 genetic units that compose each of them are identical. These 30,000 facets of a person's identity resonate identically. Electrons, protons, neutrons, and quarks are disposed in identical fashion. It is no surprise, therefore, that so many similarities, both physical and behavioral, are encountered in this population.

Yet I was impressed by an anecdote reported to me by André Langaney, Professor at the Musée de l'Homme of Paris. The problem of the comparison of twins was discussed in a television program. Often, twins are identical and there's no psychological rivalry between them. The television program brought together on the set scientists, psychologists, linguists, and a number of monozygotic twins in their thirties. The paired twins look extraordinarily alike, except for two sisters. These two twins had decided from adolescence that they wanted to be as different as possible. They dress differently. One is sexy looking with her short skirt, open-necked blouse, and blond hair cut very short. The other is almost austere-looking with her long skirt, navy pullover closed at the neck, and long, straight brown hair. One is ostentatiously made up, the other is barely made up at all. Physically, they don't want to be mixed up and they've pulled it off. André Langaney adds that he was struck by another aspect of their identity.

It occurs to him to question the guests invited on the set about the vocal timbre of the different monozygotic twins present on the set that night. The guests are blindfolded. On the set, the twins each pronounce the same test sentence. The conclusion of the scientific witnesses is implacable. The vocal imprint is identical. No one is able to differentiate between the two twin sisters. Their external appearance can mislead, but their voices can't be disguised or faked. Proof voice, with all its complexity depends on what is innate, on DNA, which once again marks us with its seal.

The human voice is unique to each of us, except in the case of monozygotic twins. It can't be duplicated. What is the impersonator's secret?

Impersonators, but not quite like the song bird

Is Man the only species that does imitations? Do animals have this ability? Birds that imitate do exist. In North America, the mockingbird sings the melodies of the blackbird. The female blackbird recognizes the faker by analyzing his acoustic signal. Acoustic spectrography has revealed differences between the faked melody and the original melody relating to the length of the musical sentence, its tonality, its punctuation, and, especially, its silences. It seems that it's mainly the difference in the length of silences that enables the female blackbird to spot the imposter. The female finch can also spot a male finch that is from a different territory, and won't let him seduce her, as if a man from Marseilles (a town in the south of France where people have a very strong accent) couldn't seduce a woman from Lilles (a town in the north of France where people also have a very strong accent, but one quite different from the Marseilles accent).

The impersonator tries, and often manages, to give the illusion that we are listening to Frank Sinatra, Charles Aznavour, Al Pacino, or Humphrey Bogart. He leads us into a fantasy world of harmonics in order to hoodwink us. He's a mystifier of the human voice. Indeed, to recognize a voice, one must first have heard it and memorized it.

The impersonator emphasizes the caricatural features of the person he is imitating. This approach is particularly impressive if you select a radio station at random, without knowing who is talking. Only by listening will you be able to specify: "That's Charles Aznavour," or "that's Louis Armstrong." The words aren't those of his songs. A few minutes later, you realize that it was an impersonator behind the microphone. In this instance, his physical appearance in no way influenced your brain, it was only the harmonics, the musicality, the rhythm, the words, the silences that misled you as to the artist's identity. It is by listening to these artists on the radio that one is best able to appreciate their talents.

A contortionist of the vocal tract

Vocal suppleness

The impersonator is an artist in every sense of the word. Contortionist of the larynx, conjurer of our hearing, he manipulates perfectly the mechanics of the voice and its intelligibility. Is his musical instrument, his larynx, different from ours? Has he, like the ventriloquist, certain peculiarities? Does he have a gift that allows him to move his vocal musical instrument in a particular way? Finally, how is he able to create the same rhythms of speech as a Jean Gabin, a Humphrey Bogart, or a Michel Simon? He can reinvent the mimics and the attitude of the person he imitates. An exceptional caricaturist, he recreates the vibratory environment in two strokes of the pencil.

His larynx, like any larynx, has two vocal cords that vibrate normally. It is not a harp! It also has the same jointed system: the arytenoids at the back, that give the vocal cords their mobility, the epiglottis poised above this vibratory anatomic space, and the resonators.

Thus, in this case, the elements that enable the imitation are the pharynx, the tongue, the soft palate, and the vocal cords. A nasal voice is required to imitate Michel Simon, a vibration in semi-tone is key to imitating Frank Sinatra or Ray Charles. Yet the majority of the impersonators that I have been able to observe have one spectacular characteristic in common.

The larynx that "squints"

Their larynx is often asymmetric. They adjust the left vocal cord in relation to the right one like an acrobat. The right vocal cord can partially overlap the left at the level of the arytenoid, or inversely. It is a "cross-eyed" larynx.

Observation of the larynx through the nasal videofibroscope, which in no way interferes with the technique of the impersonator as he practices his art, reveals the secret of his instrument:

- The vocal cords are powerful.
- The epiglottis modifies the vocal timbre.
- The ligaments between the epiglottis and the cordal joints form a laryngeal ribbed vault, a particularly powerful vocal cathedral that can adapt to every type of imitation.
- The articulator system of the vocal cords is the impersonator's orchestra leader.

These muscles, cartilages, and joints enable him to juggle with the voice, accentuating, if necessary, the laryngeal asymmetry, should it not exist naturally. The best vocal performances are underpinned by impersonators' speed of execution and precise mobility.

The original and the fake: not only the larynx

- The vocal instrument—This congenital predisposition, this acoustic gift, amounts to nothing without hard work and talent. The proper placing of the vocal instrument enables a high-pitched or low-pitched voice to be created or modified quickly and efficiently. I was surprised, when observing the musical instrument of these artists and comparing it to the original, to find that their larynx even tends to take on the same mimics as the larynx they imitate. Because he is able to lengthen the right vocal cord more than the left, for example, and is thereby able to create different harmonics at will, the impersonator can come closer to the artist he's mimicking.

Impersonators develop and make supple their pharyngolaryngeal muscles and resonators as much as possible. They contort their epiglottis, which in certain mimics moves farther back in the pharynx and closer to the arytenoids. At other times, they preserve the asymmetry that's an asset conferred to them by nature, and in a tenth of a second, they contract the soft palate, recreating the nasal voice of Michel Simon. Then in the next sequence, they become Aznavour, Gainsbourg, or Yves Montand.

• The mimics—the impersonator also applies himself to training his neck and face muscles in order to imitate more closely the person he is imitating. All artists have lip movements that are particular to them. All artists move their jaws in a characteristic way. The impersonator focuses on the mimics of the person he is imitating, accentuates the vocal characteristics of his speech, accent, or rhythm. Some try to intensify the resemblance by wearing a wig or a hat, a scarf or a jacket, or by walking on stage the same way the other person walks. This accumulation of signals allows us to imagine that the impersonator is someone else; like a child, we allow ourselves to be inveigled into this world of illusion.

He is the illusionist of the Commedia dell'arte, the artist of artists

Whereas an actor learns a text written by an author, gets under the skin of the character, and interprets the part as he sees fit, bringing his own approach and his personality to the part, not only does the impersonator have to respect the original character, he also has to gives us a caricatural illusion of him. He is the actor. He writes his own texts. He imitates the artist by underscoring aspects of his public façade, without ever being able to bring into play the artist's private self.

He does not become the other, he interprets him. He never imagines he is the other. He is the illusionist of the Commedia dell'arte. Whenever an impersonator imitates someone well known, he keeps his own personal identity. An experienced ear recognizes which artist is being portrayed, but also recognizes the impersonator hiding behind the artist or politician who is being imitated.

The impersonator is an outstanding interpreter. He is the artist of the artists! He borrows the mimics of the person he imitates. He recreates that person's expression, gestures, body posture. He models his resonators, his pharynx, his buccal cavity, his lips after him. If you need convincing, just observe French impersonators such as Michel Leeb, Patrick Sebastien, Yves Lecoq, Laurent Gerra, or Didier Gustin imitating Michel Simon.

Listening: the brain of imitation

The audiophonatory feedback: one of the clues to the imitator's art

These artists with a hundred voices have a gift for imitation that's inseparable from their gift for listening to others and to themselves. It seems that the retro-control "mouth-to-ear," or the audiophonatory loop, is perceived by the impersonator without any distortion from his own voice, which is not true for most of us. Indeed, when you record your voice on an automatic answering machine, for example, and then listen to it, is your reaction not: "But I can't recognize myself, that's not my voice!" And yet, that's how others hear you. This is a very important point. Indeed, the impersonator hears himself exactly as he speaks. This enables him to modulate his voice at will and to recreate the timbre he's after. He hears that other person's voice also as if it were himself talking.

Each impersonator has his own vocal imprint

If the impersonator has his own vocal imprint, with its own harmonics, will he create another vocal imprint, a "vocal twin" of the person he's imitating? Absolutely not. The vocal print is comparable to a fingerprint, it is specific to each impersonator. Quite simply because a voice is dependent on complex parameters: the "bellows," the vibration of the vocal cords, the resonators, the emotional heritage of our voice and our culture shape its personality.

This fine acoustic private eye keeps his personality, his own vocal print. When Michel Leeb imitates Michel Simon, you know that it is Michel Leeb, just as you would know if Yves Lecoq were imitating Michel Simon that it is Yves Lecoq. In both instances, Michel Simon exists, but his interpreter keeps his own particular vocal harmonics.

The impersonator closely observes the artist he wants to imitate. He observes the way he scrunches up his eyes, or moves his lips. Finally, he tries his best to understand the behavior and emotional rhythm of the person he is going to mimic. He makes use of the person's silences. He refines his artistic approach with tape recordings, videos, and repeated observations of artists. For example, Jacques Brel often extends both arms toward the front and swings them, Aznavour often has his head slightly inclined and turned to the right, Michel Simon hunches. Some people, though, are difficult to imitate.

Because of his technique, his vocal warm-up, his body mimics, an impersonator very rarely suffers any problem with his voice. He knows his laryngeal instrument inside out; he knows how to preserve his hearing as well as his transmitting organ.

Artist of the artists

Exploring the larynx may have revealed the secret of the impersonator's mechanics, but it has not thrown any light on this vocal achievement that combines emotion and vocal art. The impersonator isn't Faust. He isn't here to take possession of the original version. He has come to imitate him. He respects him. He merely caricatures him. Contortionist of the larynx, caricaturist of the other's voice, the impersonator is the artist of the artists. The voices of others are his landscape, his palette is his vocal instrument.

Chapter 20

The ventriloquist: magician of the voice

> *"Magician, man of a thousand hands,*
> *What you make us believe in*
> *Is more real than reality that is a dream,*
> *For in this party, you are cast in the*
> *role of chance and mystery,*
> *Your lies are preferable to you than our sad truth."*

Jean Cocteau

A voice from elsewhere

Ventriloquist: a strange word indeed! In Greek, he is called *egastrimitos*: from *gaster*, stomach and *mythos*, speech—the spoken voice of the stomach. Yet who has ever seen a stomach articulate words? His set lips give the illusion of a voice coming from elsewhere.

Jean Cocteau's verse on the magician could well describe the ventriloquist: the man with a thousand hands would become the man with a thousand voices.

His own modified voice seems to come from elsewhere, from a puppet, a ceiling, a basement, a telephone, or simply from his pocket. Ventriloquy is both a technique and an art. It has to do not with lyrical song, comedy, or theatre, but with magic. The ventriloquist is a conjurer of the voice.

His moves are just as important as his text or his improvisations in front of the public he is performing for. He can imitate animals, machinery noises, a child's voice, an adult's voice, an old man's voice. He can create the illusion that someone is locked up in a trunk and that someone else is going to come and set him free, that the door is closing with a spooky grating noise.

But what most impresses us are these voices that intermingle, that interrogate each other, that argue with each other, be it close by or from further afield. Their intermingling transports us into a mysterious universe. Yet the ventriloquist is alone on stage.

Today, this magician of the voice entertains us; yesterday, he was the representative of dark forces, he communicated with the dead who spoke through him and he predicted the future. His body possessed by spirits communicated with the beyond. This occult science was called "necromancy."

Conversing with the gods

From the Holy Book

In the first book on Samuel, we discover the story of King Saul and the sorceress Endor. Saul, terrified of the Philistine army, prays to God, but in vain. A wave of panic engulfs him. At the head of his army, with his thousands of soldiers, he already imagines himself as beaten. In despair and against the teachings of his religion, he consults the most renowned fortune teller of his epoch, Endor. She is known as "She who possesses the *obb*" or "the gift of reading in the minds of the dead." After considerable difficulty, his servants finally locate her.

King Saul and his bodyguards travel southward from Mount Thabor in the night not to raise suspicions. The sorceress lives in a small hamlet on top of the mountain where she exercises her craft. Saul walks toward her rundown house. He enters. He sees the sorceress. He asks her to question the prophet Samuel. The woman's face changes when she sees the King draped in his cape. Indeed, she fears for her life when she recognizes him. He could kill her at any moment, and she is well aware of this. He promises to spare her if she meets his request. She gets up, sees him without seeing him. Her eyes become glazed and she goes into a trance.

Saul asks her: "What do you see?" She answers: "An old man with a coat." Saul tries to recognize in this skimpy description the man who consecrated him as king when he was forty, the prophet Samuel. He insists. He wants to know the prophet's message. A voice from afar answers: "Your army will be beaten by the Philistines. You will lose your scepter." Endor's face is waxen, her lips do not move. Where does the voice come from? Saul laps up the words he's just heard. He listens desperately, almost convincing himself that he can see the ghost of the prophet. In the dark shadows, the sorceress answers the King's questions. Scared of being killed, she explains that she is but a channel between Samuel and him. She insists. "My King, I speak from my stomach that transmits the words to my throat, my lips don't move." Endor, ventriloquist and fortune teller, had just described ventriloquy for the first time to King Saul.

From Greece: the Pythia of Delphi

Hippocrates sketches an explanation of *egastrimitos*. Ventriloquy is the soul's voice uttered by an internal force. People practicing this vocal magic use their thorax more than their stomach. Thus, he repeats the description made in the Bible by Isaac, 29-4. But it is among the oracles that one encounters the powers of these magicians of the voice at their height: the Pythia of Delphi, who rendered Apollo's oracles, was a dark force.

We are in the fifth century BC, at Delphi, on Mount Parnassus, a few hundred kilometers from Athens. Diodorus of Sicily recounts that in certain places in Delphi, steam escapes from the earth. This steam troubles the spirit, perturbs the senses. A shepherd accompanying his flock of goats notices that when the goats approach these vapors, they begin to skip about, to get excited, they make unusual noises, their bleats are different. The gases escaping from these conduits have a particular composition. The shepherd's curiosity isn't satisfied yet. He lowers his head and breathes in this euphorizing steam. It is his turn now to skip about, seized by an uncommon enthusiasm. He has visions and expresses himself in a strange language. "Something divine must exist around these vents!" Indeed, the steam is intoxicating and changes the density of the air. The voice becomes odd, higher.

The news quickly spreads around the country. People like to think that divine intervention is involved. A few unfortunates rush to breathe in these strange vapors. They fall into the vents and die. The decision is taken that a woman shall become its priestess, the Pythia, priestess of the Python. She alone renders the oracles: through her intermediary, Apollo can be questioned, and he answers.

But how is she to breathe these magical ethers without also falling to the bottom of the vent? They make a three-legged stool for her (later, the tripod is considered to be the stool of priestesses and prophets). The stool is placed straddling the vent so that she may better capture the magical ethers.

The Pythia sits on this supreme seat that has a hole in its center. She is swathed in these vapors that have a surprising effect. Some attribute the effects of these essences to the fact that they pass through her most intimate parts, her sex organs. Then she turns into a prophet. Her voice changes. Her timbre is different. She is in trance. But the most stupefying part is yet to come. Her voice comes from elsewhere, her lips do not move. She is a ventriloquist. The gods speak through her. Thus the Delphi oracle was born.

More temples are built. They are made of laurel branches and beeswax. A bronze statue, a dragon called Python, guards the entrance to the temple where Themis, the goddess of Justice, rules. Egastrimitos, the ventriloquist, is practically a god. But through the voices, as really it is not him talking, he can fearlessly transmit the claims of the people and even sometimes oppose himself to reigning politicians. However, the power of the oracles remains of a spiritual order. The Pythia of Delphi is the ventriloquist who was best able to safeguard her secret. This made her impact all the more impressive, all the more powerful. Her mystery remains safe.

Nothing new in 2,000 years of history

The mystery of ventriloquy is going to be pierced in 1770

Two millennia later, at the end of the 18th century, Mr. de la Chapelle, royal censor in Paris, of the Lyon and Rouen Academies and a member of the London society, turns ventriloquy into an art and a technique rather than a mysterious witchcraft. This citizen from Saint-Germain-en-Laye is obsessed with understanding how one can form vowels without moving one's lips, how one can project sound without opening one's mouth. He is desperate to provide a scientific explanation of ventriloquy.

On February 17, 1770, Mr. de Saint-Gilles, aware of de La Chapelle's interest in ventriloquy, ushers him into a shopkeeper's back shop in the vicinity of the Château de Saint-Germain. He stands by the chimney and can't keep his eyes off the ventriloquist who is telling jokes. The ventriloquist falls silent, he looks up at the ceiling and suddenly one hears: "Mr. Abbot de La Chapelle!" The voice comes from far, very far. The Abbott is transfixed, he stares at the ceiling. Stupefied, he asks: "Is that you?" The answer is obvious, yet doubt still lingers. A few seconds go by, then again the voice: "No, don't look this way, look in the opposite direction." He looks down at the parquet floor. His surprise is even greater. This new voice now comes from the floor. Yet the lips of Mr. de Saint-Gilles have not moved. His face has also remained impassive. This meeting between these two characters makes an everlasting impression on Mr. de la Chapelle. One can understand perfectly well the strong impression the Delphi oracles made on the local population a few millennia ago. It is not really magic; no need to conjure up the gods or the scriptures, but the auditory illusion is amazing. But how does the artist pull it off?

Is the ventriloquism magical and diabolical?

The writings of a 17th century doctor, Fabrizio Aquapendene, offer an odd explanation: "Ventriloquists are people who have a well-articulated voice in their stomach and chest, their mouth and lips remaining closed. This isn't natural, it's magical and diabolical." The unknown is always unsettling. The Church remains categorically opposed to any investigation of this strange magic. One has the impression of dealing with the voice of the soul.

A doll in his pocket

Toward the end of the 18th century, on the 20th of March, 1770, another ventriloquist, the Baron von Mengen, from Austria, meets

Mr. de La Chapelle. The baron has a small rag doll in his pocket. He declares: "You bring me unsettling news." To which the rag doll answers: "Mister, slandering is easy." "Miss, don't try to be smart." "Mister, one isn't always free to attack, but one is always entitled to defend oneself." "Shut up!" and the baron returns the rag doll to his pocket. She becomes agitated and murmurs: "How typically male, because men are stronger, they like to think that authority is synonymous with justice."

The rag doll has just come to life. An Irish officer passing by seizes the baron's hand roughly and makes a grab for the pocket the rag doll is in. New moans give the impression that she's choking and squashed. The officer lets go. He thinks it must be an animal. The baron shows the young man that it's just a rag doll in the shape of a coat. The illusion had been perfect. The baron's lips had not moved, his face had expressed compassion for the doll. The quickness of the repartees between the doll and the baron had reinforced the illusion.

The baron had used two kinds of magical voices: one close to us when the doll was in the open pocket (the *near voice*), and another that seemed farther away, when the doll was choking and was "locked up" (the *distant voice*).

At the time, all sorts of hypotheses were put forward. People thought it must be a gift, or done with the lips, the teeth, the esophagus. When the baron is asked for his version, he seems to think it quite natural. He considers it a vocal art that deceives. His doll enables him to say what he can't say in person and gives him the freedom to be impertinent. The movements of his hand must be extremely fast and evoke feelings. His left hand holds the doll, and he forms its voice between his cheeks, tongue, and teeth. He doesn't have the impression that his tummy and stomach have to make any special effort, and they don't articulate any sounds. He stresses lingual mobility and breathing, also the rhythm he imposes on himself to establish the dialogue between the doll and "himself."

A closely kept secret

How is one to analyze these vocal mechanics in this game of questions and answers? Magic and technical skill are inseparable. In those days, research was difficult, there was no instrument yet with which to observe the ventriloquist's voice during his vocal utterances.

The fascination is at its height in 1876, when Fred Nieman performs with seven puppets. He therefore has eight different voices. The theatrics are amazing. His own voice gives the repartee to the seven characters he has created.

The whole art of ventriloquy consists in creating another voice from one's own voice. The ventriloquist mystifies, amuses, distracts, intrigues. He transports us into a different universe.

Freddy arrives with his tutor Christian: but who is doing what?

Christian adopts Freddy the puppet

Christian enters my office, sits down. Intrigued, I ask him how he got the idea for his puppet, Freddy, a mischievous monkey. Christian has been fascinated with ventriloquy from the age of twelve. A circus arrives in town. He attends every single performance during a week. A small chimpanzee, a live one, fascinates him. It wasn't something he could easily procure for himself. So he decides to "adopt" Freddy. His talent for ventriloquy is already known at his school. But while he explains this, Freddy is becoming impatient. He is already in place in Christian's right hand. Although Christian is as impatient as I am to discover "the double voice," he makes a few mimics that denote apprehension. "Are you going to hurt him?" Freddy asks. I'm taken by surprise, I wasn't expecting to hear him at all. Christian's lips haven't moved. "No, I won't hurt him. But don't you warm your voice up, Christian?" "He doesn't need to," Freddy answers, nodding his head, "he's too eager to hear my voice." The complicity between Freddy and Christian is baffling. It plunges us right into the heart of the matter.

The explorer and the ventriloquist

I prepare for a dynamic vocal exploration. I pass the endovideoscope into the nasal fossa and slip it through to the back of the throat past the uvula down to the roof of the larynx. This rare examination will reveal the ventriloquist's phonatory mechanism. The scope passes above the mouth, through the nose. Therefore, it doesn't interfere with the movements of his lips, tongue, jaw, or laryngeal muscles. Christian is able to talk or sing with his mouth closed; he can laugh or cough. The internal imagery of his vocal instrument will be snapped by this numeric technique. The secrets of this multiple voice are within our reach, at least I hope so (see Plate 26).

We are ready. The recording can start. Our approach is that of a detective hunting for the slightest clue, the slightest vibratory print left by Freddy or Christian. Freddy talks, he creates his own voice. Christian is the master of ceremony. Whether it is Christian or Freddy talking, the ventriloquist or his puppet, the contraction of the abdominal muscles is striking. In seasoned professional ventriloquists it's hardly visible, but in novices, their respiratory control obliges them to pause when they switch from one voice to another.

The five signs of the artist

First sign: the same exhalation, whether it's Freddy or Christian

I am struck by the speed of repartee between Freddy and Christian. They almost give the impression of speaking at the same time. Indeed, they use the same exhalation when Christian becomes Freddy and vice versa. There is no pause in between. Moreover, the inhalation is used to voice certain phonemes, dampened for sure, but perfectly intelligible. One could almost say that there is no silence between the two voices. The avalanche of words, the gestures, the stillness of the lips, then their mobility, all are key aspects of his talent and require exceptional respiratory and pharyngolaryngeal efforts.

- At times, Freddy gives us the impression of being in apnea, and blocks his Adam's apple. The hyoid bone is practically sticking to the mandible. The small muscle between the thyroid and cricoid cartilages contracts violently, which accentuates the height of the larynx. All the neck muscles are contracted.

- Christian talks, all seems relaxed and natural. But the difference between the two is hardly perceptible if you aren't forewarned.

Second sign: the vocal instrument, framework of the laryngeal acrobat

Freddy speaks. His internal landscape is surprising. All the muscles inside his throat are working at full throttle.

- The laryngeal muscles, the lateral muscles of the soft palate and the uvula play a preponderant role. They tighten and give this part of the pharynx a tubelike appearance.

- The master of this enclave is the tongue. The dome of the tongue lightly abuts the soft palate, without making proper contact. The tip of the tongue does not touch the top row of teeth either. It stays 1 to 2 mm behind them. Thus, the voicing can come out through the nose or through the mouth, giving whoever is listening, a distorted sense of its direction, which adds to the ventriloquist's powers of illusion. All these elements are put to work in perfect synchronicity and in the record time of one-tenth to one-fifteenth of a second.

Now Christian talks. The muscles change. The larynx becomes normal again, so to speak.

- It looks like an upside-down cornet once more.

- The tongue resumes its central position; it no longer pulls the larynx upward. The lips move normally again. Then, as the game of questions and answers with Freddy progresses, the process starts all over again.

Observation of the larynx using videofibroscopy is completed with three-dimensional radiology imagery. Thus, the work carried out in Paris with Doctors Albert Castro and Rodolphe Gombergh gives us a better understanding of the workings of the vocal apparatus of Christian and other ventriloquists, and of its muscular, articular, and osseous functions. Observing with a scanner, we are at liberty to focus on any specific tissue.

- We catch the muscular contractions of the tongue and pharynx, of the soft palate and lips, by modifying the transparency index.

- We reveal the jointed agility of the membrane between the thyroid and the cricoid cartilages, between the cricoid and arytenoids, within that astonishing bony trampoline, the hyoid bone, from which the heads of the lingual muscles surge upward.

I'm beginning to get a sense of ventriloquy's armature. It is taking shape.

Third sign: head voice for Freddy and chest voice for Christian

The vocal cords vibrate the same way for Freddy or his master.

- The only difference is that they are shorter when Freddy speaks, which is to be expected, as the doll speaks in a head voice that's more highly pitched than the ventriloquist's.

- Frequently, to make Freddy speak, Christian passes from the chest voice (which is a man's normal speaking voice) to the head voice, with the larynx tipped up and the voice highly perched.

- This new vocal register is accompanied by a complete change in the artist's attitude. The physical vocal profile alters as he passes from one to the other.

Spectrography provides analyses of the different acoustic prints and the speed with which the ventriloquist switches from Freddy's head voice to Christian's chest voice. In a few fifteenths of a second, two distinct spectral identities are formed, and yet they are one and the same.

The ventriloquist's lung capacity is comparable to that of great singers or great tragedians.

- The paradox here is that Freddy and Christian have two different voices, both created by the same instrument, using two different techniques and two different languages. It is the vibration of the vocal cords that gives life to Freddy's voice or to Christian's voice.

- The ventriloquist never uses his esophageal voice, a voice well known to people who have been operated on for cancer of the larynx and who no longer have a larynx with which to speak. They swallow air into their stomach and somehow exhale it to make their esophageal outlet vibrate. The resonance chamber does the rest.

- Freddy speaks: the exhalation phase is slow, it lasts over 15 seconds. The diaphragm is perfectly controlled to produce this impressively slow exhalation. This enables him to modulate the voice, but more than that, it gives him time to position the muscles of the resonators that will shape the second voice.

- Christian speaks: his phonatory exhalation lasts between 7 and 10 seconds. His muscular resistance is that of an athlete.

We now understand better the mystery of the ventriloquist mechanism: this incredible "compression" of the pharyngolaryngeal muscles. It's at its maximum in the far voice, or *distant* voice, that requires tremendous subglottic, then supraglottic strength and energy. The breathing is still abdominal, but with a fair share of thoracic and diaphragmatic breathing. This muscular mechanism imposes a well-oiled neuronal control. The permanent interplay between the ventriloquist's voice and the puppet's voice demonstrates the amazing agility of this contortionist.

Fourth sign: to manipulate vowels and consonants, cheating is often necessary

The formation of vowels and consonants depends on the shape of the buccopharyngeal and respiratory tract. This contortionist of the larynx owes his talent to his fast neurologic control over this zone, and to his lung capacity. (A reminder: the mechanical control of the pharyngolaryngeal space is governed by cranial nerves XII, V, IX, X, and VII, and the mechanical control of breathing is governed by the spinal nerves that govern the thorax, abdomen, and pelvis muscles.)

The ventriloquist can't form all the vowels and consonants the same way, so how can he cheat?

Whereas Christian smacks his lips together to voice consonants, Freddy can't benefit from this gesture. The most problematic consonants are *p*, *b*, *f*, and *m*. These professionals find *c*, *d*, *g*, *k*, *n*, *q*, *s*, and *x* relatively straightforward; whereas articulating *r*, *t*, *v*, and *z* is a bit trickier.

A genuine language evolves for the puppet: *b*arrier becomes *v*arrier. *F*ormidable becomes *h*ormidable. Your brain immediately corrects the fraudulent letter. When Freddy sings "The singer from Mexico," he pronounces it—*N*exico, but the auditory illusion is perfect, you hear "Mexico."

Lack of practice during a period of a month or so will handicap the ventriloquist. Emitting vowels is the foundation of the ventriloquist voice. They have to be clearly intelligible, yet while the ventriloquist's face must be expressive, his lips must not move and neither must his jaw. This may seem simple enough; however, the real problem starts when consonants and phonemes have to be pronounced, and worse still, when the two voices begin their game of Ping-Pong.

"Le Corbeau et le Renard": a second language

Father Rex brought to our attention a ventriloquy exercise used since 1944: it consists in reciting "Le Corbeau et le Renard" (the fable of the crow and the fox) in ventriloquy. The title becomes "Le Cor*b*eau et le Renard."

> "*N*aître Cor*b*eau sur un ar*b*re *h*erché
> —Instead of *M*aître Cor*b*eau sur un ar*b*re *p*erché
>
> Tenait en son *b*ec un *h*romage.
> —Instead of Tenait en son *b*ec un *f*romage.
>
> *N*aître Renard, *h*ar l'odeur alléché,
> —Instead of *M*aître Renard, *p*ar l'odeur alléché,
>
> Lui tint à *h*eu *h*rès ce language:
> —Instead of lui tint à *p*eu *p*rès ce language

Hé! *h*onjour, *n*onsieur du Cor*h*eau!
—Instead of Hé! *B*onjour, *M*onsieur du Cor*b*eau!

The ventriloquist learns what amounts to a second language. His reflex, when the puppet is speaking, is to replace certain consonants with others that are so close to the original ones that you don't notice the switch. Indeed, when Freddy recites for us this fable of the Crow and the Fox, we understand him perfectly. We substitute the missing consonants instinctively, subconsciously. Our left brain will understand and decode words that aren't actually those pronounced by the ventriloquist. Our left brain is able to decode these words because we know them already. We anticipate Freddy's recital. Thus, to make the illusion possible, the ventriloquist uses well-known popular songs and poems.

What we understand is more important than what we hear: the auditory illusion is based on a readjustment on our part that can go as far as verbal anticipation. But this is only possible because the sham phoneme occurs in a context that is comprehensible. It is only a link in a chain, one element in the sentence that we perceive, one element of the sense we are going to give this sentence; it's one of our phantom phonemes. (Remember the "*slide room* and *glide room*" in chapter 7 on Voice and language)

Two characters, two different languages

Thus, there are really two characters (two languages) inhabiting the artist, each with its own pharyngolaryngeal mechanism, its own characteristic phonemes, its own spoken and sung musicality. The singing voice in ventriloquy is a real technical feat as it requires the laryngeal mobility we have seen in the singer, great suppleness, and the ability to work in whatever register the ventriloquist decides to display.

Fifth sense: Freddy's teeth

The role played by our dental articulation is essential in ventriloquy: no teeth, no ventriloquist. Teeth are a pillar of our articulated language. Christian immobilizes his lips against his teeth when

Freddy interrupts him. If the dentition is altered, it alters the jaw's articulation in such a way that the emission of vowels and consonants can no longer be controlled with the required precision. The tongue can no longer place itself for the ventriloquy. Buccodental hygiene is key to avoid losing teeth, which would cause the jaw to decalcify in the longer term. It seems that if necessary, dental implants are the best solution for Freddy to avoid the risk of premature vocal aging.

Hydration for muscular strength

During this exercise, I pointed out to our ventriloquist the importance of hydration and lubrication for his vocal instrument, crucial for him given the importance of muscular and labial suppleness to the practice of his art. This level of technical agility is only possible if the degree of lubrication allows the muscles to slide and the epithelium of the vocal cords to vibrate without any previous warm-up. He also needs to wet his lips with water and moisten them regularly, because in the space of fifteen minutes, the mucous membranes of the lips and tongue dehydrate and the exercise then becomes practically impossible.

To see and to hear, who is the fastest: the cards or the echo

Examining, explaining, observing a ventriloquist is no easy endeavor. We must be wary of the mystery element. We must respect the prodigal performer. We must try to catch him in the subtleties of his art. We must unmask him when he switches from his own voice to the puppet's voice. It is a road with obstacles that we must decode.

The ventriloquist's gaze

The ventriloquist sets traps for us. Hanging on his every word, we are riveted by his talk. But we have to admit that we don't believe our eyes. Just add to this maxim: "you only believe what you hear," and the illusion is in the bag! But in this case, seeing and hearing overlap; they're separate, yet intimately connected. Our eyes, our ears scrutinize the puppet or the ventriloquist, never both. The illusion is perfect. We pass from one to the other in a few tenths of a second. Who is speaking, the puppet or the artist? Who answers, who questions, who is the genuine one, if there is one. Both characters are sincere. Is this a hoax, or is it merely the juxtaposition of two authentic protagonists?

He is two or more

The artist is at the height of his art when there is perfect harmony between his gestures and his *voices*. His right hand manipulates the puppet. He remains facing his public. His lips never move. His face, his eyes look surprised when the puppet talks. Christian cocks his head as if to better hear Freddy. And in a fraction of a second, the repartee is given.

This technical talent gives a perfect illusion of the two characters. The artist becomes "a double voice." This split-off in the cerebral integration of the voice is remarkable. This double voice exists only because it is supported by a double cerebral projection of the characters played.

We are systematically duped. Our hearing is slower than his lips. Our eyes are guided, oriented, controlled even by the artist's eyes. Consequently, our ear is mistaken as to the direction of the sound. Our hearing is not precise enough, especially when we're ten meters away from the ventriloquist. The exact identification of the origin of the emitted voicing solicits our vision, which now completes our imperfect hearing.

A real illusion

Normally, when we speak our lips move. I look at you, I hear you, and I associate the movement of your lips to the sounds I'm hearing. Therefore, I know it's you speaking. This illusion is well known in televised playback. On stage, your vision and hearing help you recognize where a sound is coming from. The ventriloquist speaks using the timbre of his choice. He is always intelligible, easy to comprehend, whether it's him or his puppet talking. He deceives your ear. His face isn't expressionless, he looks at his puppet with a questioning look. Freddy's gestures, the mobility of his lips, the surprised expression of the artist as he listens, head cocked toward the little chimpanzee, all contribute to perfect the illusion. Like Christian, we watch Freddy. Like him, we acquiesce with or share what he says. The magic is total.

When a magician does a card trick, his hand is faster than our eyes. Here, the ventriloquist's voice goes faster than our ear's ability to perceive the direction of sound. Indeed, the trajectory of the acoustic waves associates itself with the trajectory of our gaze. One could almost say that we listen with our eyes. The artist exploits this. But this artist is not alone on stage, his puppet is also an artist in its own right. He lets him talk. He breathes words into him. This private conversation between the two of them rapidly becomes a game of threesome with the public.

The magic casts its spell

- Christian asks his puppet Freddy: "How are you?"

- Silence: he looks at Freddy. The puppet starts to move. It doesn't open its lips. It looks at him. It moves. And just when Freddy's lips are about to open, Christian's vocal instrument is going to spring into action and Freddy will speak. Christian still looks questioningly at Freddy, his lips don't move. He comes closer to Freddy, opens his eyes wide, pretending he can't understand.

- When Freddy answers "Yes, I'm fine, why shouldn't I be, what about you, how are you?" The dialogue is now established.

- The spectator is trapped. He's a witness; he even identifies with the puppet for whom he will develop a soft spot. The more so since Freddy will also question the spectators. The magician of the voice has won the round. He has created a trio: puppet—ventriloquist—spectator.

The ventriloquist can never be caught. Indeed, he has extended his active visual field. When he exhibits Freddy on stage, his concentration and mobility are such that his field of vision is almost 360°. This observation was brought to me by other professionals such as James Hodges, Ron Lucas, or Valentine Vox, whose writings are classics in the field.

The ventriloquist uses his voice to dress up his puppet. He transfers to it emotion, a personality, a lifelike impression. The changes of tonality in its voice, its laughter, its tears will animate the game that is developing out of this double personality of the ventriloquist. Like any of us, he will call upon his brain's language areas.

All the ventriloquists that I have been able to observe have a common denominator: a perfect mastery of the two, even three, or four voices they use. The speed with which they switch from one to the other in their question-and-answer game is mind blowing, just amazing. When the dialogue gets going between the puppet and the ventriloquist, between Freddy and Christian, we are under their spell. But, paradoxically, and this impressed me, Christian isn't quite himself either when the little chimp is there.

Las Vegas . . . and the puppets come to life

Is there a dualism of the brain? Does ventriloquy require an apprenticeship from childhood? Is there a physical or intellectual predisposition for it? Is it a gift, or a quest for one's inner self? I got the answers to my questions in Las Vegas, in April 2001.

Ventriloquists are in the room, the doctor is on stage

At the end of the day, I arrive at the hotel in which a world congress of ventriloquists has been organized, in the center of the city of lights. The next day, around 10 AM, I am to deliver a presentation to an audience of ventriloquists. For once, the roles are reversed. I will be on stage and they will be in the hall.

I arrive in the ballroom. The hall is packed. Several hundred heads follow me from my chair to the stage. I greet them. The audience is impressive, silent and expectant, possibly wondering whether I am about to reveal their well-kept secret. I begin with a scientific exposé of the ventriloquy "phenomenon," backed by images and films. To my delight, they are fascinated, intrigued, surprised. The medical and anatomical world doesn't awe them. I have the impression I'm explaining to violinists the functional aspects of violin and bow. Their questioning eyes seem to be finding the answers to queries that have been without answer for too long.

Ventriloquists are protected by their puppets

After my presentation, Valentine Vox, the international president of the ventriloquists, asks if there are any questions. And then, believe it or not, nearly every ventriloquist brings a puppet out of a pocket, a bag, or a box. Within a few seconds, we find ourselves with twice as many characters in the room. Everyone is feverishly manipulating his or her puppet to make it ask a question.

A Mexican ventriloquist begins, but it's his puppet that does the talking, as if protecting him from his shyness. "Chico senior, says the puppet, my lifelong friend has been a ventriloquist since he was very young. Is it a gift?" I answer that the apprenticeship of ventriloquy since childhood is indispensable to facilitate the required cerebral activation and to train the larynx. Even if the gift appears later, a predisposition exists.

The ventriloquist is a multilingual interpreter

Moreover, my hypothesis—and it seems to me to correspond most closely with reality—is to consider the ventriloquist as a bilingual interpreter, someone who masters two languages. Despite the similarities, each language has its own vowels and consonants. Freddy and Christian can't always use the same consonants for the same words. Two different mechanical strategies for speech are needed. Indeed, at a conference or in a televised live transmission, the interpreter listens to what the speaker has to say, and then, within a few tenths of a second, translates the speaker's words simultaneously. The interpreter has controlled his brain in two different directions: for reception and for transmission, with extremely short latency. This faculty requires regular practice. These professionals' concentration is remarkable, and they translate into their mother tongue, of which they master perfectly the syntax and linguistic subtleties.

Does this not come close to what the ventriloquist does? I must also point out that given the resonators required for this art of the voice and of magic, a good ventriloquist must have reached puberty.

A passion and a vocation: not a job

As it happens, Chico junior is present with a small elephant for a puppet. He is four-and-a-half years old. Imagine my surprise to find that this child is already a ventriloquist. Chico, or more precisely his elephant, Dumbo, speaks to me with determination and vigor. "Of course I'm Dumbo, and my master is the ventriloquist Chico junior, who is like his father, his mother, and his grandfather: all ventriloquists." His lips barely move. I ask him to speak in his own voice. His tone is timid, awkward, uncertain. What duality since childhood! But recall when we were children we also made our toys talk; it was a form of liberation for us. Chico and his friends, Indy and Lorry, are ventriloquist children. Embarrassed, I was not sure what to answer, other than to draw an analogy with the bilingual child: Chico had acquired almost two mother tongues, his own and Dumbo's, borrowed from his father or his mother when he saw them and heard them rehearsing. In fact, once more, it was their environment in a very cohesive ventriloquist family that had provided these children with two forms of language from early childhood.

An adult resonance chamber is not a prerequisite to take up this profession and art form, to perform on stage. The suppleness of these children, especially Chico, the young ventriloquist, was astonishing. His dialogues with his puppets, the agility of his duo were as good as those of any adult ventriloquist.

Questions were still shooting back and forth, always asked by the puppets. All these ventriloquists whom I was lucky enough to meet, hailing from China, India, Japan, the United States, Germany, Belgium, or France, had started working at their gift around the age of five or six. Most of them had come from a circus or magician background. Indeed, being a ventriloquist is like being a singer or a theatrical actor. It isn't a job, it's a passion and a vocation. One or two were dilettante ventriloquists: one was a doctor, another a schoolteacher, the third a lawyer. Imagine in a court of law, having the means to make anyone you wish take the floor with the words of your choice!

The backstage of the ventriloquist:
he creates lips behind lips

Warming-up session and the center of the gravity of the voice

After the conference, that same night, the ventriloquists invited me into the wings of their show world. Before their entry on stage, they prepare themselves. Christian warms up his voice for nearly ten minutes, doing voicing with his mouth closed, then vocalizing vowels with his mouth open, finally practicing yawning exercises to help tune up the muscles of his neck, abdomen, and resonance chamber. Stretches, flexions, and extensions of the cervical verte-brae, deep breathing inhaling and exhaling, movements of the wrist and fingers to warm up the muscles that are going to bring the puppet to life, such are the muscular scales that the ventrilo-quist perforce practices before every show. In addition, he tries to loosen his back to find the center of gravity of his voice. Holding a puppet offsets the ventriloquist's vocal verticality and can cause physical asymmetries. These maintenance exercises are crucial to avoid getting into bad habits that are later difficult to correct. By warming and hydrating his voice, then the puppet's voice, the ventriloquist will avoid any hitches, or a pulled vocal cord muscle that can cause a muscular hematoma.

And, thus, it came about that I witnessed a most extraordinary demonstration of ventriloquy in a small theatre in Las Vegas (seating no more than 200 spectators). The top professionals were gathered in this temple of ventriloquy.

Two techniques of ventriloquy

Two ventriloquy techniques face up to each other. On stage, two ventriloquists and two puppets face off. The *near voice* and the *distant voice*. I closely observe the artist at work. Bearing the morning's questions in mind, I'm keen to solve the enigma of these two techniques.

But how do these techniques work? The mystery was still unsolved.

The near voice

When the ventriloquist uses his near voice, the puppet is close to him. He has the impression that his voice pierces his skin, comes from his neck, that it is a throat voice or a head voice. Yet we know that the voice is in fact more internal. It stops just before the teeth, before the lips. It is slightly more nasal that his normal voice, because it is produced in a higher register.

I was watching the pharyngolaryngeal Lego taking shape, as I had done during the fibroscopic examination of Christian. The larynx rises and falls very quickly.

Make-up of the near voice:

- It is produced by positioning the tongue in a particular way. When Christian speaks normally, his tongue is flat, the voicings pass over it, one could say, mostly flowing through the mouth and lips, partially through the nose.

- When the artists speaks using ventriloquy, he inverses these forces by arching his tongue and rounding the base of the tongue, thus bringing it into contact with the uvula and the posterior part of the soft palate.

- The tongue is shaped like a dome at the back, in contact with the soft palate. The tip of the tongue is relatively low, two to three millimeters from the lower teeth.

- Thus, the vibrations flow mostly through the nose and only partially through the mouth. This dual exit via the nose and mouth creates ambiguity in that the spectator can't tell very well where the sound is coming from, and this reinforces the sense of illusion. You can get an idea of this by pronouncing the letter *G*, as in *Gang*. This is why many puppets have a nasal voice.

Being able to switch rapidly to this alternative lingual position is something the ventriloquist has to practice over and over.

Good control of the lips also comes from regular practice. He rehearses mostly in front of a mirror. However, occasionally, if tired, he will turn his head slightly to fake the consonants *b*, *p*, *f*, *m*, *v*.

The vowels can only be produced by contorting the tongue and the buccopharyngeal muscles.

I had just understood one aspect of the enigma of how the ventriloquist forms words: he creates lips behind his lips.

The distant voice

His operational mode is different.

Make-up of the distant voice:

- He curls his tongue inside his mouth to enable the sound to echo.

- He creates a buzz, in other words a movement to and fro of the harmonics, in his buccal cavity. The voice is dampened. The vocal cords shorten, but are very rounded, and the timbre is relatively high-pitched.

- The pharyngeal muscles on each side of the larynx contract violently.

- The hyoid bone rises and is almost level with the mandible.

- The tongue is almost clamped to the roof of the mouth.

- The larynx tips forward. The frequency of the voice is variable, deep or high. It is like a breathy voice.

- Thanks to the tongue, the resonators are able to create a second resonance chamber inside the mouth, hence the echo. Due to this double resonance, the voice seems to come from elsewhere, from the depths of the abyss, from the ceiling, from the other side of the wall. The timbre is low and muffled.

- Here too, the ventriloquist creates lips behind his lips thanks to the shape he gives his tongue and to its position in relation to the soft palate and uvula.

- The contraction of the abdominal muscles is an important facilitator of his excellent control over the phonatory exhalation.

Back to Las Vegas: I witness ventriloquists' prowess

These technical skills are crucial in both ventriloquy approaches. But on stage, the ventriloquists weave a game of pretense between them, the puppets, and this public of professionals, who, despite knowing all the tricks of the trade, get caught up in the illusion, are moved, laugh to tears, and get fired up every time a character intervenes.

Then, suddenly, there are no puppets. Only the ventriloquist's gaze: he looks up, he cocks his head, his stage accomplice, the other ventriloquist, does the same, so do you. He asks: "Who is there?" His face sets and you hear: "It's me, I'm on the first floor." His whole body is angled toward the ceiling; you do likewise. The voice magician is at the height of his art! The same subterfuges will be used for a voice that comes from the floor or from behind the door or from his pocket, but without the help of a rag doll.

How to become a ventriloquist: agile brain and muscles

The ventriloquist is a bodybuilder of the larynx

The ventriloquist is used to working his muscles, joints, and phonation from childhood on. He trains his vocal suppleness, his cerebral, phonatory, and auditory agility; his memory, the speed with which he adapts from the different voices he wants to create to his own voice and back again, endow him with spectacular dexterity. But nearly all ventriloquists adhere to a healthy way of life.

The apprenticeship of ventriloquy can be compared to that of diplophonic singing. The very essence of the puppet's voice is the vibration of the vocal cords. The larynx is the ventriloquist's music instrument. The warm-up exercise known as "the bumblebee" enables him to recognize the different positions of his buccal and laryngeal muscles.

Pseudolips are created behind the lips using the tongue, the palate, and the other pharyngeal muscles. But the mandible barely moves, and this is very hard to pull off. It comes as no surprise, therefore, that one observes in ventriloquists a hypertrophied lingual muscle, powerful ligaments between the epiglottis and the arytenoids, hyperdeveloped pharyngeal muscles, and an exceptional mobility of the soft palate, the epiglottis, the tongue, of course, but also the vocal cords. These characteristics give the ventriloquist the appearance of a bodybuilder of the larynx. As a result the adaptation of these internal pseudolips for each phoneme is one of the keys of the mystery of the ventriloquist.

He needs a "double" common sense

This agility is not purely mechanical, it's also cerebral, as we've seen by analogy with the universe of bilingual children and the apprenticeship of simulated phonemes (cor*b*eau instead of cor*b*eau). To maintain a high standard of ventriloquy, vocal practice and the stimulation of memory and linguistic gestures are essential. The magic of the sounds, the game of the actor, the power of his gaze, the manipulation of the rag doll are the indispensable trump cards of these dream artists.

This magician of vibration makes us dream, yet his impressive agility has still not been entirely elucidated. His theatrical art and magic transport our spirit into the intangible dimension of the illusion of harmony.

Chapter 21

The parrot, both imitator and ventriloquist

It's in Man's nature to speak, it's in the parrot's to repeat.

My interest in parrots is somewhat unusual. It is often said that we speak with our lips. To gain a better understanding of ventriloquy, I decided to observe the parrot. Indeed, what could be more incredible than a talking beak?

The bird, a relic from the dinosaur

Birds appeared on our planet relatively recently, less than 100 million years ago. Their apparition is probably a consequence of the evolution of these fascinating reptiles that are the dinosaurs. The takeoff of an albatross is a throwback to a very distant past.

But what reptilian form can have given birth to birds? What magic enabled them to fly, and in some cases, to speak?

In birds, feathers have taken the place of scales. These feathers allow the body to remain warm. Although we know of many more extinct species of mammals and reptiles than we do live ones, thanks to the remarkable conservation of their skeletons, we have observed only 500 bird fossils out of over 20,000 known species of birds. Birds become fossilized with difficulty.

The very first bird, the one that shows us his dinosaur origins unequivocally, is *Arcgaeornis*, which appeared some 10 million years ago. He is a biped. His coat is feathered like a bird's. His cranium is already a bird's cranium. Yet his bones aren't pneumatic. He was examined for the first time in the 19th century, in Blumenberg, Germany. He presents two distinct cerebral hemispheres. When H. von Meyer discovered him in 1861, he understood that he was looking at the missing link between dinosaurs and birds.

Numerous discussions liven up the living rooms of paleontologists. In 1982, research by Gardiner discusses the descent of birds in relation to dinosaurs and reptiles. Indeed, at the end of the 19th century, Huxley's opinion that the bird descends from dinosaurs and crocodiles is generally accepted. In the 1980s, Gardiner simply observes that on a biological level, birds are very close to mammals: their body temperature is constant (homeothermia), the structure of their cerebellum is similar, their central nervous system is surrounded by a protective sheath (the pia mater) and by an arachnoidean layer in the meninges, the pineal gland is an autonomous endocrine gland. Finally, myoglobin, an essential structure, is also present in birds and shows many similarities with the myoglobin of mammals, but not of reptiles.

The parrot's cerebral power is on a scale with that of mammals, but this doesn't apply to all birds, far from it. The exact origin of the bird remains debatable, although numerous specialists in this field favor the extinct reptilian monster.

The brain and the bird

A bird's brain: far superior to reptiles'

The structure of the brain and nervous system is generally one of the most representative expressions of animal evolution, as we have observed along our voyage. The body of birds, the richness of their behavior, the ease with which they adapt, their differentiation, highly evolved in some cases, and notably, their capacity for learning how to speak, are indicative of the surprising variety in the central nervous system of certain species.

Like the mammal, birds have a spine with marrow, a spinal column with a cervical, thoracic, lumbosacral, and coccygeal portion. Their brain is far superior to reptiles'. The ratio is one to ten. The cerebral hemispheres are developed, but the cortex is small. It presents no circumvolutions.

In birds, the main cerebral function is reproduction. We have witnessed the complexity of the nuptial dances of some species. The annex centers near the brainstem are mainly concerned with vision. As in mammals, the cerebellum allows them to coordinate their movements, it regulates their balance and muscle tonus. However, proportionally it is much smaller than in mammals.

Birds must learn to sing, just as Man must learn to speak

Like Man, birds have to go through a learning process. Yet one observation is pertinent only to birds: the size of the brain and its specificity show extraordinary variability. This is not true of primates. Parrots, for example, are endowed with the most developed hemispheres of their species. Proportionally, their brain is eight times bigger than a hen's. This makes it easier for us to understand how it is that certain species of birds are good talkers or good singers, and that these specific activities can have created privileged connections and oriented their development toward whatever function they most used, which is certainly a form of intelligence. In this development, the ear will play a fundamental role for parrots. They will only be able to reproduce sounds they've heard. Birds don't chatter. Primitive song will not develop in deaf birds. It seems, therefore, that the ontogenesis of bird song is necessary to enable its apparition.

Does Man descend from the parrot?

The human child, the chimpanzee, and the parrot

For some fifty years, we've witnessed an odd infatuation for comparing the great ape with Man. It is true, there is a certain unquestionable physical resemblance, and certain attitudes and behaviors can seem comparable. Yet one of the animals closest to the human child is without doubt the Gray parrot.

Speaking is specific to Man's nature, but not exclusively so! It is also specific to the Gray parrot, and he is the most gifted of his species in this respect. DNA's evolution, all these dozen of millions of years, in no way gave rise to suppose that the parrot, descended from dinosaurs, would one day speak. Is it simply a conditioning, a derivative of the Pavlovian reflex or does the parrot merely stubbornly repeat after us? Is this just a learning aptitude? The first experiments tested his mathematical abilities, then his language abilities. He is an excellent pupil. "He" learns remarkably well. Like Man, he sulks, he can be bad-tempered. He stops eating and becomes depressed. But he can also be happy and playful, displaying a remarkable form of intelligence.

The Gray parrot learns mathematics

In 1959, Logler demonstrates that the Gray parrot is able to learn elementary math and do arithmetic, which requires concentration and a short-term memory. In 1976, Premack carried out similar tests among primates, with only relative success.

The Gray parrot, with his considerable powers of concentration, can stay perfectly still watching the world go by. He imitates and plays in the true sense of the word, like dolphins do.

Most of the Gray parrot's performances are close to those of a three-year-old child. He sorts objects, calculates succinctly. He creates sentences. But he cannot create a voice. He remains an imitator, a clever one, true, and playful with it, but his language will never produce an idea, nor will he subsequently translate this idea into his spoken language. He can't create new words and hardly any new associations between words.

He speaks, yes, but how?

Two larynges for the parrot?

But how can he speak? What organ enables this function? We have only had the answer to this since the end of the 1990s.

All birds have a syrinx, equivalent to our larynx. Its conformation is unique in the animal kingdom. We may say that the male Gray parrot has two "larynges," more exactly, a larynx combined with a syrinx. Sound is produced in the syrinx and modulated in the larynx. This pseudolarynx is located at the top of the trachea, just below the tongue; the syrinx sits below the trachea. The trachea, thus, separates them (see Plate 27).

In Greek mythology, Syrinx was the companion of Artemis. This nymph was courted by Pan. She couldn't allow herself to fall for his charm. To escape from him, she drowned herself. Zeus, god of the gods, transformed her into a bed of reeds. Pan created his flute—the Pan pipe—from these reeds to play melodies to her and palliate his sadness. His melancholy was a heavy burden for him. Henceforth, the flute was called a syrinx.

The syrinx

The syrinx is located level with the two lungs, at the point where they join the trachea. The junction between each lung and the trachea meets a system of muscles and membranes that cause vibration when they move closer to each other. A pseudovocal cord attached to this junction creates the sound. Here, only nine to twelve muscles are required. Each fold vibrates independently, on the left and on the right. Each element, on either side, is connected to its respective lung.

The singing or talking bird, therefore, produces two vibratory sounds, either in the same frequency, or in two different frequencies. This acoustic information creates a sinusoid wave that reaches our ear and gives us the vibratory illusion of a human voice. However, in parrots, as described for us by Warren, one can make out just at the back of the tongue a sort of larynx and a glottic space above the trachea. Thus, the column of air in the trachea, trapped between the larynx at the top and the syrinx below, forms a resonator that is in addition to the first one. This structure fundamentally differentiates the Gray parrot from Man.

The Jew's harp: a synthetic parrot

A strange instrument, but essential to understanding the secret of the mechanism behind the parrot's voice, the Jew's harp, or jaw's harp, is formed by a rigid half-ring within which a finger provokes the vibration of a metallic lamina. It is held between the teeth. Its small tongue is always of the same width and always has the same vibratory rhythm. The resonance cavity is not after the vibration (as it is in the human larynx), but before the vibration.

The Jew's harp is held between the teeth; therefore, its resonance cavity is the mouth. By moving the tongue, by modifying the shape of one's cheeks, palate, or lips, one can create different overtones and, therefore, a melody.

Yet the metal lamina is always the same length, and the finger that sets up the vibration of the lamina has the same original strength. It is the different lengths and shapes of the resonators that create the different frequencies. The metallic lamina itself hardly generates any sound, unless it is amplified by a resonator that receives the vibration. The vibratory dispersion produced by this metallic lamina dies in the aerial space around it if it doesn't encounter an amplifier. On its own, this vibration is too weak to be heard.

However, the vibration is perfectly audible when amplified. An amplifier, in this instance the buccopharyngeal cavity, is indispensable.

The beak is rigid, like the lips of the ventriloquist, and it says vowels

How can spoken language be possible without lips? The parrot's larynx and resonators aren't at all comparable with those of other animals. They are also different from Man's. Until now, control of the larynx and of the resonance chamber by the brain with its neuronal connections was thought to be specific to Man.

Numerous researchers spent years trying to make the chimpanzee, the animal closest to Man, speak. Their repeated attempts all ended in failure. The chimp does not talk! He looks like he should, though. But the parrot, with a vocal apparatus so different from ours, does speak. The most exhaustive research on Gray parrots was carried out by Irene Pepperberg.

With the help of the scanner and spectrography, the veil has almost completely lifted

Toward the end of the 1990s, the mystery of parrot speech is pierced. Alex can talk; therefore, he controls his vocal tract, his mechanism, his expression, with his brain. He pronounces words with consonants and vowels. He seems gifted for a certain grammar. With the help of techniques such as the scanner and magnetic resonance, the vocal mechanism of this parrot is better understood now. It is a complex process.

In Man, the vocal cords confront each other, vibrate during the exhalation, and facilitate the formation of phonemes that travel upward to the resonance chamber and the lips to allow the definitive word to be created. A spectrogram analysis shows that in certain words, Alex's formants oddly resemble those of Man.

Note that Gray parrots such as Alex, of the *Psittacus erithacus* species, have a special characteristic. The shape of their syrinx is even better suited to forming phonemes.

The walls of the syrinx, instead of being oval, as in other species, are composed of straight cartilage and positioned very anteriorly. Owing to this unusual structure, Alex has perfect control of the frequency he emits during his vocalizations. The sound is ferried by the trachea up to the larynx at the top of the latter. Thus, the tracheal column also serves as a resonance chamber for the syrinx.

What is amazing is that Alex can modify the length of his trachea, shortening it or lengthening it by 10%. This observation was made possible by magnetic resonance imaging, which clearly shows the trachea lengthening when Alex pronounces the vowel *o* and shortening when he pronounces *i*. As for the larynx, it has its own musculature.

The existence of a hyoid bone enables the insertion of very powerful lingual and jaw muscles that produce the excellent distortion of the supralaryngeal resonator.

However, it would seem that the larynx produces hardly any sound, but by changing shape, it transforms the vibrations emitted by the syrinx into intelligible phonemes.

It plays the role of lips for Alex's Herculean tongue. Thanks to the thirteen pairs of muscles that compose it, the tongue's mobility is exceptional. By opening or closing the larynx at the back of the tongue, the parrot is able to modulate sound, lengthen or shorten the trachea, and, therefore, adjust the resonance chamber perfectly to imitate the human voice as closely as possible.

However, let us not forget how important Alex's mandible is, nor its mobility, its amplitude, its mechanism, its adaptability. As for the resonance chamber, it plays a small role in the vocalization; somewhat as in Man, the outward airflow passes from the buccal cavity into the nostrils via the choanae.

In the talking bird, the spectacular strength of the tongue combines with the pseudolarynx to deliver what are in effect virtual lips. Thus, the parrot's resonance chambers contain two "echo" chambers, one tracheal and one supralaryngeal. The supralaryngeal space creates different volumes with the help of the tongue, and forms the bird's articulated language.

However, as in the case of ventriloquists, the bird is unable to pronounce certain consonants, for these require a double resonator, posteriorly and anteriorly, as in Man. These resonators enable the creation of formants 1 and 2. Alex emits vowels and formulates certain consonants by moving his mandible, by manipulating his tongue and his larynx, and by creating a vibration with his syrinx and larynx.

The parrot's vocal instrument can be considered a wind instrument that is open at both ends, but this doesn't explain everything.

How does his brain function to produce language, even only to mimic? Alex was able to establish friendly relationships with his minders. Indeed, this magician of bird language would interrupt tests imposed on him to say: "I'd like a banana" or "Scratch me." This is no longer pure mimicry, the Gray parrot is definitely capable of concrete language.

Dreams and voice

This collusion with the animal evokes the words of Nalunglaq in "the magical words":

> *In ancient times, when men and animals lived on Earth, a man could become an animal if he so wished and an animal could become a man if he so wished. There were people, there were animals, they were alike and they spoke the same language. Those were the days when words were magical.*

Chapter 22

Strange myths and voices

The voice of the force or the forcer of the voice,
the answer is in your inner self.

Voodoo: the body as medium of the voice

Lydwin

- Cotonou's Hospital

March 1997, southern Benin, Lydwin, a secretary, is eighteen years old. She's stricken by a raging fever. Unconscious and convulsive, she is transported urgently to the hospital of Cotonou, economic capital of this country of West Africa in which voodoo reigns supreme. Dr. Konrad Rippman, a doctor from Hamburg who is also an ethnologist, is on duty and takes charge of her. Her fever was caused by "bad air," a literal translation of "*mal aria*." Malaria has struck. He prescribes the appropriate treatment, her fever disappears. But her whole body hurts. She suffers from headaches. She feels increasingly tired. She sleeps badly. She loses weight. Her level of red blood cells diminishes. Her mother is worried. Her whole family, all fervent Catholics, pray for her night and day. Lydwin has been unable to work for several weeks now. Anemic, she soon hasn't got the strength even to walk unassisted. Allopathic medicine has done all that it could for her.

- She is at death's door: the power of *"vodun d'asi"*

At wits end, her mother appeals to Hounon Djalé, a priest and healer who practices voodoo. Her family is against this. How can she possibly lend herself to these pseudo-mystical rites? How can she inveigle her daughter in such an adventure? But stubbornly she takes Lydwin to see Hounon Djalé. She's at death's door. He examines her. His verdict is unshakable. She is "pre-possessed" or *"vodun d'asi."* Lydwin leaves town. After traveling a few hours, she arrives at the monastery. This building, place of worship of the voodoo healer, will be Lydwin's residence for nearly three months. The shaman will initiate her, prepare her for the rites, and deliver her from evil spirits. Two experts accompany her.

- A battle against "demons"?

Three months go by. Her mother is entreated not to visit her. When she sees Lydwin again a few weeks later, her daughter has gained weight. She is no longer tired. She has won her battle with the demons. Good has won over evil. But on her recovery path, she still has a decisive hurdle to overcome. A new Lydwin must be born again, otherwise she will relapse. Lydwin has become a voodoo adept. She must be "consecrated" to her protector god during the "ceremony" she's preparing herself for. In August 1997, Hounon Djalé explains to Dr. Konrad Rippmann that Lydwin is possessed. It hardly seems credible.

What relation could there be between *Plasmodium falciparum*, the parasite that provokes malaria, and the cause of her raging fever, and spirits? His answer is simple. Spirits promoted the infestation. They weakened Lydwin. But now that the fever is gone, the spirits still hound her. A broken love that had perturbed her was at the origin of this possession.

- "The great ceremony"

Now the evil spirit needed to be exorcised, the time had come for her to leave the boundaries of sickness and enter the world of healing. Lydwin is spending her last days in the monastery. She is preparing for a well-known rite, the "great ceremony": she takes a relaxing bath with aromatic plants, against a background of chanting and drums. She goes through different phases: agitation, depres-

sion, alternating between dance, immobility, and sideration. This is
the prepossession phase that's followed by trances.

Now the possession crisis can take place. The time is ripe for
it. It will mark the end of the initiation, allowing the old Lydwin,
possessed by evil spirits, to die. It will be her "voodoo death." She
will be reborn. D-day arrives, Houmon Djalé leads her to the circle
of voodoo dancers around the altar of the protector god who is to
look after her: Danoua-Woto, god of War and of the Wani-Wata cult.
The healer voodoo priest guides Lydwin. His eyes never leave her.
He is attentive to her every word and gesture.

- Lydwin's voice will set her free

He is waiting for her voice, mirror of her emotional state, to
speak to him, to indicate to him the path of her recovery. In this
instance, Lydwin's voice will be the key to open the door of her
freedom. The pulsing rhythm of the drums and of the dances
changes tempo. Her face is transformed. Her left leg freezes.

The trance has started. Careful! She is voicing words from a
strange language, the timbre of her voice deep. It is the voice of
her protector god, Danoua-Woto. He asks Djalé for a live hen. The
silence is awesome, then Lydwin sacrifices the hen. She emits gut-
tural sounds. Her throat contracts. Acoustic noises intended for the
god Danoua-Woto are emitted. The villagers attending the ceremony in a circle around Lydwin listen to her utterances.

Little by little, Djalé brings Lydwin back to the land of the living with his words. She emerges from her trance. The ritual is con-
cluded. Nearly an hour has elapsed.

Lydwin, healed, goes back to her mother, to her normal family,
social and spiritual environment. Now the ceremony demands that
a ritual meal be offered. The human voice acted as a channel for the
mysterious world of spirits. To an extent, one can see it as Hounon
Djalé's victory as a "healer priest" over occidental science in a
Catholic family from the big city. Indeed, in Benin, the voodoo conception of health is one of harmony between one's gods, one's
ancestors, and one's environment.

Is there an explanation?

But what exactly went on here? How does one explain this state
of trance? What physical elements led up to Lydwin's state of

possession? Dr. Rippmann provides a simple and logical explanation for this. Lydwin's intense concentration on certain parts of her body causes discharges of endorphins, the well-known excitatory hormone secreted by the hypothalamus. Fast and shallow breathing causes her to hyperventilate and leads to states of hyperactivity and exhaustion. These variations in the oxygen concentration and in endorphin levels in her organism create biochemical and bio-electric alterations in the brain, inducing sweating, dilated pupils, possibly cramps, and torpor.

The human voice, her center of hearing, the impact of the rhythmic drum beats, the particularly aggressive voices of the singers, all create such cerebral turmoil that dizziness ensues and the cerebral areas of language are stimulated. All these are rational elements that reassure us.

During her trance, Lydwin's voice revealed her deepest emotional state. She liberated herself in the Freudian sense. This story shows the impact of the human voice on the inner self, the physical impact it can have on the brain, as exemplified by sacred religious chants that can also provoke, albeit differently, a state of trance—do all these rationalizations elucidate the fact that she was restored to health?

Song punctuates the rhythm of our life, our birth, our baptism, our wedding, our death. A person can be possessed by voices. He becomes the tool of spirits and, according to beliefs that came to us from Africa, the voice of the Ancients then takes possession of the body. The most spectacular and awesome manifestation of this is tied to the peoples of Benin and neighboring territories. This region of Africa can be considered the cradle of voodoo, which was subsequently exported, notably to Haiti.

Voice and spirit

There are some 400 voodoo gods. "In the beginning, there was Olorum, god of the Skies, who reigned over the Sun that reigned over the waters; the Earth did not exist. Olorum dispatched his son Obatola, carrying a large sphere that he deposited in the sea. This sphere was the Earth. It broke, and thus were the mountains and valleys formed, encircled by water."

According to these beliefs, the gods may be far from us, but the spirits are always close by. The soul of every being participates in this spiritual universe. It never dies. It survives, first as an ancestor, then in reincarnation. The soul separates from the body. We find this notion in Africa as well as in India. It underscores the importance of possession of the body and of mediumship through the voice while in a state of trance.

The body then serves as a tool for the spirits, gods, and ancestors. The medium enters an ecstatic state, from the Greek word *ekstasis*: to be out of one's mind. This is proper to the shaman. For the shaman to be able to meet an ancestor while in this state of ecstasy, he must first prepare himself through a ritual that includes fasting, prayers, and repetitive chanting.

When the shaman is possessed by the voice of an ancestor, he reproduces not only the ancestor's voice, but also his expressions and gestures. Shamans are imitators. The medium's influence is collective, which makes it easy for religion to enter the picture. But observers are quick to spot an impostor. Simulation is easily detected. The fake shaman is revealed. When the medium is in a trance, he sweats, he burns up, he becomes agitated. His voice is transformed, taking on a strange timbre and unusual harmonics. He can engage in outlandish behavior. Experienced adepts protect him from himself. He sacrifices a hen or a ram and drinks its blood. He is impervious to fire and injury. He is in a detached state in which his utterances and gestures know few boundaries. As soon as he "awakens" from this state of possession, his timbre becomes normal again, his brain has erased all memory of the trance. He has complete amnesia of the events he has just been through. The voice liberates the inner self.

The voice: an internal force in martial arts

The kiai *and the center of energy*

One of the extreme forms the voice can take, in the literal rather than figurative sense, is well known in the martial arts. It is the *kiai*, the shout that kills. It is an awesome vocal emission, powerful and very brief. It is created by a vibration of the vocal cords that have closed together violently.

The *kiai* is brief, willful, full of purpose. According to Japanese Masters, of whom the closest to us is Okisawa, its source is considered as "cosmic energy." This internal energy can only be mobilized and concentrated after a lengthy physical and mental apprentice-ship. The *kiai* follows a controlled inhalation and deep concentra-tion. Its powers of liberation are exceptional. All one's strength, all one's muscular and mental energy are mobilized in a few tenths of a second. According to Christian Tissier and Pierre Blot: "Its strength lies in both defense and attack." It inhibits an adversary. The opponent freezes for a few seconds. He sustains the acoustic and mental impact of the *kiai* full on. The resonance it produces and the vibratory shock it causes to the ears produce waves that invade the opponent's brain.

The *kiai* is directional. It captivates the attention of the per-son it's aimed at. It immobilizes the opponent who is within fight-ing distance. During karate training, one can observe the ritual that takes place on the exercise mat. Gliding steps are suddenly inter-rupted as an opponent briefly adopts a frozen stance. He anchors himself to the ground. He is stable, purposeful. In a fifteenth of a second, he utters a *kiai* that very briefly paralyzes his opponent and gives him an opening to attack. The attack is quick and gives the impression of a photographic still at the moment of impact.

The power comes at the end of the shout, at the end of the exhalation; the fist is only the arrow that the bow has set in motion. The *kiai* annihilates any counterattack. It enables one to dominate an opponent and neutralize his strength, both physical and mental. As in the singing voice, the power of the *kiai* emanates from below the navel, where the exhalation originates. Depending on one's mental make-up, it takes one about six years to understand and begin to master the *kiai*.

This approach to an almost sacred type of voicing, this brutal vocalization that tables on a perfect synchronization of spirit and mind, of muscle power and acoustic vibration, of physical power and concentration, demonstrates that this liberating shout, as quick as lightning, is an extreme energetic form of the human voice.

The kiai: *more than a sound*

The *kiai* is an exhalation caused by a tightening of the muscles of the abdomen. The sound is created from the vocal cords. At the same time, you pronounce "HII" or "EEE." However, any sound that accompanies it tends to be of secondary importance. It should not be confused with a yell. Unlike yelling, a well-executed *kiai* will never hurt the vocal cords and you should not feel any roughness. The *kiai* provides an escape route for air during major exertion. It could be useful not only in martial arts but also, for example, in weightlifting. It is also a psychologic technique for releasing maximum energy suddenly. The *kiai* involves the philosophy of the yin and the yang, the force of our breathing and meditation.

The magic of voices and myths

Is voice beyond reality?

In the mythology of the Dogons of Mali, the supreme master is endowed with speech. He fashions the original placenta. He fertilizes the placenta and then offers it to Din, the chosen one among men. It is He, and He alone, who will develop the human voice.

The voice charms, seduces. The power of this acoustic intangible, the human voice, has limits that are difficult to define. From the first second of life, the newborn inhales and, thus, with his outward airflow, enables his first breath of life. This in and out of inhalation—exhalation, the yin and yang of our existence—is the harmony of our life on this planet, on which our last exhalation will also be our last sigh, the ultimate breath of our voice. Our voice accompanies us, even in its silences, during our entire life. Whether in babble or in talk, in song or in shouts, in laughter or in crying, the complex mechanism of our musical instrument, the larynx, and of our conductor, the brain, finds multiple modes of expression.

From Orpheus to Ulysses

Language, both spoken and sung, allows expression, but is also a medium for our inner self. Athena invents the flute, Hermes invents the lyre, Apollo plays the lyre on Olympus and charms the gods. Hermes then manufactures the shepherd's fife, with its spellbinding melody. But the Muses invent the wind and cord instrument. It is the Voice, Orpheus, born of Apollo and her mother Calliope, herself a muse with a beautiful voice, and brought up in Thrace, land of song and music.

Ulysses asks his crew to tie him solidly to the mast of his ship to stop him from following the mermaids, whose bewitching singing beckons him. His companions plug their ears so as not to hear them, not to listen, not to be hypnotized; bewitching mermaids, half women half fish, both singers and musicians. They attract sailors into their territory to conquer them and cast a spell on them.

The Argonauts are also exposed to the mermaids' charm. But Orpheus takes his lyre and plays a melody that drowns the mermaids' voices, thus saving the crew's life. Back in Thrace, her homeland, Orpheus marries Eurydice, who dies a few days later of a viper's bite. Orpheus descends into Hell to save his love and plays the lyre to charm the dog Cerberus. The wheel of Ixion no longer turns. Tears course down the faces of the Furies, goddesses of the macabre and of horror, as Orpheus sings and plays the lyre to bring Eurydice back to life. "He brought tears of steel to Pluto's cheeks and Hell granted Love's wish to bring Eurydice back to life."

Narcissus: the mirror of appearances, Echo: the mirror of vibrations

In Greek mythology, the charm of the voice, the importance of words, and the lyre's music are the ambassadors of the sacred in its most profound expression: life and the vibrations of the voice.

The echo intrigued the Greeks. How strange this sound that reflects off a surface, be it once or twenty times. The mountains speak! Echo, spouse of Narcissus, lacks the vocal and musical charisma of Orpheus. Yet her bewitching voice hypnotizes his mother Hera, who therefore doesn't realize that Zeus has a mistress. Hera is furious. Victim of the charm of her own voice, Echo is subjected to the brunt of Hera's anger, wife of Zeus. Her fate is cast: "You shall never be the first to speak, but you shall always have the last word, the one last pronounced by your interlocutor, which you shall repeat indefinitely." Henceforth, Echo is deprived of her own verbal creativity. She can but mimic others. Her voice repeats what others say to her. Reduced to mirroring the voice, she no longer is, as she no longer creates. Narcissus succumbs to the mirror of appearances, Echo to the mirror of vibrations.

For Plato: voice is the link between gods and mortals; Oracles are the proof

Zeus, the god with the most powerful voice, is master of all voices. His is the voice of authority. His word is *muthos*, the voice that has public authority, as against *ethos*, the voice that is socially less influential. He asks Hephaestus to knead the seas and the earth to give birth to Pandora. The gods endow her with a human voice. Plato's concept of the voice was naturalist, whereas Epicurus believed that articulation and a ready sense of words and sentences were innate to language in its natural state. So did Diogenes. The Greeks considered the voice to be a physical element that comes from the heart and represents our thinking. It was the only means of communication between the gods and mortals, but it was not created by the gods. It has no physical support, no physical obstacle. Its origins impose two contrary flows: as in all else, it must have its contrary, hell and paradise, night and day. The voice has a devilish origin because it strikes a blow at the air we breathe, and a divine origin because it is intangible and the bearer of messages.

The voice is particularly influential during the oracles. The sibylline oracle predicts the importance of the divine voice. It seems that her prophecies were an uninterrupted flow of words and phrases in a very high register. This vocal flow comes from the larynx. It is intelligible. It can be seductive. The sibylline priestess probably was a polyphonic singer, as she was described as having several languages in her voice simultaneously, producing concurrently multiple sounds that echoed in her mouth.

The incantations

The sorcerers and magicians of yesteryear adhere to a remarkable phonatory rule during their incantations. They have to reproduce the noises and sounds of certain deities, imitate their existence. They learn to manipulate their resonance chambers. They have to give the impression that their voice approaches the gods or moves farther away from them. They are ventriloquists and diphonic singers. Their voice has to be capable of casting a spell on the souls of those who listen to them.

They repeat the *s* to invoke Eros, the *e* for Psyche. And it is said: "Take a magnetic stone on which thou shall engrave Aphrodite, Psyche, and Eros, accompanied by magic chanting. And on the reverse side, engrave Psyche and Eros embracing with their sounds. Once the stone has been engraved and consecrated, place it under thy tongue, turn it over and pronounce the incantation." Thus, this magician has to reproduce animal sounds, the breath of life, and the human voice. He makes it possible to dialogue with the gods, he sings with mortals. Through the medium of his voice, he is the link between the divine and Man. The voice, essential part of Man, be it his inner voice or his emitted voice, is the vessel for his prayers.

The singular and diphonic chanting

Tibetan chanting

The diphonic chanting of Tibetan monks sounds very peculiar. One February morning in 1987, the scientist and artist Trân Quang Hai and his wife Bach Yên's, who also sings, telephone me wishing to understand the internal mechanics of diphonic chanting. We had met a few months earlier at the London Royal Academy of Music. His technique and artistic talent had made a strong impression on me. He had published his own conclusions on Tibetan chanting and was himself a diphonic chanter. A researcher, he had worked since 1968 in the ethnomusicology department of the Musée de l'Homme in Paris. This Saturday morning, we are both eager to discover his voice. A voice that gives the impression of several voices singing simultaneously, of a voice, or should I say of several voices, emanating from someplace else. It is the outcome of two combined sounds: the bumblebee, or fundamental note that remains constant during the entire exhalation, and its harmonics that vary but are always harmonics of the fundamental tone. This voice is a mixture of sounds from a Jew's harp and from a flute.

Ode to Joy

I examine him, I could almost say that Hai and I both examine him. Indeed, the endovideoscope allows us to follow on screen the unraveling of the mystery of diphonic chanting. The fibroscope passes through his right nasal fossa, then behind the uvula. Finally the roof of the larynx is on screen.

- Hai first sings the "Ode to Joy" in a normal voice. The pharyngolaryngeal cathedral looks perfectly normal. The soft palate, tongue, pharynx, and vocal cords are mobilized. However, the strength of the larynx resembles that of a ventriloquist.

- Then he sings the "Ode to Joy" in diphonic chant in the "*e*." The transformation is stunning. The vocal cords contract, with the ventricular bands or false vocal cords on top of them. The joints of the vocal cords (the arytenoids) tip slightly forward, practically masking the vocal ligament. My fibroscope is 8 cm above the vocal cords. To see what is going on, I'm obliged to lower the fibroscope into the vocal tract to a point 5-mm above the vocal cords and arytenoids. Hai's mastery of singing helps me enormously.

- We both observe the cordal vibration. It is not the ventricular bands that are vibrating, but the vocal cords themselves, contrary to numerous accepted theories. I carefully bring the fibroscope back up, level with the tongue and uvula.

Diphonia and ventriloquy: a similar technique

He sings the same hymn again, still in "*e*." No doubt about it, the conformations and distortions of the tongue and soft palate are the same as those observed in ventriloquists, but only in the vertical plane, from bottom to top, and in a horizontal plane, from front to back, not at all laterally, as he isn't pronouncing any syllables. The tongue flirts with the soft palate without actually touching it. It is much arched, and depending on the note emitted, it is mobilized through the creation of a second resonance chamber. Trân Quang Hai is demonstrating on the spectrograph what amounts to two fundamental tones, where you and I only have one!

This type of chanting is variably called diphonic, biformantic, or diplophonic. The bumblebee is the first fundamental tone (produced by the first resonance chamber). In a sense, one could say it provides the basic structure for the second one. Maintaining the bumblebee sound at a constant pitch, in the same frequency, with the same volume, on one single exhalation, enables the melody to develop. This melody, formed around the second fundamental tone, is dependent on the first one. This voice, produced by the vocal cords, triggers two sets of harmonics all at once. This technique has long been in the service of Buddhist philosophy. It aspires to be the instrument of immanence. We are a long way off our European civilization, often obsessed with transcendence. The Tibetan monks aren't alone in practicing this singular vocal technique, it is also found among certain Mongols, the Tuvas, among others. Tuva, in the depths of Russia, and its capital Kyzyl, is today considered to be the heartland of diphonic chanting.

In religion

In different religions, the voice is the bearer of the divine message, whatever the beliefs: from Buddhism to Islam, from Christianity to Judaism. A vessel for prayer, the timbre of the preacher's voice galvanizes the faithful. He addresses the believer, it's the individual addressing the crowd. He creates a unique atmosphere through the communion of the vibratory harmonics that he unleashes.

Voices can be unusual or sacred, nevertheless they carry the message of the vibration of the human being from generation to generation. Today, their mechanism is well known, but their source remains a mystery.

Our voice can be soft, warm, sensuous, while elsewhere it can be curt, hypnotizing, metallic, coaxing, sometimes dull or toneless. It merely reflects our present feelings. Yet this voice is in space-time continuum; it has existed, it will exist, but as soon as it is uttered, it is already of the past. In sacred contexts, it combines with music, art, and song. It has never ceased to evolve. Today, the echoes of its harmonics still fill cathedrals, temples, and churches. Our voice communicates our emotion, just as our tears betray the sadness in our heart.

Chapter 23

Voice and seduction

Is the voice in the service of seduction,
or is seduction in the service of the voice?

The sound of a light breeze rustling through leaves may seduce you. The voice has unbelievable powers of seduction. Be it men or women, their timbre, their harmonics are part of their personality. A deep voice can be a woman's voice. Musicality and choice of words are the signature of the woman's voice. Conversely, a high-pitched voice can be a man's voice.

I'm a criminal lawyer: feeling good about one's voice in the same way as one can feel good about oneself

I don't like my voice

One afternoon in April 1997, around 3 PM, a mannishly dressed woman consults me: leather jacket and black trousers, short hair, forty-seven years old, strong personality. I notice her very masculine voice from her first "Hello, Doctor."

Hers is the voice of a smoker. She seems in perfect harmony with her personality: "Doctor, I'm a criminal lawyer. I have a deep voice. Often, I'm taken for a man. I defend a lot of riff-raff, and for several years now, I've been winning nearly all my cases. But I no longer like my voice." Is there a conflict between her voice and her physique? It's true that her voice doesn't surprise me. It fits her appearance. She has charm and I can just imagine her pleading her client's case in court. She is waiting for me to comment. "True, your voice is deep, but it fits in perfectly with who you are; what has brought you here, fear of cancer, or your deep voice?" "No," she answers, "my timbre bothers me, I can't detect it anymore."

The examination reveals an important edema of her vocal cords (a polypoid cord). The swelling is visible on either side. The stroboscopic examination enables us to discard fairly certainly the possibility of a cancer. Indeed, the membrane vibrates, it isn't blocked. It is yellowish, filled with a thick fluid that's visible through the epithelium layers, there is no suspect plaque. I'm able to reassure Mrs. C. A. The state of her vocal cords is hardly surprising, she smokes fifty cigarettes a day! Plus she has a little glass of whiskey every night. She's been immersed in this universe of criminal law for years. Now she knows that if we decide to operate, it will be because of the timbre of her voice, not for fear of cancer. She still wants me to operate on her. It is certainly the only solution that will enable her to recover four or five notes in the higher register and put pay to her masculine voice. I'm not in favor, her look harmonizes perfectly with her voice.

After a few minutes of discussion, she confides that she has had a new man in her life for the past few weeks, who isn't too keen on her vocal timbre, finding it too masculine. Nevertheless, I am still not in favor. It seems to me that, if we change her vocal timbre, we'll be tinkering with her personality, with her charm, which, despite the timbre, are still feminine. She consults me again a month later. Again she asks me to operate. I refuse to give in. I ask her to give up smoking and to go to voice therapy sessions. My recommendations go unheeded. She stubbornly sticks to her guns, as you can imagine, and requests an operation.

A voice metamorphosis

Six months later, a woman enters my consulting room. She has mid-length hair, a beige muslin dress, a clear, high voice: "Hello Doctor, how are you?" I have to confess that for a few seconds, I don't recognize the patient. The woman is familiar, but I can't place her. Then I realize I have before me the lawyer, Mrs. C. A., with a new voice. "How are you, Mrs. C. A.?" The examination confirms that her vocal cords have healed well.

But how has she experienced this vocal metamorphosis? After a brief discussion, the verdict is terrible: "When I dream, I dream with my old voice. When I plead, I no longer have the zest, boldness, and conviction I used to have. I am fragile. I no longer charm with my voice. It's me, I'm on the defensive. I can't recognize myself in my voice. I feel as if my voice has become schizophrenic."

There is a duality now between her voice and her personality. Then she adds: "My boyfriend left me three months after my surgery. He couldn't bear my new voice. I stopped smoking, I've gone off my whiskey. And as if that weren't bad enough, she says, I'm losing all my cases." Surgically speaking, her vocal cords had been well operated on by a fellow specialist, "but there is a but." For all that the operation was performed at Mrs. C.A.'s request, in no way did her new voice fit her personality. "Mrs. C. A." I told her, "smoke 3 to 5 cigarettes a day again under medical supervision, it will allow the edema of the vocal cords to form again, which will deepen your voice. Do about fifteen sessions of voice therapy. You'll feel at home again with your voice, and you'll get back to feeling good about yourself." And this she did. I see her regularly. A year later, this mannish woman consults me again, dressed in slacks, with a deeper, richer voice. She's recovered the harmony of her personality, of her voice, of her charm. It's reminiscent of the charm of actresses such as Simone Signoret or Lauren Bacall.

Female voice, male voice: seduction is in the voice's musicality and in its silences

Women play with vowels, men play with exclamation marks

Timbre and seduction are intimately connected. Female voice, male voice, the ingredients are multiple. In the 20th century, the seductiveness of a voice stems from its height, its resonance, from the deep harmonics that ornament the higher pitches in a woman's voice, equally from the rhythm of its silences. The feminine voice that seduces you, be it the voice of Marlene Dietrich, Delphine Seyrig, or Jeanne Moreau, owes its charm to its deeper overtones that are barely audible, and to the sensuous breath of the vibratory emission. Sometimes it owes its charm to an edema of the vocal cords, to a small nodule or to a growth that's best left alone. This unusual frequency creates the landscape of these sensual feminine voices. Men and women have a different way of speaking, a different verbal mode of expression, a different vocabulary, a different way of punctuating their speech with their body language. The actresses just mentioned were never mistaken for men. Yet, if you were to analyze the acoustic spectra of their speech, you'd be in for a surprise. You would conclude that the frequencies are masculine, that the acoustic wave is hardly present in the higher register, that this hoarse, veiled voice is borderline pathological.

How reductionist this would be. The vocal musicality of these women is stunning! Thus her personality is wrapped up with this "something" in voice: emphasis, its intonation, its vocal rhythm. A woman's voice is melodious, almost a singsong, her spoken voice has a musicality very different from a man's; his voice is measured, almost *staccato*. He rarely makes liaisons. Women play with vowels, men play with exclamation marks.

The range of the voice is part of the seduction

A woman consults me for a hoarseness that has lasted several years, deepening her timbre. Of late, it has been getting worse. "I teach, by the end of the day I battle to give class. I smoke twenty cigarettes a day, but they're low tar." Examination of the vocal cords of this 42-year-old teacher reveals a cordal edema that looks benign and is fairly typical of someone who smokes this much. "It's all I need to know," she says, "I wanted to be sure that I don't have cancer. My deep voice doesn't bother me. I play with it. I dance circles around people with it. People like that. I'm not keen to change it." This woman had understood perfectly well that femininity and seduction are not all about vocal frequency, they are also about intonation. The emotional language of women and men is also different. Women say "I would like," men say "I want." He is decisive, she suggests.

Research at Yale University in this field has demonstrated that a man's voice is projected solely in his left brain, his logical brain, whereas a woman's voice is projected into the left and right brains, into the hemispheres of reasoning and emotion, as well as into the limbic brain, the cerebral seat of seduction. This should not surprise us in an occidental world in which man is brought up according to the precepts of a pyramidal education. He isn't allowed to cry. Brought up like a soldier, a warrior, he must take a position. She takes the middle road between order and emotion. She is allowed to show her feelings without being belittled for it.

Science and vocal art: not always on the same wavelength

A perfect voice: in relation to what?

Our voice is tied up with our sexuality. It has undeniable seductive powers. This acoustic communication with others can weaken you if it becomes hoarse or too metallic, scratchy or faint; it can make you lose confidence. The perfect voice doesn't exist. There is always a little something in the *vibrato* or in the *passagio* or again in the timbre: this is what makes a voice sublime; without this it would be the voice of a robot. Often the charm, beauty, and attraction of a voice is due to its imperfections.

A seductive voice creates a radiance that comes from within and makes the other person vibrate. It is a voice that reassures you, that comforts you, that galvanizes you. By trying too hard to pierce the mystery of vocal seductiveness, we risk breaking the secret of vocal emotion. True, we have lined up statistics, scientific, medical, and acoustic explanations, but happily, somewhere, there is an inaccessible vibration, which is that of charm. You can say of a violin: that is a Stradivarius, but unless the person playing it is a virtuoso, like Yehudi Menuhin or Isaac Stern, it won't mean much. Understanding the vocal mechanism was an obligatory step, but trying to fathom seduction is part of another galaxy.

The voice and life's scars

Life's scars can give charm to a voice, but sometimes, they can alter it. Is our voice not our acoustic shield, intangible with respect to external aggressions? There are multiple therapeutic approaches that can be envisaged when the voice is altered. Allopathic solutions, vitamins, trace elements, minerals, voice therapy, all can help in the recovery of the voice.

Nevertheless, occasionally microsurgery may be necessary as a last recourse against an alteration that is handicapping the patient and has given rise to a complex. The phonosurgeon, or surgeon of the voice, will act on something that is not merely mechanical, but has to do with the essence of the human being: our tuneful vibration. Thereafter, thanks to these various therapies, vocal charm is often restored, and the singular personality reconquered.

Some speakers, journalists, or actors seem to speak of their voice as it if were a work tool that needs to be readjusted or fine-tuned. Life's scars mold the voice of these professionals, dynamically conferring to it a strong personality that keeps evolving in step with their emotional world. There's no such thing as a vocal Venus or a vocal Apollo, it's a meaningless concept. One can certainly fall in love with a voice, and I have oftentimes been asked to give a patient Lauren Bacall's voice, a deeper voice, or a higher voice, as if these people can no longer bear the sound of their own voice. Occasionally, the request is a valid one, if the voice is bitonal or very rasping. Then indeed the voice surgeon can harmonize the voice with its physical envelope. But these cases are rare. In other cases, an inner conflict can trigger voice strain and its chain of consequences.

An erotic voice and Casanova

A vocal Casanova

A seductive voice can be an erotic, breathy voice with deep consonants and sharp dissonances. A voice can also hypnotize, coax, and perturb. In the Germanic culture, the Lorelei's voice was one that was bewitching, that could be fatal. Does the public speaker not control the crowd by communicating his individual vibration to it?

In Cyrano de Bergerac, Cyrano's lament beneath Roxana's balcony lent charm to the vocal harmony of the narrator. Yet the verbal seducer, Cyrano de Bergerac, was no vocal Casanova. His vibration was totally dedicated to loving. "Vocal Casanova" is an improbable association of words. Why? Because the voice betrays one. It is the mirror of the soul. It reveals the personality. It contains the pure light of the sun, which under the prism of the self, gives the colors of the rainbow the distribution of which is singular to each of us.

Plastic surgery of the voice: myth or reality

Although some people are prepared to go to any lengths, including plastic surgery, voice surgery can destroy a personality if it does not take into account the whole being, because feeling good about one's voice, just as feeling good about oneself, is essential for our communication with oneself and with others.

Some voices, as they age, become reassuring, seductive, caring. Others will need the help of a singing teacher, a voice therapist, or a laryngologist to recover their beauty and charm. I am struck by the growing recourse to plastic surgery these days: people have their face redone at the age of sixty so that they can look in the mirror and see a forty-year-old face—why not? But if the voice doesn't follow suit, if the timbre of an older person comes out of the mouth of this younger face, it really shocks. The voice has to be taken in hand, if necessary, through voice therapy or a lifting of the vocal cords if they have lost volume and tonus and need to be toned and rounder again, although this isn't always possible.

Seduction, sounds, and science: a remarkable story

Sex and voice have been intimately connected since time immemorial

But what is the basis of vocal seduction, what explains the excitement we can feel hearing a particular voice? By what process, since millennia, are we brought almost to ecstasy by a voice?

The answer lies far back in Man's evolution, in the evolution of Life. If two voices of opposite sexes meet, they respond to one another, they take an interest, they flirt, they seduce, sometimes they become erotic. This seduction process is inextricably bound up with acoustics. It can be a telephone message, a voice on the radio, in which case you are only a receiver of it. We know that the seductive powers of a voice are subject to the influence of testosterone. Indeed, a minimum of 150 µg of testosterone is required for a woman to have any sexual desire; in men, the minimum threshold is a little higher. This hormonal influence enables us to keep the charm in our voice.

The ancestor of this hormone is the pheromone. The first organisms, at the beginning of life on Earth, lived without oxygen. They found energy in the dissolution of sulfurous oxygen, given that no efficient photon could contribute any specific luminous energy. Nearly 3 billion years ago, our Planet underwent a revolution when the rays of the Sun became visible. These photons enabled the existence of chlorophyll, the source of our oxygenated Blue Planet. Indeed, chlorophyll in turn enables the existence of free oxygen, of carbonic gas, and, thus, the regulation of oxido-reduction in the living world. The phenomenon is a simple one. Chlorophyll captures solar photons, notably blue and green photonic units, and transforms them into the molecules from which our living world is built. Green, the color of chlorophyll, is what makes our planet blue. The oxygen thus liberated is the source of a new form of life and also of a new form of death, due to the possible formation of unstable molecules, free radicals that destroy the cellular membrane and induce apoptosis, or the suicide of the cell.

Another 2.5 billion years go by before there is sufficient oxygen on our planet, in free supply and suitably stable, to make life possible for the animals we know of. Evolution continues its course. Cells without a nucleus evolve toward cells that have a nucleus. A specific bacterium makes its appearance, one that's essential for the survival of animals, essential to Man's life. These bacteria seduce other cells to allow osmosis with them. It brings an unbeatable respiratory system. It is an exceptional energy factory. It is the Cyaonobacteria, which becomes the mitochondrion. In symbiosis with its host cell, the mitochondrion enables the survival of both. This first hurdle is followed by another, indispensable to evolution, that of the sexual cell. Seduction has just made its appearance.

Molecules and sex

The pheromone, a molecule with 15 carbon atoms, the molecule of attraction between human beings, an expert at seduction, has existed for several million years. Indeed, the pheromone's ancestor is mevalonic acid: a molecule with 6 carbon atoms that stabilizes as isoprene, an acid with 5 carbon atoms. According to Claude Gudin, it was from this original molecule that the pheromone, hormone of attraction, originated, but also our sex hormones, testosterone, estrogens, and progesterone, as well as the molecules involved with scent or food, the carotenoids.

Insects (of which there are around 400,000 species) form the number one species of the living world. They are almost as numerous as plant species on our planet. There are only 30,000 species of fish. Faced with this multitude of physical envelopes for DNA, in our world in which cloning is underway, let us not forget that the essence of charm lies in difference and sexuality. Just imagine if we began to clone the voice, that would spell the end of seduction and vocal sensuality. The history of human evolution proves this. Parthenogenesis produces viable clones that could be a thousand times more numerous than a sexual population. But uniformity forbids all evolution. 95% of the animal kingdom has chosen to be sexual, and this is no coincidence. It is the one and only way, mutation aside, of creating an individual cell that differs slightly from its mother cells. This difference stems from the mixing of genes. This genetic coupling is decisive. It enabled the creation of Man.

Sex and the evolution of the voice

Consider the example of seduction among birds. Their color vision is excellent. They possess five retinal cones for color, including ultraviolet, which we lack, but which predators have, although they see in black and white. Humans have three types of cones: red, green, and blue. This enables us to see the colors of the rainbow, but we see neither ultraviolet rays nor infrared rays. Men are less sensitive to certain colors than are women. The reason for this is simple. Chromosome X possesses green and red genes. As women are XX, they have a keener sense of these colors and therefore to certain hues. The songbird is perforce sexual, it's why he sings. There are some 8,500 species of birds, of which less than half are songbirds. Their melody attracts the female. It's the male that sings, rarely the female. An experiment was run with zebra finches, in which females injected with testosterone began to sing.

An amazing bird with an amazing singing: male and female in one

Robert Agathe makes a surprising discovery. This scientist from the University of California notices that certain zebra finches are gynandromorphic: both male and female. The right half of this bird's body is male, the left half is female. On one side "he" has a testicle, on the other side "she" has an ovary. The bird's singing is stunning. The volume and register are far more impressive than in a normal "male male" bird. The right brain is more developed than the left. It corresponds to the male half-body. Bird song depends on male hormones, hormones of acoustic seduction that are close to pheromones.

The song of the male bird seduces the female. It is the vehicle for his seduction, the vehicle for his sexuality. If the female has defective hearing, or if the male is no longer able to sing, reproduction is no longer possible and their breeding stops.

Opera of the deep blue

In another register, the humpbacked whale, or Caruso whale, sings for hours on end to seduce a female. His singing is superb. The melody presents numerous identifiable musical phrases that are elaborate, built with logical frequential sequences. If these harmonic sequences were altered, there would be no sexual communication between these cetaceans. This opera of the deep blue lasts for hours and is renewed regularly before every coupling near the coasts of Canada, Madagascar, and Argentinia.

To seduce, we must have someone to seduce: another person, or the public

At the end of the day, the groupie fan of the pianist is probably another facet of the universal seduction of the human voice. There is an element of maturity that enters into vocal seduction, just as it enters into sexual attraction. But although you can modify your body, your face, your attitude, you can't modify your voice. It is part of your present personality, of the expression of your liveliness, of the being that will seduce. This approach to the voice is increasingly widespread, no doubt because our civilizations are running out of steam. They aspire to real, natural color, far from artifice. The search for one's own vibration, for the other's vibration, is no more than a search for real harmony, which seems harder and harder to find.

Seduction does not necessarily end in coupling or in procreating, but it always leads to a certain form of pleasure, to pre-ecstasy. Seducing means having someone to seduce, it means wanting to seduce, but also it often means the other has given his or her prior consent to being seduced. The human voice is the vehicle for this walkie-talkie signal. The voice is also the seducer, through its vibrations, vibrations that trigger and solicit certain stimuli: pheromones and even secretions of sex hormones. Have you never been charmed, if not bewitched, by a voice on the radio?

Emotion and seduction are interconnected. The emotion stirred up by a voice, listening to an opera, looking at a sculpture or a painting, in turn provokes a reaction in the person with us. This vegetative reaction of our reptilian brain is followed by the emotional reaction of our limbic brain. This emotional particle of Man that is the vocal vibration is often sufficient to unleash a passionate tidal wave in the mind.

To reduce the human voice, its charm, its personality to the genes of words, to neurotransmitters, to the buccopharyngeal articulate, to vocal cords, to Broca's area or Wernicke's area in our left hemisphere, is like describing a painting and its colors without having perceived its creative harmony. It is like saying of Rodin, the sculptor, or of Michelangelo, who undresses marble to reveal Moses, that they are merely good technicians. Happily, creation is authentic and can't be faked. Even though irrefutable vocal technique and a particular anatomy are required to perform in Molière or to sing to Verdi's musical scores, the artist's creativity lies somewhere between beauty and seduction, eroticism and ecstasy, science and art.

Is the voice not the past in the present?

Chapter 24

The force of the voice

The force of our voice is immanence and transcendence.

After this long voyage on the vessel of the human voice, certain questions may still remain unanswered, but many enigmas revealed their mystery to us.

The arrow of time led us to the cell of *Homo sapiens*, then of *Homo vocalis*. His most important tool is his voice, its agility is exceptional. It is the vessel of his thinking and of his dreams. But can it be that this wonderful mechanical and emotional machinery is reaching the end of its story?

Indeed, for the past dozens of millions of years, the voice hasn't really progressed. Yet our underutilized brain seems to be in the early stages of its development. This cerebral galaxy is an impressive formation of nebulae, inborn and acquired, specific to each of us, is, above all, our communication tool.

Is the human voice still going to evolve? Will language become more and more symbolical, more and more abstract? Will telepathy remain a legend?

Today, six billion *Homo vocalis* have their own individual vibration, their own voice, their own imprint. Their voices exhibit the scars of their life and are as different as the grains of sand in the ocean. They reveal our thoughts and lift the veil on our sexuality. They wrinkle and assert our personality.

Professionals of the voice have made this vibration their instrument. Lyrical artists, popular singers, actors accomplish themselves

473

in it and through it. The performer of the voice gives his persona to the crowd as he creates his interpretation.

This interpretation exists only in the present and is distributed in space-time continuum. Indeed, despite its intangibility, its vibration marks space with its imprint.

Our voice is one of the paths of the mind and imagination of each of us. Like a scribe for our thoughts, it expresses our inner self, both in its immanence and in its transcendence.

Through its imprint in space, the voice feeds the memory of the Universe.

Afterword

The word odyssey means "an extended adventurous wandering." What better way to describe the wonders of Jean Abitbol's book, *The Odyssey of the Voice.* The human voice is both adventurous and mysterious. Despite the critical role of the voice in all of human communication, the reasons why and the mechanism of how the voice developed into the extraordinary organ representing the multiple emotions of man has remained a mystery. Jean Abitbol is perhaps the first to really look at the evolution of the voice not from the perspective of an anthropologist but from that of a physician dedicated to preserving and improving the features, characteristics, and beauty of the greatest instrument.

His descriptions of the development of voice and language read like a mystery novel, where each page leaves clues from the past, sometimes millions of years earlier, as subtle hints as to where the future will lead. The imagery entwines the evolutionary pressures to develop speech and language, how they separate us from even our closest animal lineages, and the roles that voice and language play in the development of culture. The mystery progresses to describe the unique facets of human voice, the wondrous physics and physiology that allow this tiny little part of the body to produce the magnificence of sound. The transformation of the voice with the maturation of the human body is presented as a prelude to many of the physiologic changes that occur. Abitbol's review of the impact of hormones, particularly on the female voice, is evidence of his unique background and experience with hormonal changes in the voice.

Once the development and physiology of the voice has been described and developed, the journey continues as Abitbol reveals the care that is needed to sustain this excellence. Finally, he twists his plot to present the unique and periphery of typical voice use, from twins to ventriloquists, from voodoo to the edges of the universe.

Abitbol's odyssey, his adventurous wandering, leaves the reader looking beyond, almost as if the gods were guiding the voyage. It is apropos that, in Homer's *Odyssey*, it is notOdysseus'skills as a

475

warrior, hunter, seaman, or marksman that ultimately control his destiny. Rather it is the voices of the characters that inevitably guide their paths. Odysseus tricks the Cyclops, Polyphemus, with his voice by telling him that his name is "Nobody." Later, mankind's struggle with lethal, but overwhelming appeal is represented by the Siren's irresistible songs. Odysseus is nearly driven mad as he hears their song. Finally, it is Odysseus' ability to vocally recant the stories of his adventures to the Phaeacians that ultimately wins their admiration and convinces them to return him home to Ithaca. Abitbol's book reads like the *Odyssey* with its rich language, poignant imagery and character development. The hero, however, is not an individual, but rather a part of all of us—our voices. Homer would have been proud that his legend would serve as the signature of this delightful tale of that part of us that makes us uniquely human. I am sure that like me, *Odyssey of the Voice* has inspired you to experience the marvels of your own voice.

Michael S. Benninger, M.D.
Department of Otolaryngology–Head and Neck Surgery
Henry Ford Hospital, Detroit, Michigan

Bibliography

ABITBOL, Jean. *Atlas of Laser Voice Surgery.* Singular Publishing Group, Inc. 1995.

ABITBOL, Jean. *Les Coulisses de la Voix* (from the opera *Norma).* 1994.

ABITBOL, Jean, ABITBOL, Patrick, ABITBOL, Béatrice. Sex hormones and the female voice. *Journal of Voice.* Vol. 13, No. 3, pp. 424–446. 1999.

ABITBOL, Jean. Premenstrual voice syndrome. *Genesis,* No. 62. 2001.

ABITBOL, Jean et al. Voix et ménopause: crépuscule des divas. *Journal de Contraception, Fertilité, Sexualité,* Vol. 6, No. 9, 1998.

ABITBOL, Jean, Abitbol Béatrice. Haemorrhage of the vocal fold. *Journal of Voice,* Vol. 2, 1988.

ADASHI, Eli Y., ROCK John A., ROSENWAKS Zew. *Reproducitve Endocrinology, Surgery and Technology* (Vols. 1 & 2). Lippincott, Raven Press. 1996.

ALBY, Jean-Marc, ALES, Catherine, SANSOY, Patrick. *L'esprit des Voix.* La pensée Sauvage. 1990.

ALVAREZ, Luis, ALVAREZ, Walter. *Nature.* No. 404, pp. 122–123, 2000.

ANDREA, Mario Dias Oscar. *Atlas of Rigid and Contact Endoscopy in Microlaryngeal Surgery.* Lippincott, Raven Press. 1995.

ANDREWS, Moya L. *Manual of Voice Treatment: Pediatrics Through Geriatrics.* Singular Publishing Group, Inc. 1995.

ANNOSCIA, Giuseppe. *Universalia 2003 La Politique, les Connaissances, la Culture en 2002.* Encyclopedia Universalis France S.A. 2003.

APPELMAN, Ralph D. *The Science of Vocal Pedagogy: Theory and Application.* Indiana University Press. 1967.

ARONSON, Arnold E. *Les Troubles Clinique de la Voix.* Masson. 1983.

ARTAUD, Antonin. *Le Théâtre et Son Double.* Gallimard. 1964.

AURIOL, Bernard. *La Clef des Sons: Éléments de Psychosonique.* Erès. 1994.

BADIR, Semir, PARRET, Herman. *Puissances de la Voix.* Presses Universitaires de Limoges. 2001.

BAGNOLI, Giorgio. *The La Scala Encyclopedia of the Opera.* Simon & Schuster. 1993.

BAKEN, R. J. *Clinical Measurement of Speech and Voice.* College-Hill Press. 1987.

BARRAQUE, Philippe. *A la Source du Chant Sacré, S'initier aux Chants de la Terre.* Diamantel. 1999.

BARTHELEMY, Yva. *La Voix Libérée.* Robert Laffont. 2004.

BASHEVIS SINGER, Isaac. *The Golem*. Le Seuil. 1997.

BATTA, Andras. *Opéra: Compositeurs, Oeuvres, Interprêtes*. Könemann Verlagsgesellschaft mbH. 2000.

BELHAU, Mara. *O Melhor que vi e Ouvi: Actuelizaçao em Laringe e Voz, Manisme*. Revinter. 1998.

BENICHOU, Grégory. *Le Chiffre de la Vie: Réconcilier la Génétique et L'humanisme*. du Seuil. 2002.

BENNINGER, Michaël S., JACOBSON Barbara H., JOHNSON Alex F. *Vocal Arts Medicine: The Care and Prevention of Professional Voice Disorders*. Thieme Medical Publishers, Inc. 1994.

BENOIST-MECHIN, Jacques. *Frederic de Hohenstaufen* (pp. 354-360). Librairie Académique Perrin. 1980.

BENZ, W, CAMERON, A. G. MELOSH, H. J. The origin of the moon and the single-impact hypothesis IV. *Icarus*, No. 81, pp. 113-131, 1989.

BERESNIAK, Daniel. *L'histoire étrange du Golem*. de la Maisnie. 1993.

BERGER, Natalia. *Jews and Medicine: Religion Culture Science*. The Jewish Publication Society. 1995.

BERTON, H. *De la Musique Mécanique et de la Musique Philosophique*. Alexis Eymery. 1826.

BICKERTON, Derk. *Language and Species*. University of Chicago Press. 1990.

BILLORET, Anne. *Traitements Homéopathiques des Maladies de la Voix*. Maloine.1989.

BLAKEMORE, Colin, GRIEENFIELD, Susan. *Mind Waves: Thoughts on Intelligence, Identity and Consciousness*. Basil Blackwell Ltd. 1987.

BLANCHARD, Roger, DE CANDE, Roland. *Dieux & Divas de L'Opéra: Des Origines au Romantisme*. Plon. 1986.

BLANCHARD, Roger, DE CANDE, Roland. *Dieux & Divas de L'Opéra: de 1820 à 1950: Grandeur et Décadence du Bel Canto*. Plon. 1987.

BLESS, Diane M., ABBS, James H. *Vocal Fold Physiology: Contemporary Research and Clinical Issues*. College-Hill Press. 1983.

BLIVET, Jean-Pierre. *Les Voies du Chant: Traité de Technique Vocale*. Fayard. 1999.

BONFILS, Pierre. *Pathologie ORL et Cervico-faciale: Comprendre, Agir, Traiter*. Ellipses. 1996.

BOUVIER, René. *Farinelli: Le Chanteur des Rois*. Albin Michel.1943.

BRAHIC, André. *Les Comètes*. PUF. 1993.

BRAHIC, André. *Planète et Satellites*. Vuilbert. 2001.

BRAHIC, André. *Enfants du Soleil*. Odile Jacob. 2004.

BRAHIC, André. *La plus Belle Histoire de la Terre*. du Seuil. 2004.

BROCA, Paul. *Bulletin de la Société D'anatomie de Paris. 18 Avril 1861. Publication à la Société d'Anthropologie Française de L'observation TAN*, No. 3, pp. 330-355, 1861.

BRODNITZ, Friedrich S. *Keep Your Voice Healthy.* Little, Brown and Company, Inc. 1988.

BROWN, W. S., VINSON, Betsy Partin, CRARY, Michael A. *Organic Voice Disorders: Assessment and Treatment.* Singular Publishing Group, Inc. 1996.

BRUNEL Pierre, WOLFF, Stéphane. *L'Opéra.* Bordas. 1980.

BRYSON, Bill. *A Short History of Nearly Everything.* Doubleday. 2003.

BUNCH, Meribeth. *Dynamics of the Singing Voice.* Springer-Verlag-Wien. 1982.

BUSTANY, Pierre. *Le Langage dans Essai: Art-Langage-Cerveau* (pp. 95–108). Factuel. 2000.

CANN, R. L., STONEKING, N., WILSON, A. C. Mitochondrial DNA and human evolution. *Nature.* No. 325, pp. 31–36, 1987.

CAPUTO ROSEN, Deborah, SATALOFF, Robert Thayer. *Psychology of Voice Disorders.* Singular Publishing Group, Inc. 1997.

CARTER, Rita. *Mapping the Mind.* Phoenix Paperback. 1998.

CASANOVA, Nicole. *Germaine Lubin.* Flammarion. 1974.

CASTAREDE, Marie-France. *La Voix et les Sortiléges.* Les Belles Lettres. 1991.

CHANGEUX, Jean-Pierre. *L'Homme Neuronal.* Arthème Fayard. 1983.

CHANGEUX, Jean-Pierre. *Gènes et Cultures: Enveloppe Génétique et Variabilité Culturelle.* Odile Jacob. 2003.

CHAUVIN, Bernadette, CHAUVAN, Rémy. *Le Monde des Oiseaux.* du Rocher. 1996.

CHOUARD, Claude-Henri. *"L'Oreille Musicienne: Les Chemins de la Musique de l'Oreille au Cerveau.* Gallimard. 2001.

CLAIR, Jean. *L'âme au Corps: Arts et Sciences—1793–1993.* RMN/Gallimard-Electa. 1993.

CLERICY DU COLLET, M. *La Voix Recouvrée par la Rééducation des Muscles du Larynx.* Librairie Ch. Delagrave. 1899.

COHEN, Claudine. *La Femme des Origines.* Belin Herscher. 2003.

Colloque de Mouans-Sartoux. *Art—Langage—Cerveau: La Dynamique de L'Échange.* Factuel. 2001.

COLTON, Raymond H., CASPER, Janina K. *Understanding Voice Problems: A Physiological Perspective for Diagnosis and Treatment.* Williams and Wilkins. 1990.

CONNOR, Steven. *Dumbstruck: A Cultural History of Ventriloquism.* Oxford University Press. 2000.

CONSOLAZIO, C. F., et al. Relationship between calcium in sweat, calcium balance and calcium requirements. *Journal of Nutrition,* No. 78, pp. 78–88, 1962.

COOPER, Morton. *Stop Committing Voice Suicide.* Voice and Speech Company of America. 1996.

COPPENS, Yves, PELOT, Pierre. *Le Rêve de Lucy.* du Seuil, 1990.

COPPENS, Yves, PICQ, Pascal. *Aux Origines de L'Humanité: De L'Apparition de la Vie à L'Homme Moderne.* Librairie Arthème Fayard. 2001.

COPPENS, Yves, PICQ, Pascal. *Aux Origines de L'Humanité: Le Propre de L'Homme.* Librairie Arthème Fayard. 2001.

CORNUT, Guy. *La Mécanique Respiratoire dans la Parole et le Chant.* Presses Universitaires de France. 1959.

CORNUT, Guy, *La Voix (Que sais-je?).* Presses Universitaires de France. 1983.

CRICK, F. H. C. *What Mad Pursuit: A Personal View of Science.* Basic Books, 1988.

CUTLER, A. The syllable's role in the segmentation of stress languages. *Language and Cognitive Processes,* No. 12, pp. 339–345, 1997.

CYRULNIK, B. *Si les Lions Pouvaient Parler.* Gallimard. 1999.

DAMASIO, Antonio R. *Spinoza Avait Raison: Joie et Tristesse: Le Cerveau de L'Émotion.* Odile Jacob. 2003.

DARWIN, Charles. *The Origin of the Species by Natural Selection.* 1859.

DAVIES, Garfield, JAHN, Anthony J. *Care of the Professional Voice: A Management Guide for Singers, Actors and Professional Voice Users.* Butterworth-Heinemann. 1998.

DAVIS, Pamela J., FLETCHER, Neville H. *Vocal Fold Physiology.* Singular Publishing Group, Inc. 1996.

DAWKINS, Richard. *The Selfish Gene.* Oxford University Press. 1989.

DEBRE, Patrice. *Louis Pasteur.* The Johns Hopkins University Press. 2000.

DEGROOT, Leslie J. *Endocrinology* (Vols. 1–3). W.B. Saunders Company. 1995.

DEWHURST-MADDOCK, Olivea. *La Thérapie par les Sons: L'Autoguérison par la Musique et L'Expression Vocale.* Le Courrier du Livre. 1995.

DIAMOND, Jared. *The Third Chimpanzee.* HarperPerennial. 1992.

DIAMOND, Jared M. *Guns, Germs, and Steel: The Fates of Human Societies.* W.W. Norton & Company, Ltd. 1997.

DINOUART, Abbé. *L'Art de se Taire.* Jêrome Million, 1996.

DINVILLE, Claire. *Les Troubles de la Voix et Leur Rééducation.* Masson. 1978.

DULONG, Gustave. *Pauline Viardot: Tragédienne Lyrique.* Association des Amis d'Yvan Tourgeniev, Pauline Viardot, Maria Malibran. 1987.

DUPOUX, Emmanuel. *Les Langages du Cerveau.* Odile Jacob. 2002.

DUTOIT-MARCO, Marie-Louise. *Tout Savoir sur la Voix.* Pierre-Marcel Favre, S.A. 1985.

EDWARDS, Katie, ROSEN, Brian. *From the Beginning.* Natural History Museum, London. 2004

EINSTEIN, Albert. *Relativity, The Special and the General Theory.* Crown Trade Paperback. 1995.

EMIL-BEHNKE, Kate. *The Technique of Singing.* Williams and Norgate, Ltd. 1945.

ENARD, W., et al. Molecular evolution of FOXP2, a gene involved in speech and language. *Nature,* No. 418, 2002.

Encyclopedia Universalis. La science au présent 2003. Encyclopedia Universalis S.A. 2003.

ESCHERNY (chambellan comte d'). *Fragments sur la Musique, Extraits des Mélanges de Littérature—Philosophie, Politique, Histoire et Morale.* L'Huillier et Delaunay. 1809.

ESTIENNE, Françoise. *Je Suis Bien dans Ma Voix.* Office International de Librairie S.A. (Belgique). 1980.

EZANNO-LECOUTY, Catherine. *Les Imitateurs, Comment Font-ils?* (Mémoire pour le Certificat de Capacité D'orthophoniste). 1984.

FAIN-MAUREL, M. A. *Biologie Cellulaire 1.* Bréal. 1986.

FERLITO, Alfio. *Diseases of the Larynx.* Arnold. 2000.

FINK, Raymond B. *The Human Larynx: A Functional Study.* Raven Press. 1975.

FITZGERALD, M. J. T., FOLAN-CURRAN, Jean. *Neuro-anatomie Clinique et Neurosciences Connexes.* Maloine. 2003.

FONAGY, Ivan. *La Vive Voix: Essais de Psycho-phonétique.* Payot. 1983.

FORD, Charles N., BLESS, Diane M. *Phonosurgery Assessment and Surgical Management of Voice Disorders.* Raven Press. 1991.

FORD, Gillian. *Listening to Your Hormones.* Prima. 1996.

FOSSEY, Mathieu. *Les Hormones.* Arthéme Fayard. 1959.

FOURNIER, Edouard. *Physiologie de la Voix et de la Parole.* Adrien Delahaye. 1866.

FRACHET, Bruno, et al. *La Communication: Modalités, Technologies et Symboles.* Arnette. 1991.

FRECHE, Charles, et al. *La Voix Humaine et Ses Troubles.* Arnette. 1984.

GAGNARD. Madeleine. *La Voix dans la Musique Contemporaine et Extra-européenne.* Van de Velde. 1987.

GAGO, N., et al. Progesterone and the oligodendroglial lineage: Stage-dependent biosynthesis and metabolism. *Glia,* No. 36, pp. 295–308; 2001.

GALLIEN, Claude-Louis. *Homo: Histoire Plurielle d'un Genre Très Singulier.* Presses Universitaires France. 2002.

GANDOLFI, Linda, GANDOLFI, René. *La Maladie, le Mythe et le Symbole.* du Rocher. 2001.

GARCÍA, Manuel. *Traité Complet de L'art du Chant en 1854.* Minkoff. 1985.

GARDINER, B. Cited in Janvier, P. Le divorce de l'oiseau et du crocodile. *La Recherche,* No.149, pp. 1430–1434, 1983.

GARDNER, R. A., GARDNER, B. T. Teaching sign language to a chimpanzee. *Science,* No.165, pp. 664–672, 1969.

GEISON, Gerald L. *The Private Science of Louis Pasteur.* Princeton University Press. 1995.

GESCHWIND, N., LEVITSKY, W. Human brain: left-right asymmetries in temporal speech region. *Science,* No. 161, pp. 186–187, 1968.

GILLIE-GUILBERT, Claire, FRITSCH, Lucienne. *L'Épreuve Optionnelle de Musique.* Bordas Pédagogie. 2003.

GOULD, Stephen Jay. *Ontogeny and Phylogeny.* The Belknap Press of Harvard University Press. 2002.

GOULD, Wilbur J., SATALOFF, Robert T., et al. *Voice Surgery.* Mosby. 1993.

GOURRET, Jean, LABAYLE, Jean. *L'Art du Chant et la Médecine Vocale.* Roudil S.A. 1984.

GRAIN René. *Les Bases Physiologiques du Chant.* Docteur Grain.1950.

Groupe de Recherche et D'information sur la Ménopause (GRIM). *La Ménopause et L'Ovaire.* Laboratoire Ciba-Geigy–Edimedica. 1996.

GUDIN, Claude. *Une Histoire Naturelle de la Séduction.* du Seuil. 2003.

GUILBERT, Yvette. *L'Art de Chanter une Chanson.* Bernard Grasset.1928.

GUIRAUD-CALADOU, Jean-Marie. *Musicothérapie: Paroles des Maux— Réflexions Critiques.* Van de Velde. 1983.

HAGEGE, Jean-Claude. *Le Pouvoir de Séduire.* Odile Jacob. 2003.

HALLE, P. A., BEST, C. T., LEVITT, A. Phonetics vs. phonological influences on French listeners' perception of American English approximants. *Journal of Phonetics,* No. 27, pp. 280–306, 1999.

HAMONIC, P., SCHVARTZ, E. *Manuel du Chanteur et du Professeur de Chant.* Librairie Fischbacher. 1888.

HASBROUCK, Jon M., KENEVAN, Robert. *Speech Physiology for the Head and Neck Surgeon.* American Academy of Otolaryngology–Head and Neck Surgery Foundation, Inc. 1991.

HAWKING, Stephen. *A Brief History of Time: From The Big Bang to Black Holes.* Bantam Books. 1988.

HEDON, Bernard, MADELENAT, Patrick, MILLIEZ, Jacques, PROUST, Alain. *La Femme, le Gynécologue, les Religions.* G.R.E.F. 1995.

HEUILLET-MARTIN, Geneviève, GARSON-BAVARD Hélène, LEGRE Anne. *Une Voix pour Tous: La Voix Normale et Comment l'Optimaliser.* Vol. 1. SOLAL. 1997.

HINES, Jerome. *Great Singers on Great Singing.* Limelight. 1984.

HIRANO, Minoru. *Disorders of Human Communication: Clinical Examination of Voice.* Springer-Verlag.1981.

HOEHN, M. M. The natural history of Parkinson's disease in the pre-levodopa and post-levodopa eras. *Neurology Clinics,* No. 10, pp. 331–339, 1992.

HOPPENOT, Dominique. *Le Violon Intérieur.* Van de Velde. 1981.

HOUDE, Olivier, MAZOYER, Bernard, TZOURIO-MAZOYER, Nathalie. *Cerveau et Psychologie.* Presses Universitaires de France. 2002.

HOWARD, Walter, AURAS, Irmgard. *Musique et Sexualité.* Presses Universitaires de France. 1957.

ISRAEL, Lucien. *Cerveau Droit, Cerveau Gauche: Cultures et Civilisations.* Plon. 1995.

ISSHIKI, Nobuhiko. *Phonosurgery: Theory and Practice.* Springer-Verlag/Tokyo. 1989.

JACQUARD, Albert. *La Légende de la Vie.* Flammarion. 1992.

JESSURUM, Yitzhak Rave. *L'Hébreu: La Langue de la Création: Étude sur les 22 Lettres Hébraïques.* Centre d'Etudes Juives Ohel Torah (Marseille).

JOHANSON, Donald. *Lucie, the Beginning of Human Kind.* Oxford University Press. 1996.

JORDAN, Bertrand. *Voyage Autour du Génome: Le Tour du Monde en 80 Labos.* Inserm John Libbey Eurotext. 1993.

KAJAL, Y. *Histologie du Système Nerveux de l'Homme et des Vertébrés.* Maloine. 1909.

KANSAKU, Kenji, YAMAURA, A., KITAZAWA, S. Sex differences in lateralization revealed in the posterior languages areas. *Cerebral Cortex,* No. 10, pp. 866–872, 2000.

KAPLAN, Francis. *Des Singes et des Hommes: la Frontière du Langage.* Fayard. 2001.

KAPLAN, Francis. *Le Paradoxe de la Vie.* de la Découverte. 1995.

KENT, Raymond D. *The Speech Sciences.* Singular Publishing Group, Inc. 1997.

KERDILES, Chantal. *Je Crie et Vous Ne m'Entendez Pas.* Alain Lefeuvre. 1981.

KEY, Pierre V. *Enrico Caruso.* Little, Brown, and Company. 1922.

KIM, KH, RELKIN, NR, LEE, KM, HIRSCH, SJ. Distinct cortical areas associated with native and second languages. *Nature.* No. 388, pp. 171–174, 1997.

KLEIN-DALLANT, Carine. *Les Pathologies Vocales chez l'Enfant: Rééducation Orthophonique.* Fédération Nationale des Orthophonistes. 1998.

KOESTENBAUM, Wayne. *The Queen's throat—Opera Homosexuality and the Mystery of Desire.* Vintage Books. 1993.

LAI, Cecilia S., et al. A forkhead-domain gene is mutated in a severe speech and language disorder. *Nature.* No. 413, pp. 519–523, 2001.

LAITMAN, Jeffrey T. L'Origine du langage articulé. *La Recherche,* No. 181, Vol. 17, pp. 1164–1173, 1986.

LAITMAN, Jeffrey T. The basicranium of fossil hominids as an indicator of their upper respiratory systems. *American Journal of Physical Anthropology,* No. 51, pp. 15–34, 1979.

LA MADELEINE, Stephen (de). *Théories Complètes du Chant.* Arnauld de Vresse. 1864.

LAMPERT, H. Zur Kenntnis des Platyrrhinenkehlkopfes. *Gegenbaurs Morphologisches Jahrbuch.* No. 55, pp. 607-654, 1926.

LANGANEY, André. *La Philosophie Biologique.* Belin. 1999.

LATHAM, Michael C. *Human Nutrition in the Developing World.* FAO Rome. 1997.

LE GRUSSE, Jean, WATIER, Bernadette. *Centre d'Étude et d'Information sur les Vitamines.* Roche. 1993.

LEAKEY, M. D., HARRIS, J. *A Pliocene Site in Northern Tanzania.* Oxford University Press, 1987.

LECHEVALIER, Bernard. *Le Cerveau de Mozart.* Odile Jacob. 2003.

LEDERER, Jean. *Mythes et Réalité.* Maloine. 1984.

LEE, John R. *What Your Doctor May Not Tell You about Menopause: The Breakthrough Book on Natural Progesterone.* Warner Books. 1996.

LEROI-GOURHAN, André, *Le Geste et la Parole: La Mémoire et les Rythmes.* Albin Michel S.A. 1964.

LEROI-GOURHAN, André.*Le Geste et la Parole: Technique et Langage.* Albin Michel S.A. 1964.

LEVELT, W. J. Models of word production. *Trends in Cognitive Sciences,* No. 3, pp. 223-232, 1999.

LEWIN, Roger. *L'Evolution Humaine.* Du Seuil. 1991.

LOCQUIN, Marcel. *L'Homme et son Langage.* Arppam. 2000.

LOCQUIN, Marcel. *L'Invention de l'Humanité: Petite Histoire Universelle de la Planète, des Techniques et des Idées.* La Nuée Bleue.1995.

LOCQUIN, Marcel. *Quelle Langue Parlaient nos Ancêtres Préhistoriques?* Albin Michel. 2002.

LOGER, P. Versuche zur Frage des Zähl-Vermogens an Einem Graupapagei und Vergleichsversuche and Menschon. *Zeitschrift fur Tier Psychologie,* No. 16, pp. 197-217, 1959.

LORENZ, K. Der Kumpan in der Umwelt des Vogels. *Journal of Orniththology,* No. 83, pp. 137-413, 1932.

LOUBIER, Jean-Marc. *Louis Jouvet: Le Patron.* Ramsay. 2001.

LOWE, Carl. *The Complete Vitamin Book: The Up-to-Date Information You Need for Better Nutrition and Better Health.* Berkley. 1994.

MAC LEAN, Paul. *Les Trois Cerveaux.* Robert Laffont. 1990.

MALHERBE, Henry. *La Passion de la Malibran.* Albin Michel. 1937.

MALSON, Lucien. Les enfants sauvages, suivi de mémoire et rapport. In ITARD Jean, *Mémoire et Rapport sur Victor de l'Aveyron de 1806: Mythe et Réalité.* Union générale d'Edition, Cop. (Ed. 10-18), p. 157. 1964.

MAMY, Sylvie. *Les Castrats* (Que sais-je ?). Presses Universitaires de France. 1998.

MARICHELLE H. *La Parole d'après le Tracé du Phonographe.* Ed. Librairie Ch. Delagrave. 1897.

MARTIN, R. P. *The Languages of Heroes Speech and Performance in the Iliad.* Cornell University Press. 1989.

MARTINOTY, Jean-Louis. *L'Opéra Imaginaire.* Messidor. 1991.

MCGUIRE, P. K., SILBERSWEIG, D. A., FRITH, C. D. Functional neuroanatomy of verbal self-monitoring. *Brain,* No. 119, pp. 907–917, 1996.

MEANO, Carlo. *The Human Voice in Speech and Song.* Charles C. Thomas. 1967.

MENUHIN, Yehudi. *The Violin.* Flammarion. 2000.

MILLER, Richard. "The odyssey of Orpheus: The evolution of solo singing. *Journal of Voice.* Lippincott Raven Publishers. 1996.

MOCHIZUKI, Michiko. The identification of /r/ and /l/ in natural and synthesized speech. *Journal of Phonetics,* No. 9, pp. 80–101, 1981.

MOLIERE. *Le Bourgeois Gentilhomme.* GAUTIER Henri (Nouvelle Bibliothèque Populaire).

MOLINIE J. (Société Française d'Oto-Rhino-Laryngologie—Rapports du Congrès de 1926). *Laryngologie et Chant.* Presses Universitaires de France. 1926.

MOORE, Grace. *You're Only Human Once.* Doubleday, Doran and Co., Inc. 1944.

MOREAUX, René (Société Française d'Oto-Rhino-Laryngologie—Rapports du Congrès de 1926). *Rapports de la Laryngologie et du Chant.* Presses Universitaires de France. 1926.

MORTON, J., et al. What lesson for dyslexia from Down's syndrome: Comments on Cossu, Rossini and Marshal. *Cognition,* No. 48, pp. 289–296, 1993.

MOUCHON, Jean-Pierre. *Enrico Caruso: L'Homme et l'Artiste.* Thèse. 1977.

NACHTIGALL, Werner. *La Nature Réinventée.* Plon. 1987.

NAHON, Claude. *Quand la Nuit se Finit.* La Bartavelle. 1993.

NAHON, Claude. *Le Passant du Temps ou le Temps du Passant.* La Bartavelle. 1998.

NANQUETTE, Claude. *Les Grands Interprètes Romantiques.* Arthème Fayard. 1982.

NEGUS, V. E. *The Comparative Anatomy and Physiology of the Larynx.* William Heinemann Medical Books Ltd. 1949.

NUNN, John F. *Ancient Egyptian Medicine.* John F. Nunn. 1996.

Nutrition Reviews: Knowledge in Nutrition. The Nutrition Foundation. 1984.

OHLA, A., et al. Effect of exercise on concentration of elements in the serum. *Journal of Sports Medicine.* No. 22, pp. 414–425, 1982.

OJEMANN, G., et al. Cortical language localization in left dominant hemisphere: An electrical stimulation mapping investigation in 117 patients. *Journal of Neurosurgery,* No. 71, pp. 316–326, 1989.

OSTRANOER, Sheila, et al. *Les Fantastiques Facultés du Cerveau.* Robert Laffont. 1979.

PARKER, Roger. *The Oxford Illustrated History of Opera.* Oxford University Press. 1994.

PENFIELD, W. RAMUSSENT. *The Cerebral Cortex of Man: A Clinical Study of Localization of Function.* The Mammalian Company. 1950.

PERELLO, Jorge. *Morfologia Fonoaudiologica.* Cientico-medica, Barcelona, Espana. 1978.

PEPPERBERG, Irene Maxine. *The Alex Studies.* Harvard University Press. 2002.

PERES, G. *Nutrition du Sportif (*abrégé de Médecine du sport, 8e). Ed. Masson, 2002.

PERKINS, William H., KENT, Raymond D. *Functional Anatomy of Speech, Language, and Hearing.* Little, Brown and Company. 1987.

PICQ, Pascal. *Aux Origines de L'Homme: L'Odyssée de L'Eespèce.* Tallandier. 1999.

PICQ Pascal. *Berçeaux de L'Humanité: Des Origines à L'Age de Bronze.* Larousse. 2003.

PICQ, Pascal. *Aux Commencement Était l'Homme: de Toumaï à Cro-Magnon.* Odile Jacob. 2003.

PINKER, Steven. *Comment Fonctionne L'Esprit.* Odile Jacob. 2000.

PINKER, Steven. *L'Instinct du Langage.* Odile Jacob. 1999.

PINKER, Steven. On the acquisition of grammatical morphemes. *Journal of Child Language,* No. 8, pp. 477–484, 1981.

POIZAT, Michel. *L'Opéra ou le Cri de L'Ange.* Métailié. 2001.

PORTMANN, A. *Traité de Zoologie* (Vol. 15). Pierre Grasset. 1950.

PREMACK, D. *Intelligence in Ape and Man.* Erlbaum Press. 1976.

PRIGONIE, Ilya, STENGERS, Isabelle. *La Nouvelle Alliance: Métamorphose de la Science.* Gallimard. 1979.

PRIGONIE, Ilya, STENGERS, Isabelle. *Entre le Temps et L'Éternité.* Flammarion. 1988.

PROCTOR, Donald F. *Breathing, Speech, and Song.* Springer-Verlag/Wien. 1980.

RANDOM, Michel. *La Tradition du Vivant.* du Felin. 1985.

RASMUSSEN, Knud. *Nalunglaq, Netslilik Eskimo.* Rothenberg. 1972.

RASMUSSEN, T., MILNER, B. The role of early left brain Injury in determining lateralization of cerebral speech functions. *Annals of the New York Academy of Sciences,* No. 299, pp. 355–369, 1977.

REBATET, Lucien. *Une Histoire de la Musique: Des Origines à nos Jours.* Robert Laffont. 1969.

REEVES, Hubert. *L'Heure de S'Enivrer L'Univers a-t-il un Sens?* du Seuil. 1986.

REEVES, Hubert. *Patience dans L'Azur: L'Evolution Cosmique.* du Seuil. 1988.

RIDLEY, Matt. *Genome: The Autobiography of Species in 23 Chapters.* Crown Trade Paperbacks. 2000.

RONDAL, Jean-Adolphe. *Le Langage: de L'Animal aux Origines du Langage Humain.* Pierre Mardaga. 2000.

ROSSING, Thomas D. *The Science of Sound.* Addison-Wesley Pubishing Company, Inc. 1990.

RUBIN, John S., SATALOFF, Robert T., KOROVIN, Gwen S. *Diagnosis and Treatment of Voice Disorders* (3rd edition). Plural Publishing Inc. 2006.

SAPPHO. *Poèmes et Fragments.* La Délirante. 1989.

SATALOFF, Robert, T. *Professional Voice: The Science and Art of Clinical Care* (3rd ed.) Plural Publishing, Inc., 2005.

SATALOFF Robert, T., HAWKSHAW, Mary. *Chaos in Medicine: Source Readings.* Singular–Thomson Learning. 2001.

SAXON, Keith G., SCHNEIDER, Carole M. *Vocal Exercise Physiology.* Singular Publishing Group, Inc. 1995.

SEBILEAU, Pierre, TRUFFERT, Paul. *Le Carrefour Aéro-digestif: Le Larynx—Le Pharynx.* Librairie Louis Arnette. 1924.

SEIKEL, Anthony J., KING, Douglas W., DRUMRIGHT, David G. *Anatomy and Physiology for Speech, Language, and Hearing.* Singular Publishing Group, Inc. 1997.

SHAYWITZ, Bennett, et al. Sex differences in the functional organization of the brain for language. *Nature,* No. 373, pp. 607–609, 1995.

SHELDRAKE, Rupert. *The Presence of the Past; Morphic Resonance and the Habits of Nature.* Vintage Paperbacks. 1999.

SIBLEY, Charles, G., et al. Avian phylogeny reconstructed from comparisons of the genetics material, DNA. In PATTERSON, C. *Molecules and Morphology in Evolution: Conflict or Compromise.* Cambridge University Press. 1987.

SIDPIS, J., et al. Connective interaction after staged callosal section: Evidence for transfer of semantic activation. *Science,* No. 212, pp. 344–346, 1981.

SINGH, Sadanand, SINGH Kala S. *Phonetics: Principles and Practices.* University Park Press. 1982.

SOULI, Sophia A. *Mythologie Grecque.* Michalis Toubis S.A. 1995.

SPEROFF, Leon, et al. *Clinical Gynaecologic Endocrinology and Infertility.* Williams and Wilkins. 1994.

STANISKAVSKI, Constantin. *La Formation de l'Acteur.* Petite Bibliothéque, Payot. 1998.

SULLIVAN, Jane. *The Natural Way PMS: A Comprehensive Guide to Effective Treatment.* Element. 1996.

SUNDBERG, Johan. *The Science of the Singing Voice.* Northern Illinois University Press. 1987.

TARNEAUD, Jean, SEEMAN, Miloslav. *La Voix et la Parole: Études Cliniques et Thérapeutiques.* Maloine. 1950.

TARNEAUD, Jean. *Le Chant, sa Construction, sa Destruction.* Maloine. 1946.

TARNEAUD, Jean. *Laryngite Chronique et Laryngopathie.* Maloine. 1944.

TARNEAUD, Jean. *Rapports de la Stomatologie et de la Phoniatrie* (extrait de la *Revue Odontologique*). 1942.

TARNEAUD, Jean. *Traité Pratique de Phonologie et de Phoniatrie: La Voix, la Parole, le Chant.* Maloine. 1941.

TARNEAUD, Jean. *Le Nodule de la Corde Vocale.* Maloine. 1935

TITZE, Ingo R. *Vocal Fold Physiology: Frontiers in Basic Science.* Singular Publishing Group, Inc. 1993.

TITZE, Ingo R. *Principles of Voice Production.* Prentice-Hall, Inc. 1994.

TITZE, Ingo R., SCHERER, Ronald C. *Vocal Fold Physiology: Biomechanics, Acoustics and Phonatory Control.* The Denver Center for the Performing Arts, Inc. 1983.

TRAN QUANG, Hai. *Musiques du Monde.* Fuzeau. 1993.

Transcripts of the Eight-Symposium Care of the Professional Voice. The Voice Foundation. June 1979, June 1980, June 1982, June 1985.

TRINH XUAN Thuan. *Le Chaos et L'Harmonie: La Fabrication du Réél.* Arthème Fayard. 1998.

TUCKER, Wallace, TUCKER, Karen. *The Dark Matter : Contemporary Science's Quest for the Mass Hidden in Our Universe.* William Morrow and Company. 1988.

TUCKER, Harvey. *The Larynx.* Thieme Medical. 1993.

UZIEL Alain, GUERRIER, Yves. *Physiologie des Voixes Aéro-digestives Supérieures.* Masson. 1983.

VALDARNINI, Umberto. *Bel Canto.* Janus. 1956.

VANNIER, Henri. *L'Homéopathie Française.* G. Doin et Cie. 1980.

VAUCLAIR, J. *L'Intelligence de L'Animal* Point Sciences. Seuil. 1999.

VERMEIL, Jean. *Le Journal de L'Opéra.* du Félin. 1995.

VINOD, Goel. The seat of reason? An imaging study of deductive and interactive reasoning. *Neuroreport*, No. 8, pp. 1305-1310, 1997.

VOX, Valentine. *I Can See Your Lips Moving.* Plato Publishing in association with Players Press, Inc. 1993.

WAILLY, Philippe (de). *"L'Amateur des Oiseaux de Cage et de Volière.* J. B. Baillière et Fils. 1964.

WAILLY, Philippe (de). *Nos Amis nos Animaux: Perruches, Perroquets et Autres Oiseaux Parleurs.* Solar. 1994.

WAILLY, Philippe (de). *Les Preuves D'Aamour de nos Animaux.* du Rocher. 2004.

WARD, W. R., et al. Origin of the moon's orbital inclination from resonant disk interactions. *Nature,* No. 403, pp. 741–743, 2000.

WARREN, D. K., et al. Mechanisms of American English vowel production in a grey parrot. *AUK,* No. 113, pp. 41–58, 2001.

WATSON, James D. *The Double Helix: A Personal Account of the Discovery of the Structure of DNA.* Atheneum. 1980 (first published in 1968).

WATSON, James D., Crick, F. H. Molecular structure of nucleic acids. *Nature,* No. 171, pp. 737–738, 1953.

WERKER, J., TEES, R. Cross-language Speech Perception: Evidence for perceptual reorganization during the first year of life. *Infant Behaviour and Development,* No. 7, pp. 49–63, 1984.

WERNICKE, Carl. *Der aphasische Symptomenkomplex.* Thesis. 1874.

WHIPPLE, Fred L. Background of modern comet theory. *Nature,* No. 263, pp. 15–19, 1976.

WHIPPLE, Fred L. Of comets and meteors. *Science,* No. 289, p. 728, 2000.

WHIPPLE, Fred L. The earth as part of the universe. *Annual Revue of Earth Planetary Science,* No. 6, pp. 1–8, 1978.

WICART, A. *Les Puissances Vocales: Le Chanteur* (Vol. 1, Vol. 2). Philippe Ortiz. 1931.

WILLIAMS, Peter L. *Gray's Anatomy.* Churchill Livingstone. 1995.

WYATT, Gertrude L. *La Relation Mère-Enfant et L'Acquisition du Langage.* Dessart. 1969.

WYSS, Colette. *Ce que Chanter Veut Dire: Initiation à L'Art du Chant.* Musicales. 1961.

ZEMLIN, Willard R. *Speech and Hearing Science: Anatomy and Physiology.* Allyn & Bacon. 1998.